CLINICAL EXAMINATION

CLINICAL EXAMINATION

A Systematic Guide to Physical Diagnosis

THIRD EDITION

Nicholas J Talley

MD, PhD, FRACP, FRCP (Edin), FACP, FACG, FAFPHM

Professor of Medicine,
The University of Sydney
Nepean Hospital
Sydney, Australia

Simon O'Connor

FRACP, DDU

Cardiologist
Woden Valley Hospital
Canberra, Australia

Blackwell
Science

© 1996 MacLennan & Petty Pty Limited
809 Botany Road, Rosebery, NSW 2018, Australia

First published 1988
Reprinted 1989, 1990, 1991
Second edition 1992
Reprinted 1994, 1995
Indonesian edition 1994
Chinese edition 1996
Third edition 1996
Reprinted 1998

Distributed in the United Kingdom and Europe by
Blackwell Science Ltd
Osney Mead, Oxford OX2 OEL
Orders should be addressed to:
Marston Book Services Ltd
PO Box 269, Abingdon
Oxon OX14 4YN
Tel: +44 1235 465500
Fax: +44 1235 465555

A catalogue record for this title is available from the
British Library and the Library of Congress

ISBN: 0-86542-689-9

Printed and bound in Hong Kong

FOREWORDS

With the breathtaking advances in biomedical science in recent years, especially in areas such as molecular and cell biology, molecular genetics and organ imaging, there is a disturbing trend by some clinicians to short-cut the history and examination and proceed directly to 'appropriate' (in fact often inappropriate) investigations. This often leads not only to unnecessary expense, but often to misdiagnosis and potential harm for the patient.

This trend has created an even greater need for a comprehensive, yet reader-friendly guide to the clinical history and physical examination. These techniques are now more important than ever for understanding patients' problems and for reaching an accurate diagnosis in the most cost-effective manner. In short, the ability to undertake an accurate clinical history and physical examination remains the most important hallmark of a good clinician.

In this Third Edition of *Clinical Examination* Talley and O'Connor present what is arguably the most systematic and comprehensive approach to the clinical evaluation. The book is extremely well illustrated and learning is made even more enjoyable by pertinent quotations and a nice touch of humour.

I predict that this edition will be even more popular than the first two editions. I am sure William Osler would have strongly commended it when he exhorted his students to: 'Read to understand and analyse your cases'.

Lawrie W Powell MD, AC
Professor of Medicine
University of Queensland
December 1995

The diagnosis of a patient's illness and his subsequent investigation and treatment depend upon a detailed history and careful examination. Great advances have been made in recent years with technological investigations of structural and physiological changes, but only two procedures are common to all patients: namely, a history and an examination. This is so whether they are seen in their homes or in a teaching hospital.

As undergraduates, students are expected to acquire a factual knowledge of disease and to be able to detect and interpret commoner symptoms and signs. Despite their apparent simplicity, the obtaining of a history and the performance of a physical examination often turn out to be the most difficult problems facing medical students. The purpose of this book by Drs Talley and O'Connor is to facilitate both these procedures. The authors give an excellent outline of how to obtain a history and perform a physical examination. As well, in order to make both exercises more memorable and interesting, they have described the mechanisms and significance of common symptoms and signs.

Even at the postgraduate level, no one doctor can be expert in all branches of medicine. To compensate for this the authors have had every chapter reviewed by specialists within each field.

Overall, an outstanding publication has been produced. It will be a valuable addition to the library of all students, and will supplement the previous publication by the authors.

D W Piper MD, FRACP, FRCP
Emeritus Professor of Medicine
University of Sydney
September 1987

That a carefully taken history and a thorough physical examination have always been, and will always be, the foundation upon which efficient diagnosis rests should not need to be said. However, unfortunately for society and for medicine, the point is not well enough appreciated. Thus, failure to utilise adequately the wealth of information available from these simple and inexpensive approaches is surely one reason for the recent logarithmic growth of medical costs. In this regard, the guide to historical and physical diagnosis by Drs Talley and O'Connor should, in my view, attract a readership beyond the medical students for whom it is primarily intended. The message needs to be reinforced even to those who have long since forsaken the teaching hospital for practice. I was pleased to see that the scope and detail of the material included begins at the student level but, by the inclusion of comprehensive tabulations of disease, should also appeal to and be valuable for more senior people. There are lessons here for us all, and I hope the book commands a diverse readership.

S F Phillips MD, FRACP, FRCP
Professor of Medicine
Mayo Medical School
Rochester, Minnesota
September 1987

PREFACE TO THE THIRD EDITION

Despite the increasing sophistication (and expense) of medical tests, the history and physical examination continue to be the foundation of medicine. Physical examination is an area of medicine that is less subject to change, but new problems still arise and old problems re-emerge that continue to challenge modern medical practice. For example, human immunodeficiency virus (HIV) infection and its related immunosuppression, which was not recognised 15 years ago, now affects all areas of medicine including history taking and physical examination.

In this third edition, the entire text has been revised and updated to reflect current concepts. New photographs and tables have been included to increase the clarity of the text. A chapter on psychiatric history taking and the mental state examination is included for the first time. Amusing anecdotes and classical references and quotations are featured again in the hope that they will make the facts easier to remember. A complementary question and answer book (*Multiple Choice Questions in Clinical Examination*) has also been prepared to help with understanding and revision.

To ensure that the text is current and accurate in all areas, we have again invited experts in their respective fields to review all parts of the book.

N J Talley
S O'Connor
February 1996

PREFACE TO THE SECOND EDITION

*Clinical diagnosis is an art, and the mastery of an art has no end;
you can always be a better diagnostician.*

Logan Clendering (1884–1945)

The preparation of a second edition has enabled us to undertake a major revision of the text; we have updated the entire book and have included important additional details in the form of tables and figures. In this edition our aims remain the same; to present a truly *systematic* and *comprehensive* approach to the clinical evaluation. We have also tried to make the book simple to read and even amusing, as we believe this aids the learning process. The widespread acceptance of the first edition suggests that not only medical students but also postgraduates have found the material useful and the format a success, and therefore, this is retained. As obtaining a medical history remains an essential skill, the general principles are summarised in Chapter 1, and specific details of history taking are also covered system by system. In addition, we have included some common and important surgical symptoms and signs in this edition to help ensure that the book represents a more complete text for undergraduates. We are very grateful for the positive comments and helpful suggestions that we have received from the many consultants who have reviewed the book. We hope that you will find the second edition of *Clinical Examination* to be a useful textbook.

N J Talley
S O'Connor
November 1991

PREFACE TO THE
FIRST EDITION

*A few observations and much reasoning leads to error,
many observations and a little reasoning to truth.*

Alexis Carrel (1873–1944)

Despite the sophistication of modern investigations, clinical methods remain the cornerstone of medical practice, as diagnosis depends largely on history and physical examination.

The aim of this book is to provide a modern, comprehensive, systematic account of clinical methods in internal medicine. In particular, physical examination is emphasised. This is because most students and clinicians find this part the most testing. In viva-voce examinations, candidates must examine systematically. In such examinations, the candidate needs to convey the impression that he is competent. This book will help promote such an approach.

We have designed this text to make comprehension and studying easier. The clinical methods are described in a systematic manner. Numerous tables of important facts are included. Areas of most difficulty (such as cardiology or neurology) are covered in the greatest depth. The basic pathophysiological mechanisms of physical signs are emphasised to increase understanding and to help answer those questions viva-voce examiners often like to ask. Illustrations of key examination techniques, important diseases and essential background information are incorporated. Interesting pieces of historical information are included to put current knowledge in perspective. Suggestions for further reading are found at the end of each chapter.

Bedside clinical investigations are also discussed. How to perform, for example, a sigmoidoscopy, examine the urine sediment or the blood film, and how to interpret common abnormalities, remain essential clinical skills. Also included is a systematic approach to reading and interpreting chest and plain abdominal X-ray films, as this important skill is often not emphasised. On the other hand, the electrocardiograph (ECG) is not discussed, nor is paediatric or gynaecological examination, as several textbooks (referenced in suggested reading) are available. Summaries are included at the end of most chapters.

To avoid the pitfalls of multi-author books, most of the text was written by the two authors working in close collaboration, thus making the style uniform and minimising repetition. In a few special areas, experts made short contributions which were integrated into the text. Subsequently, eminent specialists in every field reviewed the appropriate sections, to ensure the book's accuracy and relevance.

This book contains more than enough information for undergraduates. Postgraduates studying for the MRCP, FRACP, or other examinations in internal medicine, should also find this book very useful.

N J Talley
S O'Connor
September 1987

ACKNOWLEDGMENTS

We are very grateful to **Professor P Boyce** MD, FRANZCP, Professor of Psychiatry, University of Sydney at Nepean Hospital and Wentworth Area Director of Mental Health, Sydney, who provided the new chapter on psychiatric assessment for this edition, and to **Dr L Schreiber** MD, FRACP, Associate Professor of Medicine and Head, Department of Rheumatology, Royal North Shore Hospital, Sydney, who provided the new section on soft tissue rheumatology.

The following eminent specialists reviewed appropriate chapters of this book. We are very grateful for their comments and advice, but we take responsibility for any errors or omissions.

Cardiology

Dr D Coulshed FRACP, Senior Lecturer in Medicine and Staff Specialist in Cardiology, Nepean Hospital, Sydney

Respiratory Medicine

Dr M Hurwitz FCP(SA), FRACP, FCCP, Staff Specialist in Thoracic Medicine, Woden Valley Hospital, Canberra

Gastroenterology

Dr M A Kamm MD, FRCP, FRACP, Consultant Physician and Gastroenterologist, St Mark's Hospital, London, UK

Genitourinary

Professor J Stewart FRACP, Associate Dean, The University of Sydney, Western Clinical School, Nepean Hospital, Sydney

Dr C A Pollock PhD, FRACP, Senior Lecturer in Medicine, Royal North Shore Hospital, Sydney

Haematology

Dr J Isbister FRACP, FRCPA, Staff Specialist in Haematology, Royal North Shore Hospital, Sydney

Dr A Manoharan FRACP, FRCPA, Staff Physician in Clinical Haematology, St George Hospital, Sydney

Endocrinology

Dr R Coles MD, FRACP, Consultant Endocrinologist, Nepean Hospital, Sydney

Rheumatology

Dr L McGuigan MD, FRACP, Consultant Rheumatologist, St George Hospital, Sydney

Neurology

Dr P McManis FRACP, Senior Lecturer in Medicine and Staff Specialist in Neurology, Nepean Hospital, Sydney

Dr M H Silber MD, Consultant Neurologist, Mayo Clinic, Rochester, Minnesota, USA

Infectious Diseases

Dr B Frankum FRACP, Lecturer in Medical Education, University of Sydney Nepean Hospital, Sydney

General Medicine

Dr J D G Watson D.Phil, FRACP, Senior Lecturer in Medicine, Royal Prince Alfred Hospital, Sydney

Dr S Coulshed FRACP, Senior Medical Registrar, Royal North Shore Hospital, Sydney

Dr N A Talley FRACP, Consultant Physician, St George Hospital, Sydney

General Surgery

Dr M Cox FRACS, Senior Lecturer in Surgery and Staff Specialist Surgeon, Nepean Hospital, Sydney

Gynaecology

Dr B Spurrett MD, FRACOG, Associate Professor of Obstetrics and Gynaecology, Nepean Hospital, Sydney

Dermatology

Dr G Fisher, Consultant Dermatologist, Nepean Hospital, Sydney

Dr G Briggs very kindly provided the original X-ray material. Dr A Cooper prepared the original chapter on the skin for which we remain very grateful. Dr A Manoharan and Dr J Isbister provided the blood film photographs and the accompanying text. Associate Professor S Posen, Associate Professor I P C Murray, Dr G Bauer, Dr E Wilmshurst, Dr J Stiel, and Dr J Webb helped us obtain many of the original photographs, Mr D S Pady in the History of Medicine Library at Mayo Clinic assisted us with obtaining biographical information. The dermatology illustrations in Chapter 12 are reproduced with permission from *Clinical Dermatology Illustrated*: *A Regional Approach (second edition)* by John R T Reeves and Howard Maibach, published by MacLennan & Petty, Sydney, 1991. Professor John Reeves kindly lent us his transparencies. The retinal photographs were kindly provided by Dr Chris Kennedy and Professor Ian Constable (copyright Lion's Eye Institute). The text was reviewed by several medical students in the United Kindom and Australia, and their advice and assistance are also gratefully acknowledged.

CONTENTS

Chapter 5
The Gastrointestinal System

Chapter 10

The Nervous System   330

CLINICAL METHODS:
AN HISTORICAL PERSPECTIVE

*The best physician is the one who is able to differentiate
the possible and the impossible.*

Herophilus of Alexandria

From classical Greek times interrogation of the patient has been considered most important because disease was, and still is, viewed in terms of the discomfort it causes. However, the current emphasis on the use of history taking and physical examination for diagnosis developed only in the last century. Although the terms 'symptoms and signs' have been part of the medical vocabulary since the revival of classical medicine, they were until relatively recently used synonymously.

During the 19th Century, the distinction between *symptoms* (subjective complaints, which the clinician learns from the patient's account of his or her feelings) and *signs* (objective morbid changes detectable by the clinician) evolved.

Until the 19th Century, diagnosis was empirical and based on the classical Greek beliefs that all disease had a single cause, an imbalance of the four humours (yellow bile, black bile, blood and phlegm). Indeed the Royal College of Physicians, founded in London in 1518, believed that clinical experience without classical learning was useless and physicians who were College members were fined if they ascribed to any other view.

At the time of Hippocrates (460–375 BC) observation (inspection) and feeling (palpation) had a place in the examination of patients. The ancient Greeks, for example, noticed that patients with jaundice often had an enlarged liver that was firm and irregular. Shaking a patient and listening for a fluid splash was also recognised by the Greeks.

Herophilus of Alexandria (335–280 BC) described a method of taking the pulse in the 4th Century BC. However, it was Galen of Pergamum (AD 130–200) who established the pulse as one of the major physical signs, and it continued to have this important role up to the 18th Century, with minute variations being recorded. These variations were erroneously considered to indicate changes in the body's harmony.

William Harvey's (1578–1657) studies of the human circulation, published in 1628, had little effect on the general understanding of the value of the pulse as a sign. Sanctorius (1561–1636) was the first to time the pulse using a clock, while John Floyer (1649–1734) in 1707 invented the pulse watch and made regular observations of the pulse rate. Abnormalities in heart rate were described in diabetes mellitus in 1776 and in thyrotoxicosis in 1786.

Fever was studied by Hippocrates and was originally regarded as an entity rather than a sign of disease. The thermoscope was devised by Sanctorius in 1625. In association with Gabriel Fahrenheit (1686–1736), Hermann Boerhaave (1668–1738) introduced the thermometer as a research instrument and this was produced commercially in the middle of the 18th Century.

In the 13th Century Johannes Actuarius (?–1283) used a graduated glass to examine the urine. In Harvey's time a specimen of urine was sometimes looked at (inspected) and even tasted, and was considered to reveal secrets about the body. Harvey recorded that sugar diabetes (mellitus) and dropsy (oedema) could be diagnosed in this way. The detection of protein in the urine, which Frederik Dekkers (1644–1720) first described in 1673, was ignored until Richard Bright (1789–1858) demonstrated its importance in renal disease. Although weighing a patient was described by and measuring intake and output was valued by Celsus (25 BC–AD 50) these methods only became widely used in the 20th Century.

A renaissance in clinical methods began with the concept of Battista Morgagni (1682–1771) that disease was not generalised but arose in organs, a conclusion published in 1761. Leopold Auenbrugger invented chest tapping (percussion) to detect disease in the same year. Van Swieten, his teacher, in fact used percussion to detect ascites. The technique was forgotten for nearly half a century until Jean Corvisart (1755–1821) translated Auenbrugger's work in 1808.

The next big step occurred with René Laënnec (1781–1826), a student of Corvisart. He invented the stethoscope in 1816 (at first merely a roll of stiff paper) as an aid to diagnosing heart and lung disease by listening (auscultation). This revolutionised chest examination, partly because it made the chest accessible in patients too modest to allow a direct application of the examiner's ear to the chest wall, as well as allowing accurate clinicopathological correlations. William Stokes (1804–1878) published the first treatise in English on the use of the stethoscope in 1825. Josef Skoda's (1805–1881) investigations of the value of these clinical methods led to their widespread and enthusiastic adoption after he published his results in 1839.

These advances helped lead to a change in the practice of medicine. Bedside teaching was first introduced in the Renaissance by Montanus (1498–1552) in Padua in 1543. In the 17th Century, physicians based their opinion on a history provided by an apothecary (assistant) and rarely saw the patients themselves. Thomas Sydenham (1624–1689) began to practise more modern bedside medicine, basing his treatment on experience and not theory, but it was not until a century later that the scientific method brought a systematic approach to clinical diagnosis.

This change began in the hospitals of Paris after the French Revolution with recognition of the work of Morgagni, Corvisart, Laënnec and others. Influenced by the philosophy of the enlightenment, which suggested that a rational approach to all problems was possible, the Paris Clinical School combined physical examination with autopsy as the basis of clinical medicine. The methods of this school were first applied abroad in Dublin, where Robert Graves (1796–1853) and William Stokes worked. Later at Guy's Hospital in London the famous trio of Richard Bright, Thomas Addison (1793–1860) and Thomas Hodgkin (1798–1866) made their important contributions. In 1869 Samuel Wilks (1824–1911) wrote on the nail changes in disease and the signs he described remain important. Carl Wunderlich's

(1815–1877) work changed the concept of temperature from a disease in itself to a symptom of disease.

Spectacular advances in physiology, pathology, pharmacology and the discovery of microbiology in the latter half of the 19th Century led to the development of the new 'clinical and laboratory medicine' which is the rapidly advancing medicine of the present day. The modern systematic approach to diagnosis, with which this book deals, is still, however, based on taking the history and examining the patient by looking (inspecting), feeling (palpating), tapping (percussing) and listening (auscultating).

Suggested Reading

Reiser SJ. The clinical record in medicine. Part I: Learning from cases. *Ann Intern Med* 1991; 114: 902–907.

Bordage G, Where are the history and the physical? *Can Med Assoc J* 1995; 152: 1595–8.

McDonald C. Medical heuristics: the silent adjudicators of clinical practice. *Ann Intern Med* 1996; 124: 56–62.

THE HIPPOCRATIC* OATH

I swear by Apollo the physician, and Aesculapius, and Hygieia, and Panacea, and all the gods and goddesses that, according to my ability and judgment, I will keep this Oath and this stipulation:

To reckon him who taught me this Art equally dear to me as my parents, to share my substance with him and relieve his necessities if required; to look upon his offspring in the same footing as my own brother, and to teach them this Art, if they shall wish to learn it, without fee or stipulation, and that by precept, lecture, and every other mode of instruction, I will impart a knowledge of the Art to my own sons and those of my teachers, and to disciples bound by a stipulation and oath according to the law of medicine, but to none others.

I will follow that system of regimen which, according to my ability and judgment, I consider for the benefit of my patients, and abstain from whatever is deleterious and mischievous. I will give no deadly medicine to any if asked, nor suggest any such counsel; and in like manner I will not give a woman a pessary to produce abortion.

With purity and with holiness I will pass my life and practise my Art. I will not cut persons labouring under the stone, but will leave this to be done by men who are practitioners of this work. Into whatever houses I enter I will go into them for the benefit of the sick and will abstain from every voluntary act of mischief and corruption; and further from the seduction of females or males, of freemen and slaves.

Whatever, in connection with my professional practice, or not in connection with it, I may see or hear in the lives of men which ought not to be spoken of abroad I will not divulge, as reckoning that all such should be kept secret.

While I continue to keep this Oath unviolated may it be granted to me to enjoy life and the practice of the Art, respected by all men, in all times! But should I trespass and violate this Oath, may the reverse be my lot!

Many of these statements remain relevant, while others, such as euthanasia and abortion, remain controversial. The seduction of slaves, however, is less of a problem today.

---

* Hippocrates, born on the Island of Cos (460–375 BC). Agreed by everyone to be the Father of Medicine.

xxiv

Chapter 1

THE GENERAL PRINCIPLES OF HISTORY TAKING

Medicine is learned by the bedside and not in the classroom.

Sir William Osler (1849–1919)

An extensive knowledge of medical facts is not useful unless a doctor is able to extract accurate and succinct information from a sick person about his or her illness. The development of a rational plan of management depends on a correct diagnostic appraisal in all branches of medicine. Except for patients who are extremely ill, the taking of a careful medical history should precede both examination and treatment. A medical history is the first step in making a diagnosis; it will often help direct the physical examination and usually will determine what investigations are appropriate. More often than not, an accurate history suggests the correct diagnosis, whereas the physical examination and subsequent investigations merely serve to confirm this impression. The history is also, of course, the least expensive way of making a diagnosis.

Bedside Manner

History taking requires a lot of practice and depends very much on the doctor/patient relationship. It is important to try to put the patient at ease immediately, because unless a rapport is established between these two people the history taking is likely to be unrewarding.

There is no doubt that one's treatment of a patient begins the moment one reaches the bedside. The patient's first impressions of a doctor's professional manner will have a lasting effect. One of the axioms of the medical profession is *primum non nocere* (the first thing is to cause no harm). An unkind and thoughtless approach to questioning and examining a patient can cause harm before any treatment has had the opportunity to do so. One should aim to leave the patient feeling better for one's visit. This is a difficult thing to teach and each doctor has to develop his or her own method, guided by experience gained from clinical teachers and patients.

Obtaining the History

It is useful to make rough notes while questioning the patient. At the end of the history and examination a detailed record is made. This record must be a sequen-

1

tial, accurate account of the development and course of the illness or illnesses of the patient (Appendix I). A sick patient will sometimes emphasise irrelevant facts and forget about very important symptoms. For this reason, a systematic approach to history taking and recording is crucial (Table 1.1).

Introductory Questions

Introduce yourself to the patient and shake his or her hand (page 335). It is important to establish rapport. The clinician should sit down either beside the patient or even on the bed so as to be close to eye level and give the impression that the interview will be an unhurried one. The next step should be to find out the patient's major complaint or complaints. Asking the patient 'What brought you here today?' can be unwise as it often promotes the reply 'an ambulance' or 'a car'. This little joke wears thin after some years in clinical practice. It is best to attempt a conversational approach and ask the patient 'What has been the trouble or problem recently?' or 'When were you last quite well?' Encourage patients to tell their story in their own words from the onset of the first symptom to the present time. However, some direction may be necessary to keep a garrulous patient on the track later during the interview.

The Presenting (Principal) Symptom

Not uncommonly, a patient has many symptoms. An attempt must be made to decide which led the patient to present. It must be remembered that the patient's and the doctor's idea of what constitutes a serious problem may differ. A patient

Table 1.1 *History Taking Sequence*

Presenting (Principal) Symptom (PS)

History of Presenting Illness (HPI)
Details of current illnesses and treatments
Menstrual and reproductive history for women
Details of previous similar episodes
Extent of functional disability

Past History (PH)
Past illnesses and surgical operations
Past treatments
Allergies
Blood transfusions

Social History (SH)
Occupation, education
Smoking, alcohol, analgesic use
Overseas travel, immunisation
Marital status, social support
Living conditions

Family History (FH)

Systems Review (SR)
Table 1.4

Also refer to Appendix I (page 418).

with symptoms of a cold, who also, in passing, mentions that he has recently had severe crushing retrosternal chest pain, needs more attention to his heart than to his nose. Record each presenting symptom in the patient's own words, avoiding technical terms.

History of the Presenting Illness

Each of the presenting problems has to be talked about in detail with the patient. When writing down the history of the presenting illness, the events should be placed in chronological order or, if numerous systems are affected, in chronological order for each system.

Current Symptoms

In general, a number of facts have to be uncovered about each symptom. These include the time of onset and duration; the mode of onset; the site and radiation, especially of pain; the character; the severity; aggravating or relieving factors; and associated symptoms.

Time Course

Find out when the symptom first began and try to date this as accurately as possible. For example, ask the patient what was the first thing he or she noticed that was 'unusual' or 'wrong'. Ask whether the patient has had a similar illness in the past. It is often helpful to ask patients when they last felt entirely well. In a patient with long-standing symptoms, ask why he or she decided to come and see the doctor at this time.

Mode of Onset and Pattern

Find out whether the symptom came on rapidly, gradually or instantaneously. Ask whether the symptom has been present continuously or intermittently. Determine if the symptom is getting worse or better, and if so, when the change occurred. Find out what the patient was doing at the time the symptom began.

Site and Radiation

Ask where the symptom is exactly and whether it is localised or diffuse. Ask the patient to point to the actual site on the body. Also determine if the symptom, if localised, radiates. This mainly applies if the symptom is pain. Other symptoms such as cough, dyspnoea, change in weight or dizziness are not localised.

Character

Here it is necessary to ask the patient what is meant by the symptom. If the patient complains of dizziness, does this mean the room spins around (vertigo) or is it more a feeling of lightheadedness? Does indigestion mean abdominal pain, heartburn, excess wind or a change in bowel habit? If there is pain, is it sharp, dull, stabbing, boring, burning or cramp-like? Remember most such descriptions of the character of pain are difficult to interpret.

Severity

This is subjective. The best way to assess severity is to ask the patient if the symptom interferes with normal activities or sleep. Severity can be graded from mild to very severe. A mild symptom can be ignored, while a moderate symptom cannot be ignored but does not interfere with daily activities. A severe symptom interferes with daily activities, while a very severe symptom markedly interferes with most activities.

Aggravating or Relieving Factors

Ask if anything makes the symptom worse or better. For example, exertion may bring on chest pain and rest may relieve it, which suggests the diagnosis is angina (page 25).

Associated Symptoms

Here an attempt is made to uncover in a systematic way symptoms which might be expected to be associated with disease of a particular area. Initial and most thorough attention must be given to the system which includes the presenting complaint (see Systems Review, page 9). Remember that while a single symptom may provide the clue which leads to the correct diagnosis, usually it is the combination of characteristic symptoms that most reliably suggests the diagnosis.

Current Treatment

Ask the patient if he or she is currently taking any tablets or medicines (the use of the word 'drug' may cause alarm), which will often be described by colour or size rather than by name and dose. Then ask the patient to show you all his or her medications, if possible, and list them. Note the dose, length of use, and the indication for each drug. This list may provide a useful clue to current problems otherwise forgotten. Ask whether the drugs were taken as prescribed. Also ask the patient if he or she is taking any over-the-counter preparations (e.g, aspirin, antihistamines, vitamins). Always ask specifically if a woman is taking the contraceptive pill, because it is not considered a medicine or tablet by many who take it.

Sexual History

The sexual history is important, particularly if there is a history of urethral discharge, dysuria, vaginal discharge, a genital ulcer or rash, abdominal pain, pain on intercourse or anorectal symptoms, or if the acquired immunodeficiency syndrome (AIDS) or hepatitis is suspected. Determine the last date of intercourse, number of contacts, homosexual or bisexual partners, and contacts with prostitutes. The type of sexual practice may also be important: for example, oro-anal contact may predispose to colonic infection, and perirectal contact to hepatitis B, C or AIDS, while inserting objects into the rectum may cause trauma.

Menstrual History

In all cases a menstrual history should be obtained; it is particularly relevant for a patient with abdominal pain, a suspected endocrine disease or genitourinary symptoms (page 205). Write down the date of the last menstrual period. Ask about the age at which menstruation began, if the periods are regular, or whether menopause has occurred. Ask if the symptoms are related to the periods. Do not forget to ask a woman in the childbearing years if there is a possibility of pregnancy; this, for example, may preclude the use of certain investigations or drugs.

The Impact of the Illness

It is worthwhile determining the effect of the illness on the patient. Find out if the patient has seen a doctor before for the same problem and whether there has been previous diagnostic testing or treatment. Ask why the patient with a chronic complaint chose to come to the doctor now. Also ask what effect the symptoms have had on his or her life.

The Past History

Past Illnesses

Ask the patient if he or she has had any serious illnesses or operations or admissions to hospital in the past. Don't forget to inquire about childhood illnesses and about any obstetric or gynaecological problems. Previous illnesses or operations may have a direct bearing on the current health of the patient.

The patient may think he or she has had a particular diagnosis made in the past, but careful questioning may make this unlikely. For example, the patient may mention a previous duodenal ulcer, but not have had any investigations or treatment for this, which makes the diagnosis less certain. Therefore it is important to obtain the particulars of each past illness, including the symptoms experienced, tests performed and treatment prescribed.

Past Treatment and Allergic History

There are some medications or treatments the patient may have had in the past which remain relevant; these include corticosteroids, oral contraceptives, antihypertensive agents, chemotherapy and radiotherapy.

Note any adverse reactions which have occurred in the past. One should also ask about any allergy to drugs, and what the allergic reaction actually involved. Often the patient confuses an allergy with a side effect of a drug.

The Social and Personal History

This history includes the whole economic, social, domestic and industrial situation of the patient. Ask first about the place of birth and residence, and the level of education obtained. Race is important in some diseases, such as thalassaemia and sickle cell anaemia. Recent migrants may have been exposed to various illnesses like rheumatic fever during childhood.

Occupation and Education

Ask the patient about present occupation and education. Sometimes finding out exactly what the patient does at work can be helpful (page 102). Note particularly any work exposure to dusts, chemicals or disease; for example, mine workers may have the disease asbestosis. Find out if any similar complaints have affected fellow workers. Checking on hobbies can also be informative (e.g., bird fanciers and lung disease).

Social Habits

This is the time when possibly awkward questions about the patient's habits should be asked. It is important that you do not display a personal bias while asking these questions. Convey the impression you are interested and understand; you are there to help, not criticise.

Smoking

The patient may claim to be a non-smoker if he or she stopped smoking that morning. Therefore, one must ask if the patient has ever smoked and, if so, how many cigarettes (or cigars or pipes) were smoked a day and for how many years. Cigarette smoking is a risk factor for vascular disease, chronic lung disease, several cancers and peptic ulceration, and may damage the fetus (Table 1.2). Cigar and pipe smokers typically inhale less smoke than cigarette smokers, and overall mortality rates are correspondingly less in this group except for carcinoma of the oral cavity, larynx and oesophagus (page 102).

Alcohol

Ask if the patient drinks alcohol. If he or she does, ask what type, how much and how often. If the patient claims to be a social drinker find out what this means exactly. In a glass of wine, a nip (or shot) of spirits, a glass of port or sherry, or a 7oz glass of beer, there is approximately 10 grams of alcohol. Alcohol becomes a

Table 1.2 *Smoking and Clinical Associations**

1. **Cardiovascular disease**

   Premature coronary artery disease
   Peripheral vascular disease
   Cerebrovascular disease

2. **Respiratory disease**

   Lung cancer
   Chronic airflow limitation (Chronic obstructive pulmonary disease)
   Increased incidence of respiratory infection
   Increased incidence of postoperative respiratory complications

3. **Other cancers**

   Larynx, oral cavity, oesophagus, nasopharynx, bladder, kidney, pancreas, stomach, uterine cervix

4. **Gastrointestinal disease**

   Peptic ulceration

5. **Pregnancy**

   Increased risk of spontaneous abortion, fetal death, neonatal death, sudden infant death syndrome

6. **Drug interactions**

   Induces hepatic microsomal enzyme systems, e.g., increased metabolism of propranolol, theophylline

*   Individual risk is influenced by the duration, intensity and type of smoke exposure, as well as by genetic and other environmental factors. Passive smoking seems increasingly to be associated with respiratory disease.

major risk factor for liver and other diseases in men if more than 60g, or in women if more than 40g, is taken daily for five years or more. Alcoholics are notoriously unreliable about their alcohol intake, so it may be important to talk to the relatives.

Certain questions can be helpful in making a diagnosis of alcoholism; these are referred to as the CAGE questions:

1. Have you ever felt you ought to *cut* down on your drinking?
2. Have people *annoyed* you by criticising your drinking?
3. Have you every felt bad or *guilty* about your drinking?
4. Have you ever had a drink first thing in the morning to steady your nerves or get rid of a hangover (*eye* opener)?

A 'yes' to any of these questions suggests that there may be a serious drinking problem, and further inquiry into the history of this is important. The complications of alcoholism are summarised in Table 1.3.

Analgesics

If the patient has not already volunteered information about the use of analgesics, inquire about this. Again, note the type (aspirin and other non-steroidal anti-inflammatory drugs (NSAIDs), paracetamol (acetaminophen), phenacetin, or combinations), the dose taken and duration of use. It has been shown that APC (combined aspirin, phenacetin and caffeine) use is responsible for the renal disease analgesic nephropathy. The minimum dose required to produce renal scarring is 2kg of phenacetin in total, or 1g per day over one to three years in combination with other analgesics. Aspirin and other NSAIDs (but not paracetamol) can cause gastrointestinal bleeding.

Overseas Travel and Immunisation

If an infectious disease is a possibility, ask about recent overseas travel, destinations reached, and how the patient lived when away (for example, did he or she drink unbottled water and eat local foods, or dine at expensive international hotels). Ask about the immunisation status of the patient and whether any prophylactic drugs (for example, for malaria) were taken during the travels.

Marital Status, Social Support and Living Conditions

Inquire about the patient's marital status and ask discreet questions about the satisfactoriness of this arrangement. Find out the health of the spouse and of any children. Check if there are any other household members. Discreet questions about sexual activity may be very relevant. For example, impotence may occur in neurological conditions, debilitating illness or psychiatric disease. Questions about living arrangements are particularly important for chronic or disabling illnesses where one needs to know what social support is available and whether the patient is able to manage at home (for example, the number of steps required for access to the house, or the location of the toilet).

Ask about the adequacy of the patient's diet. Also ask about the amount of physical activity undertaken. Pets in the home may be important if infections or allergies are suspected.

Table 1.3 *Ethanol Abuse: Complications*

Gastrointestinal System
- Oesophagitis
- Acute gastric erosions
- Gastrointestinal bleeding from varices, erosions, Mallory-Weiss tear, peptic ulceration
- Pancreatitis (acute, recurrent or chronic)
- Diarrhoea (watery, due to alcohol itself, or steatorrhoea from chronic alcoholic pancreatitis or rarely liver disease)
- Hepatomegaly (fatty liver, chronic liver disease)
- Chronic liver disease (alcoholic hepatitis, cirrhosis) and associated complications
- Cancer (oesophagus, cardia of stomach, liver, pancreas)

Cardiovascular System
- Cardiomyopathy
- Arrhythmias
- Hypertension

Nervous System
- 'Blackouts'
- Nutrition-related conditions, e.g., Wernicke's encephalopathy, Korsakoff's psychosis, peripheral neuropathy (thiamine deficiency), pellagra (dementia, dermatitis and diarrhoea from niacin deficiency)
- Withdrawal syndromes, e.g., tremor, hallucinations, 'rum fits', delirium tremens
- Cerebellar degeneration
- Alcoholic dementia
- Alcoholic myopathy
- Autonomic neuropathy

Haematopoietic System
- Anaemia (dietary folate deficiency, iron deficiency from blood loss, direct toxic suppression of the bone marrow, rarely B_{12} deficiency with chronic pancreatitis, or sideroblastic anaemia)
- Thrombocytopenia (from bone marrow suppression or hypersplenism)

Genitourinary System
- Impotence, testicular atrophy in men
- Amenorrhoea, infertility, spontaneous abortion, fetal alcohol syndrome in women

Other Effects
- Increased risk of fractures and osteonecrosis of the femoral head

The Family History

Many diseases run in families. For example, ischaemic heart disease in parents who developed this at a young age is a major risk factor for ischaemic heart disease in the offspring. Various malignancies, such as breast and large bowel carcinoma, are more common in certain families. Both genetic and common environmental exposures may explain these familial associations. Some diseases are directly inherited (e.g., haemophilia).

Ask about any history of a similar illness in the family. Inquire about the health and, if relevant, the causes of death and ages of death of the parents and siblings.

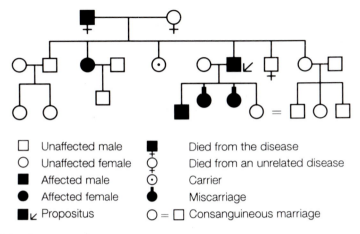

Figure 1.1 *Preparing a family tree: note the symbols used for the documentation.*

From Bouchier IAD, Morris JS, editors. Clinical skills: a system of clinical examination. 2nd ed. London: WB Saunders, 1992, with permission.

However, if there is any suggestion of an hereditary disease, a complete family tree should be constructed showing all members affected (Figure 1.1). Patients can be reluctant to mention that they have relatives with mental illnesses, epilepsy or cancer, so ask tactfully about these diseases. Consanguinity (usually first cousins marrying) increases the probability of autosomal recessive abnormalities in the children; ask about this if the pedigree is suggestive.

Systems Review

As well as detailed questioning in the system likely to be diseased, asking about important symptoms and disorders in other systems is essential (Table 1.4); otherwise important diseases may be missed. Major presenting symptoms in each system are described in the subsequent chapters. Examples of supplementary important questions to ask in the past history, social history and family history in each system are also given. Refer to the major textbooks for more details about these areas (see Suggested Reading). When recording the systems review, list important negative answers. Remember, if other recent symptoms are unmasked more details must be sought; relevant information is then added to the history of the presenting illness. Before completing the history, it is often valuable to ask what the patient thinks is wrong with him or her, and what he or she is most concerned about. Surprisingly useful facts may emerge with this approach.

Skills in History Taking

In summary, several skills are important in obtaining a useful and accurate history. First, establish rapport and understanding. Second, ask questions in a logical sequence. Listen to the answers and adjust your interview accordingly. Third, observe non-verbal clues carefully. Fourth, proper interpretation of the

Table 1.4   *The Systems Review*

Inquire about common symptoms and three or four of the common disorders in each
   major system:

Cardiovascular System

Have you had any pain or pressure in your chest, neck or arm?
Are you short of breath on exertion? How much exertion is necessary?
Have you ever been woken at night short of breath?
Can you lie flat without feeling breathless?
Have you had swelling of your ankles?
Have you noticed your heart racing or beating irregularly?
Do you have pain in your legs on exercise?
Do you have cold or blue hands or feet?
Have you ever had rheumatic fever, a heart attack, or high blood pressure?

Respiratory System

Are you ever short of breath?
Have you had any cough?
Do you cough up anything?
Have you coughed up blood?
Do you snore loudly?
Do you ever have wheezing when you are short of breath?
Have you had fevers?
Do you have night sweats?
Have you ever had pneumonia or tuberculosis?
Have you had a recent chest X-ray?
Have you had any bleeding or discharge from your breasts or felt any lumps there?

Gastrointestinal System

Are you troubled by indigestion?
Have you had pain or discomfort in your belly?
Have you had any abdominal bloating or distension?
Has your bowel habit changed recently?
How many bowel motions a week do you usually pass?
Have you lost control of your bowels or had accidents (faecal incontinence)?
Have you seen blood in your motions or vomited blood?
Have your bowel motions been black?
Have you had any difficulty swallowing?
Have your appetite or weight changed?
Do you have heartburn?
Have your eyes or skin ever been yellow?
Have you ever had hepatitis, peptic ulceration, colitis, or bowel cancer?
Tell me about your diet recently.

Genitourinary System

Do you have difficulty or pain on passing urine?
Is your urine stream as good as it used to be?
Is there a delay before you start to pass urine?   } (Applies mostly to men)
Is there dribbling at the end?
Do you have to get up at night to pass urine?
Are you passing larger or smaller amounts of urine?
Has the urine colour changed?
Have you seen blood in the urine?
Have you any problems with your sex life?

—continued

Table 1.4 *The Systems Review (continued)*

Have you noticed any rashes or lumps on your genitals?
Have you ever had venereal disease?
Have you ever had a urinary tract infection or kidney stone?
Are your periods regular?
Do you have excessive pain or bleeding with your periods?

Haematological System

Do you bruise easily?
Have you had fevers or shivers and shakes (rigors)?
Do you have difficulty stopping a small cut from bleeding?
Have you noticed any lumps under your arms, or in your neck or groin?
Have you ever had blood clots in your legs or in the lungs?

Musculoskeletal System

Do you have painful or stiff joints?
Are your joints ever swollen?
Have you had a skin rash recently?
Do you have any back or neck pain?
Have your eyes been dry or red?
Have you ever had a dry mouth or mouth ulcers?
Have you been diagnosed as having rheumatoid arthritis or gout?
Do your fingers ever become painful and become white and blue in the cold?

Endocrine System

Have you noticed any swelling in your neck?
Do your hands tremble?
Do you prefer hot or cold weather?
Have you had a thyroid problem or diabetes?
Have you noticed increased sweating?
Have you been troubled by fatigue?
Have you noticed any change in your appearance or hair, skin or voice?
Have you been unusually thirsty lately?

Reproductive History

Have you had any miscarriages?
Have you had high blood pressure or diabetes in pregnancy?

Neurological System and Mental State

Do you get headaches?
Have you had memory problems or trouble concentrating?
Have you had fainting episodes, fits or blackouts?
Do you have trouble seeing or hearing?
Are you dizzy?
Have you had weakness or numbness or clumsiness in your arms or legs?
Have you ever had a stroke or head injury?
Have you had difficulty sleeping?
Do you feel sad or depressed or have problems with your 'nerves'?
Is there anything else you would like to talk about?

history is crucial. Your aim should be to obtain information that will help establish the likely anatomical and physiological disturbances present, the aetiology of the presenting symptoms and the impact of the symptoms on the patient's ability to function. This type of information will help you plan the diagnostic investigations and treatment. First, however, a comprehensive and systematic physical examination is required.

These skills can only be obtained and maintained by practice.

Suggested Reading

Original and Review Articles

Beckman H, Markakis K, Suchman A, Frankel R, Getting the most from a 20-minute visit. *Am J Gastroenterol* 1994; 89: 662–4.

Beresford TP, Blow FC, Hill E, Singer K, Lucey MR. Comparison of CAGE questionnaire and computer-assisted laboratory profiles in screening for covert alcoholism. *Lancet* 1990; 336: 482–485.

Boland BJ, Wollan PC, Silverstein MD, Review of systems, physical examination, and routine test for case-finding in ambulatory patients. *Am J Med Sci* 1995; 309: 194–200.

Brewin T. Primum non nocere? *Lancet* 1994; 344: 1487–1488.

Furner V, Ross M. Lifestyle clues in the recognition of HIV infection. How to take a sexual history. *Med J Aust* 1993; 158: 40–41.

Kee F, Tiret L, Robo JY, Nicaud V, McCrum E, Evans A, Cambien F, Reliability of reported family history of myocardial infarction. *BMJ* 1993; 307: 1528–30.

Kehoe R, Wu SY, Leske MC, Chylack LT Jr, Comparing self-reported and physician-reported medical history. *Am J Epid* 1994; 139: 813–8.

Kitchens JM, Does this patient have an alcohol problem? *JAMA* 1994; 272: 1782–7.

Kroenke K. The case presentation: stumbling blocks and stepping stones. *Am J Med* 1985; 79: 605–608.

Longson D. The clinical consultation. *J R Coll Physicians Lond* 1983; 17: 192–195.

Nardone DA, Johnson GK, Faryna A, Coulehan JL, Parrino TA, A model for the diagnostic medical interview: nonverbal, verbal, and cognitive assessments. *J Gen Intern med* 1992; 7: 437–42.

Ness DE, Ende J, Denial in the medical interview. Recongnition and management. *JAMA* 1994; 272: 1777–81.

Newman LS, Occupational illness. *New Engl J Med* 1995; 333: 1128–34.

Platt FW, McMath JC. Clinical hypocompetence: the interview. *Ann Intern Med* 1979; 91: 898–902.

Short D, History taking. *Brit J Hosp Med* 1993; 50: 337–9.

Smith RC, Hoppe RB. The patient's story: integrating the patient- and physician-centered approaches to interviewing. *Ann Intern Med* 1991; 115: 470–477.

Stewart MA, Effective physician-patient communication and health outcomesia review. *Can med Assoc J* 1995; 152: 1423–33.

Textbooks

Billings JA, Stoeckl JD. The clinical encounter: a guide to the medical interview and case presentation. St Louis: Mosby Year Book Medical Publishers, 1989.

Cohen-Cole SA. The medical interview: the three-function approach. St Louis: Mosby, 1990.

Coulehan JL, Block MR. The medical interview: a primer for students of the art. 2nd ed. Philadelphia: FA Davis Company, 1992.

Isselbacher KJ, Wilson JD, Braunwald E, et al, editors. Harrison's principles of internal medicine. 13th ed. New York: McGraw Hill, 1994.

Kraytman M. The complete patient history. 2nd ed. New York: McGraw Hill, 1991.

Myerscough PR. Talking with patients. A basic clinical skill. Oxford: Oxford University Press, 1992.

Paton A, editor. ABC of alcohol. 3rd ed. London: BMJ Publishing Group, 1994.

Talley NJ, O'Connor S. Examination medicine: A guide to physician training. 3rd ed. Sydney: MacLennan and Petty, 1996.

Chapter 2

THE GENERAL PRINCIPLES OF PHYSICAL EXAMINATION

More mistakes are made from want of a proper examination than for any other reason.

Russell John Howard (1875–1942)

Students beginning their training in physical examination will be surprised at the formal way this examination is taught and performed. There are, however, a number of reasons for this formal approach. The first is that it ensures the examination is thorough and that important signs are not overlooked because of a haphazard method. The second is that the most convenient methods of examining patients in bed, and for particular conditions in various other postures, have evolved with time. By convention, patients are always examined from the right side of the bed, even though this may only be more convenient for right-handed people. When students learn this they often feel safer standing on the left side of the bed with their colleagues in tutorial groups, but many tutors are aware of this device, particularly when they notice all students standing as far away from the right side of the bed as possible. For clinical viva-voce (with live voice) examinations, the examiners expect all candidates to have a polished and thorough examination method.

This formal approach leads to the examination of parts of the body in systems. For example, examination of the cardiovascular system, which includes the heart and all the major accessible blood vessels, begins with positioning the patient correctly. This is followed by a quick general inspection and then, rather surprisingly for the uninitiated, seemingly prolonged study of the patient's fingernails. From there a set series of manoeuvres brings the doctor to the heart. This type of approach applies to all major systems and is designed to discover peripheral signs of disease in the system under scrutiny. The attention of the examining doctor is directed particularly towards those systems identified in the history as possibly being diseased, but of course proper physical examination requires that all the systems be examined.

The danger of a systematic approach is that time is not taken to stand back and look at the patient's *general appearance*, which may give many clues to the diagnosis.

Doctors must be observant, like a detective (Conan Doyle based his character Sherlock Holmes on an outstanding Scottish surgeon).

13

Taking the time to make an appraisal of the patient's general appearance, including the face hands and body, conveys the impression to the patient (and to the examiners) that the doctor or student is interested in the person as much as the disease.

Diagnosis has been defined as 'the crucial process that labels patients and classifies their illnesses, that identifies (and sometimes seals) their likely fates or prognoses and that propels us towards specific treatments in the confidence (often unfounded) that they will do more good than harm'.[1]

Within each of the examining systems one can describe four elements which comprise the main parts of the physical examination: looking—**inspection**; feeling—**palpation**; tapping—**percussion**; and listening—**auscultation**. Measuring is also relevant in some systems. These will each be discussed in detail in the following chapters.

First Impressions

First impressions of a patient's condition must be deliberately sought; they cannot be passively acquired. The specific changes that occur in particular illnesses, for example myxoedema, will be discussed in detail in the appropriate chapters. However, certain abnormalities should be obvious to the trained or training doctor.

First decide how sick the patient seems to be: that is, does he or she look generally ill or well. The cheerful woman sitting up in bed reading Proust is unlikely to require urgent attention to save her life. At the other extreme, the patient on the verge of death may be described as *in extremis* or moribund. The patient in this case may be lying still in bed and seem unaware of the surroundings. The face may be sunken and expressionless, respiration may be shallow and laboured, and at the end of life respiration often becomes slow and intermittent, with longer and longer pauses between rattling breaths.

Apart from one's general impression of a patient's state of health, certain general physical signs must be sought.

Vital Signs

Certain important measurements must be made during the assessment of the patient. These relate primarily to cardiac and respiratory function and include pulse, blood pressure, temperature and respiratory rate. These vital signs must be assessed at once if a patient appears unwell. Inpatients in hospital wards have these measurements taken regularly and charted. They provide important basic physiological information (Figures 2.1 and 2.2).

Facies

A specific diagnosis can sometimes be made by inspecting the face, its appearance giving the clue to the likely diagnosis. Other physical signs must usually be sought to confirm the diagnosis. Some facial characteristics are so typical of certain diseases that they immediately suggest the diagnosis and are called the diagnostic

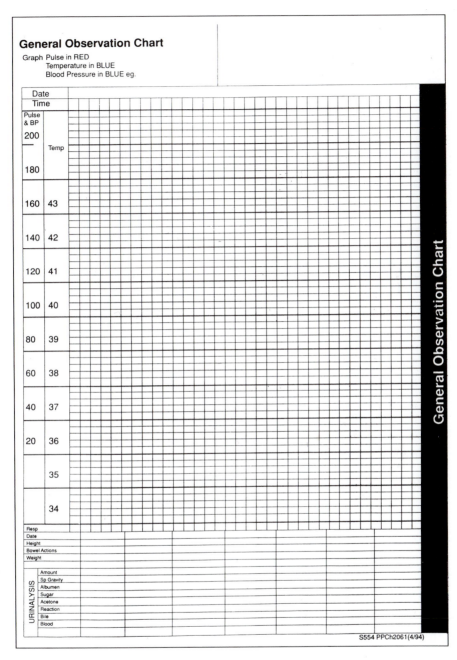

Figure 2.1   *A General Observation Chart. Regular measurements of the pulse rate, temperature and blood pressure are made for patients in hospital and recorded on this type of chart. The
frequency of the measurements depends on how ill the patient is. In appropriate patients
measurements are made of weight, urine output, fluid intake and urinalysis.*

Reproduced with thanks to Woden Valley Hospital.

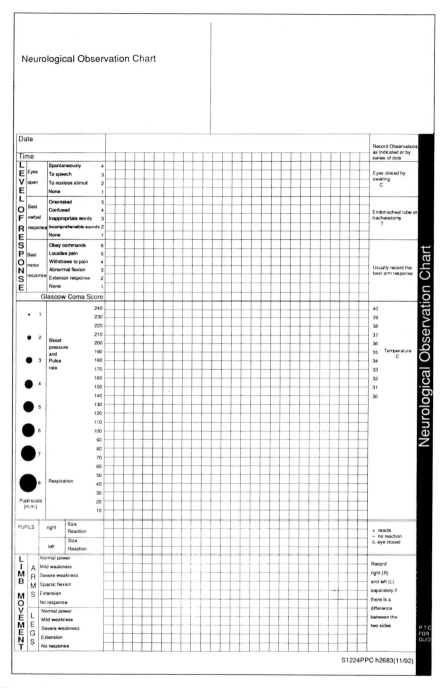

Figure 2.2 *A Neurological Observation Chart. Important information about the patient's neurological state is recorded. This is obtained from regular assessment of neurological 'vital signs'.*

Reproduced with thanks to Woden Valley Hospital.

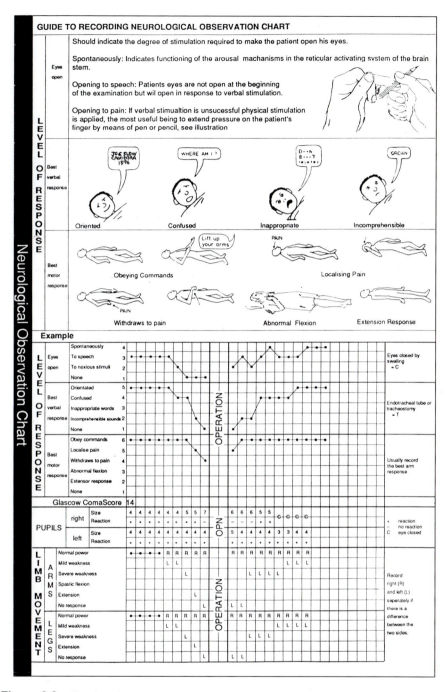

Figure 2.2   *Continued*

facies (Table 2.1). Apart from these, there are several other important abnormalities that must be looked for in the face.

Jaundice

When the serum bilirubin level rises to about twice the upper limit of normal, bilirubin is deposited in the tissues of the body and particularly in those tissues which contain elastin. It then affects the colour of the skin and more dramatically the colour of the sclerae, which are rich in elastin fibres. The sclerae are rarely affected by other pigment changes. In fact, jaundice is the only condition causing yellow sclerae. Other causes of yellow discoloration of the skin, but where the sclerae remain normal, are carotenaemia (usually due to excess consumption of carotene, often from intemperate eating of carrots or mangoes), acriflavine, fluorescein and picric acid ingestion.

Jaundice may be the result of excess production of bilirubin, usually from excessive destruction of red blood cells (termed haemolytic anaemia), when it can produce a pale lemon-yellow scleral discoloration. Alternatively, jaundice may be due to obstruction to bile flow from the liver, which if severe produces a dark yellow or orange tint. Scratch marks may be prominent due to associated itch (pruritus). The other main cause of jaundice is hepatocellular failure. Jaundice is discussed in more detail in Chapter 5 (page 184).

Cyanosis

This refers to a blue discoloration of the skin and mucous membranes; it is due to the presence of deoxygenated haemoglobin in superficial blood vessels. The haemoglobin molecule changes colour from blue to red when oxygen is added to it in the lungs. If more than 50 g/L of deoxygenated haemoglobin is present in the blood, the skin will have a bluish tinge. Cyanosis does *not* occur in anaemic hypoxia because the total haemoglobin content is low.

Central cyanosis means that there is an abnormal amount of deoxygenated haemoglobin in the arteries and that a blue discoloration is present in parts of the

Table 2.1 *Some Important Diagnostic Facies*

Acromegalic (page 307)
Cushingoid (page 311)
Down's syndrome (page 317)
Hippocratic (advanced peritonitis)—eyes are sunken, temples collapsed, nose is pinched
    with crusts on the lips and the forehead is clammy
Marfanoid (page 33)
Mitral (page 43)
Myopathic (page 369)
Myotonic (page 406)
Myxoedematous (page 304)
Pagetic (page 326)
Parkinsonian (page 410)
Ricketic (page 318)
Thyrotoxic (page 300)
Turner's syndrome (page 317)
Virile facies (page 318)

body with a good circulation, such as the tongue. This must be distinguished from *peripheral cyanosis* which occurs when the blood supply to a certain part of the body is reduced and the tissues extract more oxygen than normal from the circulating blood: for example, the lips in cold weather are often blue, but the tongue is spared. The presence of central cyanosis should lead one to a careful examination of the cardiovascular (Chapter 3) and respiratory (Chapter 4) systems (Table 2.2).

Pallor

A deficiency of haemoglobin (*anaemia*) can produce pallor of the skin and should be noticeable especially in the mucous membranes of the sclerae and mouth if the anaemia is severe (less than 70 g/L of haemoglobin). However, this is at best a crude indication of anaemia. It should be emphasised that pallor is a sign, whilst anaemia is based on laboratory results.

Facial pallor may also be found in *shock*, which is usually defined as a reduction of cardiac output, such that the oxygen demands of the tissues are not being met (Table 2.3). These patients usually appear clammy and cold and are significantly

Table 2.2 *Causes of Cyanosis*

Central Cyanosis
1. Decreased arterial oxygen saturation
   - Decreased concentration of inspired oxygen: high altitude
   - Lung disease: chronic obstructive pulmonary disease with cor pulmonale (page 122), massive pulmonary embolism (page 126)
   - Right-to-left cardiac shunt (cyanotic congenital heart disease) (page 83)
2. Polycythaemia (page 241)
3. Haemoglobin abnormalities (rare): methaemoglobinaemia, sulphaemoglobinaemia

Peripheral Cyanosis
1. All causes of central cyanosis cause peripheral cyanosis
2. Exposure to cold
3. Reduced cardiac output: left ventricular failure (page 65) or shock
4. Arterial or venous obstruction (page 64)

Table 2.3 *Causes of Shock*

1. Hypovolaemia
   - External fluid loss, e.g., blood, vomitus, diarrhoea, urine, burns, excess sweating
   - Sequestration of body fluids in the abdomen (e.g., ascites), chest (e.g., haemothorax) or limbs (e.g., fracture)
2. Cardiac
   - Pump failure, e.g., myocardial infarction, acute mitral regurgitation
   - Cardiac tamponade
   - Dissecting aortic aneurysm
   - Arrhythmia
3. Massive pulmonary embolus
4. Sepsis, e.g., Gram-negative bacteria (endotoxin)
5. Anaphylaxis
6. Endocrine failure, e.g., adrenal failure, hypothyroidism
7. Neuropathic—from drugs (e.g., antihypertensives, anaesthesia), spinal cord injury or autonomic neuropathy

hypotensive (page 19). Pallor may also be a normal variant due to a deep-lying venous system and opaque skin.

Hair

Bearded or bald ladies and hairless men not uncommonly present to doctors. These conditions may be abnormal, and occasionally are due to endocrine disease (Chapter 9).

Weight, Body Habitus and Posture

Look specifically for obesity. This is most objectively assessed by calculation of the body mass index (BMI) = weight in kilograms divided by height in metres squared. Normal is less than $25 \, kg/m^2$. A BMI > 30 indicates frank obesity.

A number of body shapes are almost diagnostic of different conditions (Table 2.4). Look for wasting of the muscles, which may be due to neurological or debilitating disease, such as malignancy.

Note excessively short or tall stature which may be rather difficult to judge when the patient is lying in bed (page 315). Inspect for limb deformity or missing limbs (rather embarrassing if missed in viva-voce examinations) and observe if the physique is consistent with the patient's stated chronological age.

If the patient walks into the examining room the opportunity to examine gait should not be lost; the full testing of gait is described in Chapter 10.

Hydration

Although this is not easy to assess, all doctors must be able to estimate the approximate state of hydration of a patient. For example, a severely dehydrated patient is at risk of death from developing acute renal failure (page 203), while an overhydrated patient may develop pulmonary oedema (page 65).

To assess dehydration (Table 2.5), inspect for sunken orbits, dry mucous membranes and the moribund appearance of severe dehydration. Reduced skin turgor

Table 2.4 *Some Body Habitus Syndromes*

Endocrine
Acromegaly (Figure 9.7)
Cushing's syndrome (Figure 9.9)
Hypopituitarism (page 30)
Pseudohypoparathyroidism (Figure 9.12)
Rickets (Figure 9.15)
Paget's disease (Figure 9.21)

Musculoskeletal
Marfan's syndrome (Figure 3.2)
Turner's syndrome (Figure 9.13)
Klinefelter's syndrome (page 319)
Achondroplasia (page 318)

Table 2.5   *Physical Signs of Dehydration*

Mild (<5%): ≈ 2.5L deficit

Mild thirst
Dry mucous membranes
Concentrated urine

Moderate (5% to 8%): ≈ 4L deficit

As above
Moderate thirst
Reduced skin turgor (elasticity), especially arms, forehead, chest, abdomen
Tachycardia

Severe (9% to 12%): ≈ 6L deficit

As above
Great thirst
Reduced skin turgor and decreased eyeball pressure
Collapsed veins, sunken eyes, 'gaunt' face
Postural hypotension
Oliguria (<400mL urine/24 hours)

Very Severe (>12%): >6L deficit

As above
Comatose
Moribund
Signs of shock

Total body water in a man of 70kg is about 40L.

(pinch the skin: normal skin returns immediately on being released) occurs in moderate and severe dehydration. Take the blood pressure (page 40) and look for a fall in blood pressure when the patient sits or stands up after lying down. This is called postural hypotension. Weigh the patient. Following the body weight daily is the best way to determine changes in hydration over time. For example, a 5% decrease in body weight over 24 hours indicates that about 5% of body water has been lost.

Remember that assessment of the patient's jugular venous pressure is one of the most sensitive ways of judging intravascular volume overload (Chapter 3).

The Hands

Changes occur in the hands in many different diseases. It is useful as an introduction to shake a patient's hand when meeting him or her. Apart from being polite, this may help make the diagnosis of dystrophia myotonica, a rare muscle disease in which the patient may be unable to let go (page 403). There is probably no subspeciality of internal medicine in which examination of the hands is not rewarding. The shape of the nails may change in some cardiac and respiratory diseases, the whole size of the hand may increase in acromegaly (page 308), gross distortion of the hands' architecture occurs in some forms of arthritis (page 257), tremor or muscle wasting may represent neurological disease (page 411), and pallor of the palmar creases may indicate anaemia (page 224). These and other changes in the hands await you later in the book.

Table 2.6 *Nail Signs in Systemic Disease*

Nail Sign	Some Causes	Page No.
Blue nails	Cyanosis, Wilson's disease, ochronosis	18
Red nails	Polycythaemia (reddish-blue), carbon monoxide poisoning (cherry-red)	241
Yellow nails	Yellow nail syndrome	120
Clubbing	Lung cancer, chronic pulmonary suppuration, infective endocarditis, cyanotic heart disease, congenital	34
Splinter haemorrhages	Infective endocarditis, vasculitis	35
Koilonychia (spoon-shaped nails)	Iron deficiency	224
Pale nail bed	Anaemia	224
Onycholysis	Thyrotoxicosis, psoriasis	299
Non-pigmented transverse bands (Beau's lines)	Fever, cachexia, malnutrition	207
Leuconychia (white nails)	Hypoalbuminaemia	153
Transverse opaque bands (Muehrke's lines)	Hypoalbuminaemia (also caused by chemotherapy or severe illness)	207
Single transverse white band (Mees' lines)	Arsenic poisoning, renal failure (also caused by chemotherapy or severe illness)	207
Nail fold erythema and telangiectasia	Systemic lupus erythematosus	279
'Half and half nails' (proximal portion white to pink and distal portion red or brown: Terry's nails)	Chronic renal failure, cirrhosis	207

The Nails

Changes in the nails can prove very helpful in diagnosis of systemic disease (Table 2.6). Nail changes are described in detail in the subsequent chapters.

Temperature

The temperature should always be recorded as part of the initial clinical examination of the patient. The normal temperature ranges from 36.6°C to 37.2°C (98°F to 99°F). In very hot weather the temperature may rise up to 0.5°C higher. The oral temperature is normally lower than the rectal temperature by 0.2°C to 0.5°C. Axillary temperature may be 0.5°C lower than the oral reading. There is a diurnal variation: body temperature is lowest in the morning and reaches a peak between 6.00 and 10.00 pm. The febrile pattern of most diseases follows this diurnal variation. The pattern of the fever (pyrexia) may be helpful in diagnosis (Table 2.7).

Table 2.7   *Types of Fever*

Type	Character	Examples
Continued	Does not remit	Typhoid fever, typhus, drug fever, malignant hyperthermia
Intermittent	Temperature falls to normal each day	Pyogenic infections, lymphomas, miliary tuberculosis
Remittent	Daily fluctuations >2°C, temperature does not return to normal	Not characteristic of any particular disease
Relapsing	Temperature returns to normal for days before rising again	Malaria: Tertian—3 day pattern, fever peaks every other day (*Plasmodium vivax, P. ovale*) Quartan—4 day pattern, fever peaks every 3rd day (*P. malariae*) Lymphoma: Pel*–Ebstein† fever of Hodgkin's disease (very rare) Pyogenic infection

* Pieter Pel (1859–1919), Professor of Medicine, Amsterdam.
† Wilhelm Ebstein (1836–1912), German physician.
Note: The use of antipyretic and antibiotic drugs has made these patterns unusual today.

Very high temperatures (*hyperpyrexia*, defined as above 41.6°C) are a serious problem and may result in death. The causes include heat stroke from exposure or excessive exertion, for example in marathon runners; malignant hyperthermia (a group of genetically determined disorders in which hyperpyrexia occurs in response to various anaesthetic agents [e.g., halothane] or muscle relaxants [e.g., suxamethonium]); the neuroleptic malignant syndrome; and hypothalamic disease.

Hypothermia is defined as a temperature less than 35°C. Normal thermometers do not record below 35°C and therefore special low-reading thermometers must be used if hypothermia is suspected. Causes of hypothermia include prolonged exposure to cold and hypothyroidism (page 302).

Preparing the Patient for Examination

An accurate physical examination is best performed when the examining conditions are ideal. This means that if possible the patient should be in a well-lit room (preferably daylight) from which distracting noises and interruptions have been excluded (rarely possible in busy hospital wards). To simulate more realistic conditions, keen students have been known to try listening to patients' hearts while the floor around the bed is being polished with a large electric polishing machine.

The patient must be undressed so that the parts to be examined are accessible. Modesty requires that a woman's breasts be covered temporarily with a towel or sheet while other parts of the body are being examined. Men and women should both have the groin covered, for example during the examination of the legs.

However, important physical signs will be missed in some patients if excessive attention is paid to modesty. The position of the patient in bed or elsewhere should depend on what system is to be examined. For example, a patient's abdomen is best examined if he or she lies completely flat so that the abdominal muscles are relaxed. This is discussed in detail in subsequent chapters.

Reference

1. Sackett DL, Haynes RB, Tugwell P. Clinical epidemiology. A basic science for clinical medicine. Boston: Little, Brown & Co, 1985.

Suggested Reading

Original and Review Articles

Detsky AS, Smalley PS, Chang J, Is this patient malnourished? *JAMA* 1994; 271: 54–8.

Fitzgerald FT, Tierney LM Jr. The bedside Sherlock Holmes. *West J Med* 1982; 137: 169–175.

Hayden GF. Olfactory diagnosis in medicine. *Postgrad Med* 1980; 67: 110–115, 118.

Sackett DL. A primer on the precision and accuracy of the clinical examination. *JAMA* 1992; 267: 2638–2644.

Textbooks

Beaven DW, Brooks SE. Color atlas of the nail in clinical diagnosis. Chicago: Year Book Medical Publishers, 1984.

Browse NL. An introduction to the symptoms and signs of surgical disease. 2nd ed. London: Edward Arnold, 1990.

Clain A, editor. Hamilton Bailey's demonstrations of physical signs in clinical surgery. 17th ed. Bristol: Wright, 1986.

Sapira JD. The art and science of bedside diagnosis. Baltimore: Urban and Schwartzenberg, 1990.

Zatouroff M. Color atlas of physical signs in general medicine. Chicago: Mosby Year Book, 1985.

Chapter 3

THE CARDIOVASCULAR SYSTEM

The heart . . . moves of itself and does not stop unless for ever.

Leonardo da Vinci (1452–1519)

This chapter deals with the history and the examination of the heart and blood vessels, as well as other parts of the body where symptoms and signs of heart disease may appear. Not only is this fundamental to the assessment of any patient but it is also an extremely common system tested in viva examinations. It is believed by cardiologists to be the most important system in the body.

The Cardiovascular History

Presenting Symptoms (Table 3.1)

Chest Pain

The mention of chest pain by a patient tends to provoke more urgent attention than other symptoms (Table 3.2). The surprised patient may find himself whisked into an emergency ward with the rapid appearance of worried looking doctors. This is because ischaemic heart disease, which may be a life-threatening condition, often presents in this manner. The pain of angina and myocardial infarction tends to be similar; it may be due to the accumulation of metabolites from ischaemic muscle following complete or partial obstruction of a coronary artery leading to stimulation of the cardiac sympathetic nerves. Patients with cardiac transplants who develop coronary disease in the transplanted heart do not feel angina, presumably because the heart is denervated.

To help determine the cause of chest pain, it is important to ascertain the duration, location, quality, precipitating and aggravating factors, means of relief and accompanying symptoms.

Angina comes from the Latin word meaning 'choking', and the patient may complain of crushing pain, heaviness, discomfort or a choking sensation in the retrosternal area or in the throat. It is best to ask if the patient experiences chest 'discomfort' rather than 'pain', because angina is often dull and aching in character and may not be perceived as pain. The pain or discomfort is usually central rather than left sided. The patient may dismiss his or her pain as non-cardiac because it is not felt over the heart on the left side. It may radiate to the jaw or to the arms but very rarely travels below the umbilicus. The severity of the pain varies. Angina

Table 3.1 *Cardiovascular History*

Major Symptoms

Chest pain or heaviness

Dyspnoea: exertional (note degree of exercise necessary), orthopnoea, paroxysmal
    nocturnal dyspnoea

Ankle swelling

Palpitations

Syncope

Intermittent claudication

Fatigue

Past History

Rheumatic fever, chorea, sexually transmitted disease, recent dental work, thyroid
    disease

Prior medical examination revealing heart disease (e.g., military, school, insurance)

Drugs

Social History

Tobacco and alcohol use

Occupation

Family History

Myocardial infarcts, cardiomyopathy, congenital heart disease, mitral valve prolapse,
    Marfan's syndrome

Coronary Artery Disease Risk Factors

Hyperlipidaemia

Smoking

Hypertension

Family history of coronary artery disease

Diabetes mellitus

Obesity and physical inactivity

Male sex and advanced age

Functional Status in Established Heart Disease*

Class I—angina or dyspnoea during unusually intense activity

Class II—angina or dyspnoea during ordinary activity

Class III—angina or dyspnoea during less than ordinary activity

Class IV—angina or dyspnoea at rest

*   New York Heart Association classification

characteristically occurs with exertion, with rapid relief once the patient rests or slows down. The amount of exertion necessary to produce the pain may be predictable to the patient. A change in the pattern of onset of previously stable angina must be taken very seriously. Although angina typically occurs on exertion, it may also occur at rest or wake a patient from sleep. Ischaemic chest pain is usually unaffected by respiration. The use of sublingual nitrates characteristically brings relief within a couple of minutes, but this is not specific since nitrates may also relieve oesophageal spasm.

The pain of myocardial infarction often comes on at rest, is usually more severe and lasts much longer. Pain present for more than half an hour is more likely to be

Table 3.2 *Causes of Chest Pain*

Cardiac pain	Myocardial ischaemia or infarction
Vascular pain	Aortic dissection
	Aortic aneurysm
Pleuropericardial pain	Pericarditis
	Infective pleurisy
	Pneumothorax
	Pneumonia
	Autoimmune disease
	Mesothelioma
	Metastatic tumour
Chest wall pain	Persistent cough
	Muscular strains
	Intercostal myositis
	Thoracic herpes zoster
	Coxsackie B infection
	Thoracic nerve compression or infiltration
	Rib fracture
	Rib tumour, primary or metastatic
	Tietze's syndrome
	Slipping rib syndrome
Gastrointestinal pain	Gastro-oesophageal reflux (common)
	Oesophageal spasm (uncommon)
Airway pain	Tracheitis
	Intubation
	Central bronchial carcinoma
	Inhaled foreign body
Mediastinal pain	Mediastinitis
	Sarcoid adenopathy
	Lymphoma

due to myocardial infarction than to angina, but pain present continuously for many days is unlikely to be either. Associated symptoms of myocardial infarction include dyspnoea, sweating, anxiety, nausea and faintness.

Other causes of retrosternal pain are listed in Table 3.2. Chest pain made worse by inspiration is called *pleuritic pain*. This may be due to pleurisy (page 114) or pericarditis (page 67). This pain is not usually brought on by exertion and is often relieved by sitting up and leaning forward. It is caused by the movement of inflamed pleural or pericardial surfaces on one another.

Chest wall pain is usually localised to a small area of the chest wall, is sharp and is associated with respiration or movement of the shoulders rather than with exertion. It may last only a few seconds or be present for prolonged periods. Disease of the *cervical or upper thoracic spine* may also cause pain associated with movement. This pain tends to radiate around from the back towards the front of the chest.

Pain due to a *dissecting aneurysm* of the aorta is usually very severe and may be described as tearing. This pain is usually greatest at the moment of onset and radiates to the back.

Massive pulmonary embolism causes pain of very sudden onset which may be retrosternal and associated with collapse, dyspnoea and cyanosis (page 126). It is often pleuritic, but can be identical to anginal pain especially if associated with right ventricular ischaemia.

Spontaneous pneumothorax may result in pain and severe dyspnoea (page 121). The pain is sharp and localised to one part of the chest.

Oesophageal spasm may cause retrosternal chest pain or discomfort and can be quite difficult to distinguish from angina but is rare. The pain may come on after eating or drinking hot or cold fluids, may be associated with dysphagia (difficulty swallowing) and may be relieved by nitrates. It is rare. *Gastro-oesophageal reflux*, however, can quite commonly cause angina-like pain without heartburn.

Cholecystitis can cause chest pain and be confused with myocardial infarction. Right upper quadrant abdominal tenderness is usually present (page 140).

Dyspnoea

Shortness of breath may be due to cardiac disease. Dyspnoea (Greek *dys* = bad, *pnoia* = breathing) is often defined as an unexpected awareness of breathing. It occurs whenever the work of breathing is excessive, but the mechanism is uncertain. It is probably due to a sensation of increased force required of the respiratory muscles to produce a volume change in the lungs, due to reduction in compliance of the lungs or increased resistance to air flow. Cardiac dyspnoea is typically chronic and occurs with exertion because of failure of the left ventricular output to rise with exercise; this in turn leads to an acute rise in left ventricular end diastolic pressure, raised pulmonary venous pressure, interstitial fluid leakage and thus reduced lung compliance. Left ventricular function may be impaired because of ischaemia, fibrosis or hypertrophy. As it becomes more severe cardiac dyspnoea occurs at rest. Orthopnoea (Greek *ortho* = straight), or dyspnoea that develops when a patient is supine, occurs because in an upright position the patient's interstitial oedema is redistributed; the lower zones of the lungs become worse and the upper zones better. This allows improved overall blood oxygenation. Patients with severe orthopnoea spend the night sitting up in a chair or propped up on numerous pillows in bed.

Paroxysmal nocturnal dyspnoea is severe dyspnoea which wakes the patient from sleep so that he or she is forced to get up gasping for breath. This occurs because of a sudden failure of left ventricular output with an acute rise in pulmonary venous and capillary pressures; this leads to transudation of fluid into the interstitial tissues which increases the work of breathing. The sequence may be precipitated by resorption of peripheral oedema at night whilst supine. Acute cardiac dyspnoea may also occur with acute pulmonary oedema or a pulmonary embolus.

Cardiac dyspnoea can be difficult to distinguish from that due to lung disease or other causes (page 99). One should inquire particularly about a history of any cardiac disease which could be responsible for the onset of cardiac failure. For example, a patient with a number of known previous myocardial infarctions who develops dyspnoea is likely to have decreased left ventricular contractility. A patient with a history of hypertension or a very heavy alcohol intake may have hypertensive heart disease or an alcoholic cardiomyopathy. The presence of orthopnoea or paroxysmal nocturnal dyspnoea is more suggestive of cardiac failure than lung disease.

Ankle Swelling

Some patients present with ankle swelling due to oedema from cardiac failure. Ankle oedema is usually symmetrical and worst in the evenings, with improvement during the night. It may be a symptom of biventricular failure or right ventricular failure secondary to chronic lung disease. As failure progresses, oedema ascends to involve the legs, thighs, genitalia and abdomen. There are usually other symptoms or signs of heart disease. It is important to find out whether the patient is taking a vasodilating drug (e.g., a calcium channel blocker) which can cause peripheral oedema. There are other common causes of ankle oedema that also need to be considered (page 60).

Palpitations

This is not a very precise term. It is usually taken to mean an unexpected awareness of the heartbeat. Ask the patient to describe exactly what he or she notices and whether the palpitations are slow or fast, regular or irregular and how long they last. There may be the sensation of a missed beat followed by a particularly heavy beat; this can be due to an atrial or ventricular premature contraction (which produces little cardiac output) followed by a compensating pause and then a normally conducted beat (which is more forceful than usual because there has been a longer diastolic filling period for the ventricle). If the patient complains of a rapid heartbeat, it is important to find out whether the palpitations are of sudden or gradual onset and offset. Cardiac arrhythmias are usually instantaneous in onset and offset, whereas the onset and offset of sinus tachycardia is more gradual. A completely irregular rhythm is suggestive of atrial fibrillation, particularly if it is rapid. It may be helpful to ask the patient to tap with his or her finger the rate and rhythm of the palpitations. Associated features including pain, dyspnoea or faintness must be inquired about. The awareness of rapid palpitations followed by syncope suggests ventricular tachycardia. Any rapid rhythm may precipitate angina in a patient with ischaemic heart disease.

Patients may have learned manoeuvres which will return the rhythm to normal. Attacks of supraventricular tachycardia may be suddenly terminated by increasing vagal tone with the Valsalva manoeuvre (page 59), by coughing, or by swallowing cold water or ice cubes.

Syncope and Dizziness

Syncope is a transient loss of consciousness resulting from cerebral anoxia, usually due to inadequate blood flow.

Syncope may represent a simple faint or be a symptom of cardiac or neurological disease. One must establish whether the patient actually loses consciousness and under what circumstances the syncope occurred (e.g., on standing for prolonged periods or standing up suddenly (postural syncope), while passing urine (micturition syncope), on coughing (tussive syncope) or with sudden emotional stress (vasovagal syncope)). Find out whether there is any warning, e.g., dizziness or palpitations, and how long the episodes last. Recovery may be spontaneous or the patient may require attention from bystanders. Bystanders may also have noticed abnormal movements if the patient has epilepsy (page 332), but these can also occur in primary syncope. If the patient's symptoms appear to be postural, inquire about the use of antihypertensive or anti-anginal drugs and other medications which may induce postural hypotension. If the episode is vasovagal, it may be precipitated by something unpleasant like the sight of blood or occur in a crowded, hot room; patients often feel nauseated and sweaty before fainting and may have had prior similar episodes, especially during adolescence and young adulthood.

If syncope is due to an arrhythmia there is often a sudden loss of consciousness regardless of the patient's posture; chest pain may also occur if the patient has ischaemic heart disease or aortic stenosis. Exertional syncope may occur with obstruction to left ventricular outflow by aortic stenosis or hypertrophic cardiomyopathy.

Dizziness which occurs even when the patient is lying down or which is made worse by movements of the head is more likely to be of neurological origin, although recurrent tachyarrhythmias may occasionally cause dizziness in any position. One should attempt to decide whether the dizziness is really vertiginous, or whether it is a presyncopal feeling.

Intermittent Claudication

The word 'claudication'* comes from Latin meaning to limp. Patients with claudication notice pain in one or both calves, thighs or buttocks when they walk more than a certain distance. This distance is called the claudication distance. The claudication distance may be shorter when patients walk up hills. A history of claudication suggests peripheral vascular disease with a poor blood supply to the affected muscles. The most important risk factor is smoking, and a history of vascular disease elsewhere in the body, including cerebrovascular disease and ischaemic heart disease, is common.

Fatigue

Fatigue is a common symptom of cardiac failure. It may be associated with a reduced cardiac output and poor blood supply to the skeletal muscles. There are many other causes of fatigue, including anaemia and depression (page 293).

Risk Factors for Coronary Artery Disease

An essential part of the cardiac history involves obtaining detailed information about a patient's risk factors.

Hypercholesterolaemia is the most important risk factor for ischaemic heart disease. Many patients now know their serum cholesterol levels because widespread testing has become fashionable. The total serum cholesterol is a useful screening test, and levels above 5.2mmol/L are considered undesirable. An elevated total cholesterol level is even more significant if the high density lipoprotein (HDL) level is low (less than 1.0mmol/L). Significant elevation of the triglyceride level may be a coronary risk factor in its own right and certainly adds to the risk if the total cholesterol is high. If a patient already has coronary disease hyperlipidaemia is even more important. Control of risk factors for these patients

---

*   The Roman Emperor Tiberius Claudius Drusus Nero Germanicus (10 BC–AD 54) limped due to some form of paralysis. The words, however, are etymologically unrelated, which seems rather a cruel coincidence for Claudius. 'Claudicant' first appeared in English in 1624.

is called secondary prevention. If the patient's cholesterol is known to be high, it is worth obtaining a dietary history. This can be very trying. It is important to remember that not only foods containing cholesterol but those containing saturated fats contribute to the serum cholesterol level. High alcohol consumption and obesity are associated with hypertriglyceridaemia.

Smoking is probably the next most important risk factor for cardiovascular disease and peripheral vascular disease. Some patients describe themselves as non-smokers even though they stopped smoking only a few hours before. The number of years the patient has smoked and the number of cigarettes per day are both very important. The significance of a history of smoking for a patient who has not smoked for many years is controversial. The risk of symptomatic ischaemic heart disease falls gradually over the years after smoking has been stopped although it probably does not return completely to normal.

Hypertension is another important risk factor for coronary artery disease. Find out when hypertension was first diagnosed and what treatment, if any, has been instituted. The treatment of hypertension probably does reduce the risk of ischaemic heart disease, and certainly reduces the risk of hypertensive heart disease, cardiac failure and cerebrovascular disease. Treatment of hypertension has also been shown to reverse left ventricular hypertrophy.

A family history of coronary artery disease increases a patient's risk, particularly if it has been present in first-degree relatives (parents or siblings) and if it has affected these people below the age of 60. Not all heart disease, however, is ischaemic; a patient whose relatives suffered from rheumatic heart disease is at no greater risk of ischaemic heart disease than anybody else.

A history of *diabetes mellitus* increases the risk of ischaemic heart disease substantially. It is important to find out how long a patient has been diabetic and whether insulin treatment has been required. Good control of the blood sugar level of diabetics probably reduces this risk. An attempt should therefore be made to find out how well a patient's diabetes has been controlled (page 320).

The presence of multiple risk factors makes control of each one more important.

Past History

Patients with a history of definite previous angina or myocardial infarction remain at high risk for further ischaemic events. It is very useful at this stage to find out how a diagnosis of ischaemic heart disease was made and in particular what investigations were undertaken. The patient may well remember exercise testing or a coronary angiogram, and some patients can even remember how many coronary arteries were narrowed.

Patients may recall a diagnosis of rheumatic fever in their childhood but many were labelled as having 'growing pains'. A patient who was put to bed for a long period as a child may well have had rheumatic fever (page 284). A history of rheumatic fever places patients at risk of rheumatic valvular disease.

Treatment

The drugs a patient is taking often give a good clue to the diagnosis. Find out about any ill effects from current or previous drugs. The surgical history must also be elicited. The patient may have had a previous angioplasty or coronary artery bypass grafting, and may know how many arteries were dilated or bypassed.

Social History

Both ischaemic heart disease and rheumatic heart disease are chronic conditions which may affect a patient's ability to function normally. It is therefore important to find out whether the patient's condition has prevented his or her working and over what period. Patients with severe cardiac failure, for example, may need to make adjustments to their living arrangements so that they are not required to walk up and down stairs at home.

The Cardiovascular Examination

The cardiovascular system lends itself particularly well to the formal examination approach. There are a number of equally satisfactory methods, but the precise approach used is not as important as having a method which is comprehensive, gives the impression of proficiency and ensures that no important part of the examination is omitted.

First one should position the patient properly and pause to get an impression of the general appearance. Then detailed examination begins with the hands and pulses and progresses smoothly to the neck, face, and then on to the praecordium (from the Latin *prae* in front of, *cor* heart).

A summary of a suggested method of examination is found at the end of this chapter.

Positioning the Patient

It is important to have the patient lying in bed with enough pillows to support him or her at 45 degrees (Figure 3.1). This is the usual position in which the jugular venous pressure is assessed. During auscultation, optimal examination requires further positioning of the patient, as will be discussed later.

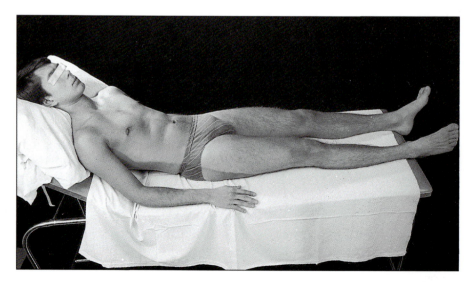

Figure 3.1 *Cardiovascular examination: positioning the patient.*

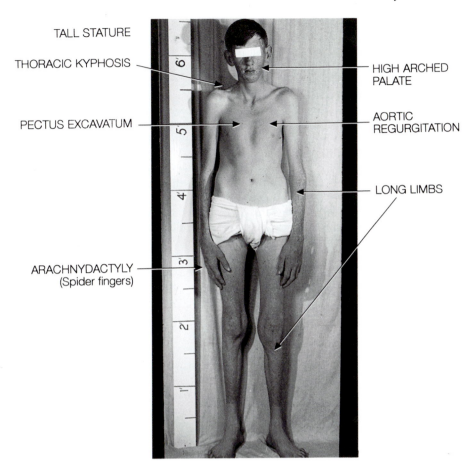

TALL STATURE

THORACIC KYPHOSIS

PECTUS EXCAVATUM

ARACHNYDACTYLY
(Spider fingers)

HIGH ARCHED
PALATE

AORTIC
REGURGITATION

LONG LIMBS

Figure 3.2 *Marfan's syndrome: tall stature, thoracic kyphosis, pectus excavatum, arachnodactyly (spider fingers), long limbs, aortic regurgitation, and a high arched palate.*

General Appearance

Look at the general state of health. Does the patient appear to be ill? If he or she looks ill try to decide why you have formed that impression. Note whether the patient at rest has rapid and laboured respiration, suggesting dyspnoea (Table 4.3, page 99).

The patient may look *cachectic*; that is, there may be severe loss of weight and muscle wasting. This is commonly caused by malignant disease, but severe cardiac failure may also have this effect (cardiac cachexia). It probably results from a combination of anorexia (due to congestive enlargement of the liver) and impaired intestinal absorption (due to congested intestinal veins).

There are also some syndromes which are associated with specific cardiac disease. Marfan's syndrome (Figure 3.2),* Down's syndrome (page 317)[†] and Turner's syndrome (page 316)[‡] are important examples.

---

*   Bernard-Jean Antonin Marfan (1858–1942), French physician in Paris.

[†]   John Langdon Down (1828–1896), English physician, described the clinical picture of mongolism.

[‡]   Henry Hubert Turner (b. 1892), described the syndrome in 1938.

The Hands

Pick up the right hand. Look first at the nails. Now is the time for a decision as to the presence or absence of clubbing. Clubbing is an increase in the soft tissue of the distal part of the fingers or toes. The causes of clubbing are surprisingly varied (Table 3.3). The mechanism is unknown but there are, of course, several theories. One theory is that, in response to arterial hypoxaemia, an unknown humoral substance causes dilatation of the vessels of the fingertips or toes. Platelet-derived growth factor, released from megakaryocyte and platelet emboli in the nail beds, has been implicated in the pathogenesis.

Proper examination for clubbing involves inspecting the fingernails (and toe-nails) from the side to determine if there is loss of the angle between the nail bed and the finger (Figure 3.3). A subtle sign may be an increased sponginess of the proximal nail bed. One should test this by compressing the nail bed and rocking it with one's finger. Eventually, the distal phalanx becomes enlarged due to soft

Table 3.3 *Causes of Clubbing*

Common
Cardiovascular
Cyanotic congenital heart disease
Infective endocarditis
Respiratory
Lung carcinoma (usually *not* small cell carcinoma)
Chronic pulmonary suppuration:
Bronchiectasis
Lung abscess
Empyema
Idiopathic pulmonary fibrosis
Uncommon
Respiratory
Cystic fibrosis
Asbestosis
Pleural mesothelioma (benign fibrous type) or pleural fibroma
Gastrointestinal
Cirrhosis (especially biliary cirrhosis)
Inflammatory bowel disease
Coeliac disease
Thyrotoxicosis
Familial (usually before puberty) or idiopathic
Rare
Neurogenic diaphragmatic tumours
Pregnancy
Unilateral Clubbing
Bronchial arteriovenous aneurysm
Axillary artery aneurysm

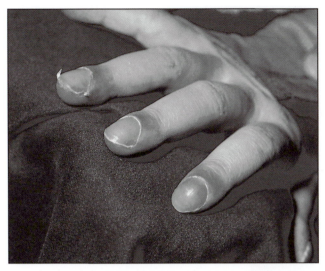

Figure 3.3
Finger clubbing.

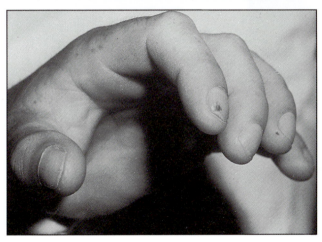

Figure 3.4
*Splinter haemorrhages
(index finger) and
vasculitic lesion (fourth
finger) due to infective
endocarditis.*

tissue swelling. Patients hardly ever notice that they have clubbing, even when it is
severe. They often express surprise at their doctor's interest in such an unlikely
part of their anatomy.

Before leaving the nails, look for splinter haemorrhages in the nail beds (Figure
3.4). These are linear haemorrhages lying parallel to the long axis of the nail. They
are most often due to trauma, particularly in manual workers. However, an important cause is infective endocarditis (page 67) which is a bacterial or other infection
of the heart valves or part of the endocardium. In this disease splinter haemorrhages are probably the result of a vasculitis in the nail bed, but this is controversial. Other rare causes of splinter haemorrhages include vasculitis, as in
rheumatoid arthritis (page 271), or polyarteritis nodosa (page 286), sepsis elsewhere in the body, haematological malignancy or profound anaemia.

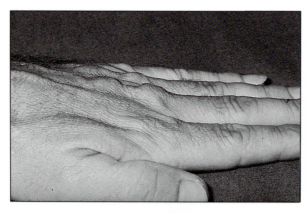

Figure 3.5
*Tendon xanthomata on the
dorsum of the hand.*

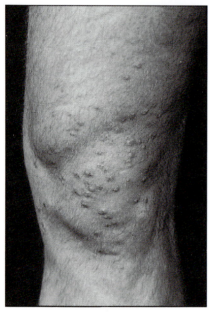

Figure 3.6
Tuboeruptive xanthomata of the knee.

Osler's nodes* are a rare manifestation of infective endocarditis. These are red, raised tender nodules on the pulps of the fingers (or toes), or on the thenar or hypothenar eminences. Janeway lesions[†] are non-tender erythematous maculo-papular lesions containing bacteria, which occur very rarely on the palms or pulps of the fingers in patients with infective endocarditis.

Tendon xanthomata are yellow or orange deposits of lipid in the tendons which occur in Type II hyperlipidaemia. These can be seen over the tendons of the hand and arm (Figure 3.5). Palmar xanthomata, and tuboeruptive xanthomata over the

---

*   Sir William Osler (1849–1919), Canadian physician, famous Regius Professor of Medicine at Oxford and renowned medical historian.
†   Edward Janeway (1841–1911), American physician.

elbows and knees, are characteristic of Type III hyperlipidaemia (Figure 3.6) (Table 3.4).

The Arterial Pulse

The accomplished clinician is able, while inspecting the hands, to palpate the radial artery at the wrist. Although the radial pulse is distant from the central arteries, certain useful information may be gained from examining it. The pulse is usually felt just medial to the radius using the forefinger and middle finger pulps of the examining hand. The following observations should be made: (i) rate of pulse; (ii) rhythm; and (iii) presence or absence of delay of the femoral pulse compared with the radial pulse (radiofemoral delay). The character and volume of the pulse are better assessed from palpation of the brachial or carotid arteries.

Rate of Pulse

Practised observers can estimate the rate quickly. Formal counting over 30 seconds is accurate and requires only simple mathematics to obtain the rate per minute. The normal resting heart rate in adults is between 60 and 100 beats per minute. Bradycardia (Greek *bradus* slow, *kardia* heart) is defined as a heart rate less than 60 beats per minute. Tachycardia (Greek *takhus* swift, *kardia* heart) is defined as a heart rate over 100 beats per minute. The causes of bradycardia and tachycardia are listed in Table 3.5.

Rhythm

The rhythm of the pulse can be regular or irregular. An irregular rhythm can be completely irregular with no pattern; this is usually due to atrial fibrillation (Table 3.5). In atrial fibrillation coordinated atrial contraction is lost and chaotic electrical activity occurs with bombardment of the atrioventricular (AV) node with impulses at a rate of over 600 per minute. Only a variable proportion of these is conducted to the ventricles because the AV node is unable to conduct at such high rates. In this way, the ventricles are protected from very rapid rates, but beat irregularly, usually at rates between 150 and 180 a minute. The pulse also varies in amplitude from beat to beat in atrial fibrillation because of differing diastolic filling times. This type of pulse can occasionally be simulated by frequent irregularly occurring supraventricular or ventricular ectopic beats.

An irregular rhythm can also be regularly irregular. For example, in sinus arrhythmia the pulse rate increases with each inspiration and decreases with each expiration. It is associated with changes in venous return to the heart. A pattern of irregularity is also detectable in the Wenckebach* phenomenon. Here the AV nodal conduction time increases progressively until a non-conducted atrial systole occurs. Following this the AV conduction time shortens and the cycle begins again.

Radiofemoral Delay

This is an important sign, and often neglected. While palpating the radial pulse one places the fingers of the other hand over the femoral pulse, which is situated below the inguinal ligament, one-third of the way up from the pubic tubercle. A noticeable delay in the arrival of the femoral pulse wave suggests the diagnosis of

---

* Karel Frederik Wenckebach (1864–1940), Dutch physician who practised in Vienna.

Table 3.4 *Clinical Features of the Hyperlipoproteinaemias*

Type	Lipoprotein Elevated	Electrophoretic Mobility	Mechanism	Primary	Secondary Causes	Clinical Features	Associations
I Familial hyperchylomicronaemia	Chylomicrons	Origin	Deficiency of extrahepatic lipoprotein lipase or apoC II deficiency	Yes	Rarely SLE	Eruptive xanthomata Lipaemia retinalis	Pancreatitis
IIa Familial or diet-induced hypercholesterolaemia	LDL	β	Receptor defect or other	Yes	Cushing's syndrome Myxoedema Cholestasis Nephrotic syndrome	Xanthelasma Corneal arcus Tendon xanthomata	Coronary artery disease Peripheral vascular disease
IIb Mixed	LDL VLDL	β & pre β	Hepatic oversynthesis of apo-β-containing particles	Yes			
III Broad beta disease	IDL	Broad β	Oversynthesis and/or abnormal apoprotein E	Yes	Renal or hepatic disease	Palmar crease xanthomata Tuboeruptive xanthomata Xanthelasma	Coronary artery disease Peripheral vascular disease
IV Familial or diet-induced hypertriglyceridaemia	VLDL	Preβ	Oversynthesis and/or undercatabolism of VLDL	Yes	Diabetes mellitus Alcoholism Chronic renal failure	Usually no xanthomata	Coronary artery disease (low HDL, positive family history)
V (Combination IV & I)	VLDL Chylomicrons	Origin & pre β	Saturation of lipoprotein lipase by VLDL so dietary fat cannot be metabolised	Yes	Diabetes mellitus Alcoholism Chronic renal failure (as for IV)	Eruptive xanthomata Lipaemia retinalis (as for I)	Pancreatitis (as for I)

LDL = low density lipoproteins. IDL = intermediate density lipoproteins. SLE = systemic lupus erythematosus. VLDL = very low density lipoproteins. HDL = high density lipoproteins.

coarctation of the aorta, where a congenital narrowing in the aortic isthmus occurs at the level where the ductus arteriosus joins the descending aorta. This is just distal to the origin of the subclavian artery. This lesion can cause upper limb hypertension (page 69).

Table 3.5 *Causes of Bradycardia and Tachycardia*

Bradycardia

Regular Rhythm

Physiological (athletes, during sleep: due to increased vagal tone)
Drugs (e.g., beta-blockers, digoxin, amiodarone)
Hypothyroidism (decreased sympathetic activity secondary to thyroid hormone deficiency)
Hypothermia
Jaundice (in severe cases only, due to deposition of bilirubin in the conducting system)
Raised intracranial pressure (because of an effect on central sympathetic outflow)—a late
    sign
Third degree atrioventricular (AV) block, or second degree (type 2) AV block
Myocardial infarction
Paroxysmal bradycardia: Vasovagal syncope
                        Acute hypoxia or hypercapnia
                        Acute hypertension

Regularly Irregular Rhythm

Sinus arrhythmia (normal slowing of the pulse with expiration)
Second degree AV block (type 1)

Irregularly Irregular Rhythm

Atrial fibrillation, with atrioventricular (AV) nodal disease or drugs (e.g., digoxin)
Frequent extrasystoles

Apparent

Pulse deficit* (atrial fibrillation, ventricular bigeminy)

Tachycardia

Regular Rhythm

Hyperdynamic circulation, due to:

- exercise or emotion (e.g., anxiety)
- fever (allow 15 to 20 beats/min per degree C above normal)
- pregnancy
- thyrotoxicosis
- anaemia
- arteriovenous fistula (e.g., Paget's disease or hepatic failure)
- beri beri (thiamine deficiency)

Congestive cardiac failure
Constrictive pericarditis
Drugs (e.g., salbutamol and other sympathomimetics, atropine)
Normal variant
The denervated heart of diabetes has a resting rate of 106 to 120 beats per minute
Hypovolaemic shock
Supraventricular tachycardia
Atrial flutter with regular 2:1 AV block
Ventricular tachycardia

—continued

Table 3.5 *Causes of Bradycardia and Tachycardia (continued)*

Irregular Rhythm

Atrial fibrillation, due to:

- myocardial ischaemia
- mitral valve disease or any cause of left atrial enlargement
- thyrotoxicosis
- hypertensive heart disease
- sick sinus syndrome
- pulmonary embolism
- myocarditis
- fever, acute hypoxia or hypercapnia (paroxysmal)
- other: alcohol, post-thoracotomy, idiopathic

Multifocal atrial tachycardia
Atrial flutter with variable block

*   This is the difference between the heart rate counted over the praecordium and that observed at the periphery. In beats where diastole is too short for adequate filling of the heart, too small a volume of blood is ejected during systole for a pulse to be appreciated at the wrist.

It is also useful to palpate both radial pulses together to detect radial-radial inequality in timing or volume, usually due to a large arterial occlusion by an atherosclerotic plaque or aneurysm.

Character and Volume

These are poorly assessed by palpating the radial pulse; the carotid or brachial arteries should be used to determine the character and volume of the pulse as these more accurately reflect the form of the aortic pressure wave. However, the collapsing (bounding) pulse of aortic regurgitation, and pulsus alternans of left ventricular failure, may be readily apparent in the radial pulse.

Condition of the Vessel Wall

Only changes in the medial layer of the radial artery can be assessed by palpation. Thickening or tortuosity will be detected commonly in the arteries of elderly people. These changes, however, do not indicate the presence of luminal narrowing due to atherosclerosis. Therefore, this sign is of little clinical value.

The Blood Pressure

Measurement of the arterial blood pressure is essential. Usually indirect measurements of the systolic and diastolic pressures are obtained with a sphygmomanometer (Greek *sphygmos* pulsing, *manos* thin). The systolic blood pressure is the peak pressure that occurs in the artery following ventricular systole and the diastolic blood pressure is the level to which the arterial blood pressure falls during ventricular diastole. Normal blood pressure is defined as a systolic reading of less than 140 *and* a diastolic reading of less than 90mm/Hg. In some circumstances (for example, in pregnancy) lower pressures may be considered normal.

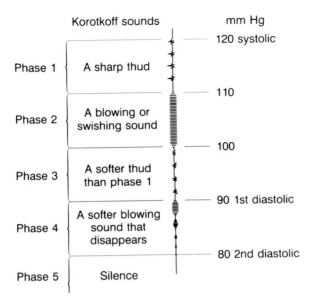

Figure 3.7 *Korotkoff sounds—systolic pressure is determined by the appearance of the first audible sound, and diastolic pressure is determined by its disappearance.*

From Burnside JW, McGlynn TJ. Physical Diagnosis. 17th ed. Baltimore: Williams & Wilkins, 1987. With permission.

Measuring the Blood Pressure with the Sphygmomanometer

The usual blood pressure cuff width is 12.5 cm. This is suitable for a normal-sized adult forearm. However, in obese patients with large arms, the normal-sized cuff will overestimate the blood pressure and therefore a large cuff must be used. A range of smaller sizes is available for children.

The cuff is wrapped around the upper arm with the bladder centred over the brachial artery. This is found in the antecubital fossa one-third of the way over from the medial epicondyle. For an approximate estimation of the systolic blood pressure, the cuff is fully inflated and then deflated slowly (3 to 4 mmHg per second) until the radial pulse returns. Then for a more accurate estimation of the blood pressure, this manoeuvre is repeated with the diaphragm of the stethoscope placed over the brachial artery, slipped underneath the distal end of the cuff's bladder.

Five different sounds will be heard as the cuff is slowly released (Figure 3.7). These are called the Korotkoff* sounds. The pressure at which a sound is first heard over the artery is the systolic blood pressure (Korotkoff I). As deflation of the cuff continues the sound increases in intensity (K II), then decreases (K III), becomes muffled (Korotkoff IV) and then disappears (K V). Different observers have used KIV and KV to indicate the level of the diastolic pressure. KV is

---

* Nikolai Korotkoff (b. 1874), a St Petersburg surgeon, described the auscultatory method of determining blood pressure in 1905, although his findings were scoffed at.

Table 3.6   *Causes of Postural Hypotension*

Hypovolaemia (e.g., dehydration, bleeding)
Drugs (e.g., vasodilators, tricyclic antidepressants, diuretics, antipsychotics)
Addison's* disease (page 312)
Hypopituitarism (page 304)
Autonomic neuropathy (e.g., diabetes mellitus (page 320), amyloidosis, Shy-Drager syndrome)
Idiopathic orthostatic hypotension (rare progressive degeneration of the autonomic nervous system, usually in elderly men)

* Thomas Addison (b. 1793), London physician.

probably the best measure. However, this provides a slight underestimate of the arterial diastolic blood pressure. Although diastolic pressure usually corresponds most closely to KV, in severe aortic regurgitation KIV is a more accurate indication (page 76). KV is absent in some normal people and KIV must be used.

Occasionally, there will be an auscultatory gap (the sounds disappear just below the systolic pressure and reappear before the diastolic pressure) in healthy people.

The systolic blood pressure may normally vary between the arms by up to 10 mmHg; in the legs the blood pressure is normally higher than in the arms.

During inspiration, the systolic and diastolic blood pressure normally decrease (because intrathoracic pressure becomes more negative, blood pools in the pulmonary vessels, so left heart filling is reduced). When this normal reduction in blood pressure with inspiration is *exaggerated*, it is termed *pulsus paradoxus*. Kussmaul meant by this that there was a fall in blood pressure and a paradoxical rise in pulse rate. A fall in arterial pulse pressure on inspiration of more than 10 mmHg is abnormal and may occur with constrictive pericarditis, pericardial effusion, or severe asthma.

High Blood Pressure

This is difficult to define. The most helpful definitions of hypertension are based on an estimation of the level associated with an increased risk of vascular disease. In this case, recordings above 145/90 mmHg may be considered abnormal; such levels may occur in up to 20% of the adult population.*

Postural Blood Pressure

The blood pressure should routinely be taken with the patient lying and standing. A fall of more than 15 mmHg in systolic blood pressure or 10 mmHg in diastolic blood pressure on standing is abnormal and is called postural hypotension (Table 3.6). It may not be associated with symptoms.

The Face

Inspect the sclerae for jaundice (page 18). This can occur with severe congestive cardiac failure and hepatic congestion. Prosthetic heart valve-induced haemolysis

---

*   In pseudohypertension, the blood pressure as measured by the sphygmomanometer is artificially high because of arterial wall calcification. Osler's manoeuvre can detect this condition: inflate the cuff above systolic pressure and palpate the radial artery, which in pseudohypertension may be palpable despite being pulseless.

of red blood cells, due to excessive turbulence, is an uncommon cause of jaundice. Xanthelasma (Figure 3.8) are intracutaneous yellow cholesterol deposits around the eyes and are relatively common. These may be a normal variant or may indicate Type II or III hyperlipidaemia (page 38).

Next look for the presence of a mitral facies, which refers to rosy cheeks with a bluish tinge, due to dilatation of the malar capillaries. This is associated with pulmonary hypertension and a low cardiac output such as occurs in severe mitral stenosis.

Now look in the mouth using a torch to see if there is a high arched palate. This occurs in Marfan's syndrome (page 33), a condition which is associated with congenital heart disease, including aortic regurgitation secondary to aortic root dilatation, and also mitral regurgitation due to mitral valve prolapse. Notice whether the teeth look diseased, as they can be a source of organisms responsible for infective endocarditis. Look at the tongue and lips for central cyanosis. Inspect the mucosa for petechiae that may indicate infective endocarditis.

The Neck

Oddly enough this small area of the body is packed with cardiovascular signs which must be elicited with great care and skill.

Carotid Arteries

The carotids are not only easily accessible, medial to the sternomastoid muscles (Figure 3.9), but provide a great deal of information about the wave form of the aortic pulse, which is affected by many cardiac abnormalities. Never palpate both carotid arteries together since they provide much of the blood supply to the brain (a vital organ). Evaluation of the pulse wave form (the amplitude, shape and volume) is important in the diagnosis of various underlying cardiac diseases and in assessing their severity. It takes considerable practice to distinguish the different important types of carotid wave forms (Table 3.7).

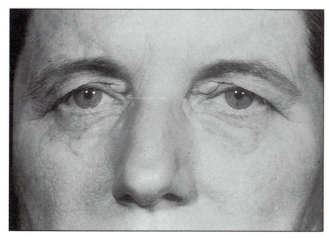

Figure 3.8
Xanthelasma.

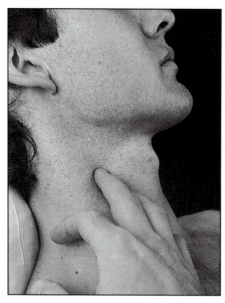

Figure 3.9
Palpating the carotid pulse.

Table 3.7   *Arterial Pulse Character*

Type of pulse	Cause(s)
Anacrotic 　Small volume, slow uptake, notched 　wave on upstroke	Aortic stenosis
Plateau 　Slow upstroke	Aortic stenosis
Bisferiens 　Anacrotic and collapsing	Aortic stenosis *and* regurgitation
Collapsing	Aortic regurgitation Hyperdynamic circulation (page 40) Patent ductus arteriosus Peripheral arteriovenous fistula Arteriosclerotic aorta (elderly patients in 　particular)
Small volume	Aortic stenosis Pericardial effusion
Alternans 　Alternating strong and weak beats	Left ventricular failure
Jerky	Hypertrophic cardiomyopathy

Jugular Venous Pressure (JVP)

Just as the carotid pulse tells us about the aorta and left ventricular function, the jugular venous pressure (JVP) (Figure 3.10) tells us about right atrial and right ventricular function. The positioning of the patient and lighting are important for this examination to be done properly. The patient must be lying down at 45 degrees to the horizontal with his or her head on pillows and in good lighting conditions. The internal jugular vein is medial to the sternomastoid muscle, while the external jugular vein is lateral to it. Although the external jugular vein is more readily visible, this is subject to compression as it enters the chest because of its tortuous course. It should therefore not be relied on to assess the position or wave form of the JVP. The internal jugular vein is more reliable. Pulsations which occur there reflect movements of the top of a column of blood which extends into the right atrium. The column of blood may be used as a manometer and enables us to observe pressure changes in the right atrium. By convention the sternal angle is taken as the zero point and the maximum height of pulsations in the internal jugular vein, which are visible above this level when the patient is at 45 degrees, can be measured in centimetres. In the average person the centre of the right atrium lies 5 cm below this zero point.

When the patient is lying at 45 degrees the sternal angle is also roughly in line with the base of the neck (Figure 3.10). This provides a convenient zero point from which to measure the vertical height of the column of blood in the jugular vein.

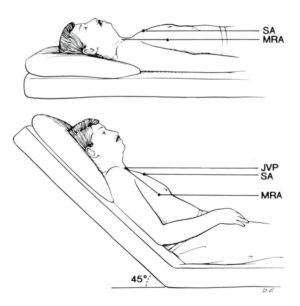

Figure 3.10   *The relationship of the normal internal jugular venous pressure (JVP) to the sternal angle (SA) (manubriosternal joint) and the clavicle with the subject in different positions. The vertical distance between the sternal angle and the mid right atrium (MRA) remains relatively constant. When the patient lies at 45° to the horizontal, venous pulsation is normally seen just above the clavicle.*

Adapted with permission from Bouchier IAD, Morris JS, editors. Clinical skills—A system of clinical examination. 2nd ed. London: WB Saunders, 1982.

The jugular venous pulsation can be distinguished from the arterial pulse because: (i) it is visible but not palpable; (ii) it has a complex wave form, usually seen to flicker twice with each cardiac cycle (if the patient is in sinus rhythm); (iii) it moves on respiration—normally the JVP decreases on inspiration; and (iv) it is at first obliterated and then filled from above when light pressure is applied at the base of the neck.

The JVP must be assessed for *height* and *character*.

Height

When the JVP is more than 3 cm above the zero point, the right heart filling pressure is raised. This may be a sign of right ventricular failure or of volume overload.

Character

The assessment of the character of JVP is difficult even for experienced clinicians.

There are two positive waves in the normal JVP. The first is called the *a wave* and coincides with right atrial systole. It is due to atrial contraction. The *a* wave also coincides with the first heart sound and precedes the carotid pulsation. The second impulse is called the *v wave* and is due to atrial filling, in the period when the tricuspid valve remains closed during ventricular systole. Between the *a* and *v* waves there is a trough caused by atrial relaxation. This is called the *x descent*. It is interrupted by the *c point* which is due to transmitted carotid pulsation, and coincides with tricuspid valve closure. It is not usually visible. Following the *v* wave, the tricuspid valve opens and rapid ventricular filling occurs; this results in the *y descent* (Figure 3.11).

In Table 3.8 characteristic changes in the JVP are described. Any condition in which right ventricular filling is limited (for example, constrictive pericarditis, cardiac tamponade or right ventricular infarction) can cause elevation of the

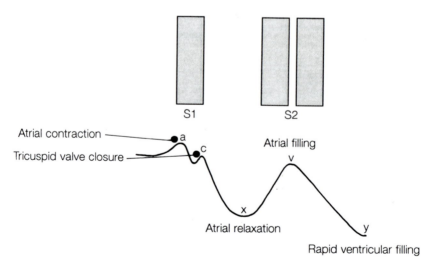

Figure 3.11   *The jugular venous pressure, and its relationship to the first (S1) and second (S2) heart sounds.*

Table 3.8 *Jugular Venous Pressure*

Causes of an Elevated Central Venous Pressure

Right ventricular failure
Tricuspid stenosis or regurgitation
Pericardial effusion or constrictive pericarditis
Superior vena caval obstruction
Fluid overload
Hyperdynamic circulation

Wave Form

*Causes of a Dominant **a** Wave*

Tricuspid stenosis (also causing a slow *y* descent)
Pulmonary stenosis
Pulmonary hypertension

*Causes of Cannon **a** Waves*

Complete heart block
Paroxysmal nodal tachycardia with retrograde atrial conduction
Ventricular tachycardia with retrograde atrial conduction or atrioventricular dissociation

*Cause of a Dominant **v** Wave*

Tricuspid regurgitation

***x** Descent*

Absent: atrial fibrillation
Exaggerated: acute cardiac tamponade
                    constrictive pericarditis

***y** Descent*

Sharp: severe tricuspid regurgitation, constrictive pericarditis
Slow: tricuspid stenosis
          right atrial myxoma

venous pressure, which is more marked on inspiration when venous return to the heart increases. This rise in the JVP on inspiration, called Kussmaul's* sign, is the opposite of what normally happens. This sign is best elicited with the patient sitting up at 90 degrees and breathing quietly through the mouth.

Pressure exerted over the liver for 15 seconds will also increase venous return to the right atrium. The JVP normally rises transiently following this manoeuvre, the *hepatojugular reflex*. If there is right ventricular failure, it may remain elevated.

Cannon a waves occur when the right atrium contracts against the closed tricuspid valve. This occurs intermittently in complete heart block where the two chambers beat independently.

Giant a waves are large but not explosive *a* waves with each beat. They occur when right atrial pressures are raised because of obstruction to outflow (tricuspid stenosis) or elevated pressures in the pulmonary circulation.

The *large v waves* of tricuspid regurgitation should never be missed.

---

*   Adolf Kussmaul (1822–1902), German physician who also described laboured breathing in diabetic coma and was the first to use an oesophagoscope.

The Praecordium

Now at last the examiner has reached the praecordium.

Inspection

Inspect first for scars. Previous cardiac operations will have left scars on the chest wall. The position of the scar can be a clue to the valve lesion that has been operated on. Most valve surgery requires cardiopulmonary bypass and for this a median sternotomy (a cut down the middle of the sternum) is very commonly used. This type of scar is occasionally hidden under a forest of chest hair. It is not specifically helpful as it may also be a result of previous coronary artery bypass grafting. Alternatively, left or even right sided lateral thoracotomy scars, which may be hidden under a pendulous breast, may indicate a previous closed mitral valvotomy. In this operation a stenosed mitral valve is opened through an incision made in the left atrial appendage. Cardiopulmonary bypass is not required.

Skeletal abnormalities such as *pectus excavatum* (funnel chest (page 108)) or kyphoscoliosis (Greek *kyphos* hunch-backed, *skolios* curved), a curvature of the vertebral column (page 107), may be present. Skeletal abnormalities such as these, which may be part of Marfan's syndrome, can cause distortion of the position of the heart and great vessels in the chest and thus alter the position of the apex beat. Severe deformity can interfere with pulmonary function and cause pulmonary hypertension (page 70).

Another surgical 'abnormality' that must not be missed, if only to avoid embarrassment, is a pacemaker box. These are usually under the right or left pectoral muscle, are easily palpable and obviously metallic.

The apex beat must be looked for. Its normal position is in the fifth left intercostal space 1cm medial to the midclavicular line (Figure 3.12). It is due primarily to recoil of the apex of the heart as blood is expelled in systole. There may be other visible pulsations, for example over the pulmonary artery in cases of severe pulmonary hypertension.

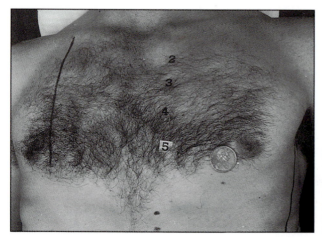

Figure 3.12

The apex beat: coin is over the apex, intercostal spaces are numbered, vertical lines show right midclavicular and left anterior axillary lines.

Palpation

The *apex beat* must be palpated. It is important to count down the number of interspaces. The first palpable interspace is the second. It lies just below the manubriosternal angle. The position of the apex beat is defined as the most lateral and inferior point at which the palpating fingers are raised with each systole. The normal apex is felt over an area the size of a 20 cent (50p) coin (Figure 3.12). An apex beat displaced laterally or inferiorly or both usually indicates enlargement, but may occasionally be due to chest wall deformity, or pleural or pulmonary disease (page 109).

The character of the apex beat may provide the examiner with vital diagnostic clues. The normal apex beat gently lifts the palpating fingers. There are a number of types of abnormal apex beats. The *pressure loaded* (hyperdynamic or systolic overloaded) apex beat is a forceful and sustained impulse. This occurs with aortic stenosis or hypertension. The *volume loaded* (hyperkinetic or diastolic over-loaded) apex beat is an uncoordinated impulse felt over a larger area than normal in the praecordium and is usually due to left ventricular dysfunction (for example, anterior myocardial infarction). The *double impulse* apex beat, where two distinct impulses are felt with each systole, is characteristic of hypertrophic cardio-myopathy (page 79). The *tapping* apex beat will be felt when the first heart sound is actually palpable (heart sounds are not palpable in health) and indicates mitral or rarely tricuspid stenosis (page 71, 78).

In some cases the apex beat may not be palpable. This is most often due to a thick chest wall, emphysema, pericardial effusion, shock (or death) and rarely to dextrocardia (where there is inversion of the heart and great vessels). The apex beat will be palpable to the right of the sternum in many cases of dextrocardia.

Other praecordial impulses may be palpable in patients with heart disease. A *parasternal impulse* may be felt when the heel of the hand is rested just to the left of the sternum with the fingers lifted slightly off the chest (Figure 3.13). In cases of right ventricular enlargement or severe left atrial enlargement, where the right

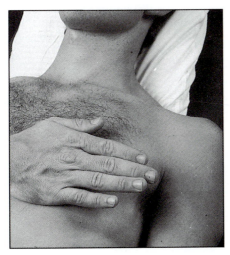

Figure 3.13
Feeling for the parasternal impulse.

ventricle is pushed anteriorly, the heel of the hand is lifted off the chest wall with each systole. Palpation with the fingers over the pulmonary area may reveal the palpable *tap of pulmonary valve closure* (P2) in cases of pulmonary hypertension.

Turbulent blood flow, which causes cardiac murmurs on auscultation, may sometimes be palpable. These palpable murmurs are called *thrills*. The praecordium should be systematically palpated for thrills with the flat of the hand, first over the apex and left sternal edge, and then over the base of the heart (Figure 3.14).

Apical thrills can be more easily felt with the patient rolled over to the left side (the left lateral position) as this brings the apex closer to the chest wall. Thrills may also be palpable over the *base of the heart* (this is the upper part of the chest and includes the aortic and pulmonary areas). These may be maximal over the pulmonary or aortic areas, depending on the underlying cause, and are best felt with the patient sitting up leaning forward and in full expiration. In this position the base of the heart is moved closer to the chest wall. A thrill which coincides in time with the apex beat is called a *systolic thrill*; one which does not coincide with the apex beat is called a *diastolic thrill*.

The presence of a thrill usually indicates an organic lesion. Careful palpation for thrills is an extremely useful, but often neglected, part of the cardiovascular examination.

Percussion

It is possible to define the cardiac outline by means of percussion (page 110) but little additional information is gained. In the cardiovascular system percussion is usually a wasteful expenditure of time.

Auscultation

Now at last the stethoscope is required. However, in some cases the diagnosis should already be fairly clear. In the viva-voce examination, the examiners may occasionally stop a candidate before auscultation and ask for an opinion.

Auscultation of the heart begins in the mitral area with the bell of the stethoscope (Figures 3.15 and 3.16). The bell is designed as a resonating chamber and is particularly efficient in amplifying low pitched sounds, such as the diastolic murmur of mitral stenosis or a third heart sound. It must be applied lightly to the chest

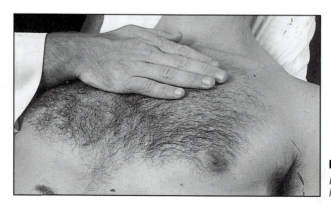

Figure 3.14

Palpating the base of the heart.

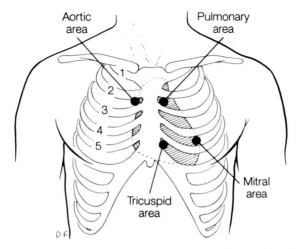

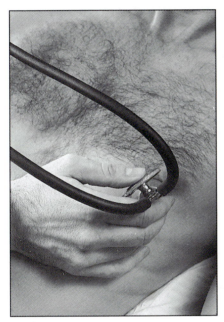

Figure 3.15 *The areas best for auscultation do not exactly correlate with the anatomical location of the valves.*

Figure 3.16

Auscultation in the mitral area with the bell of the stethoscope: listening for mitral stenosis in the left lateral position.

wall because forceful application will stretch the skin under the bell so that it forms a diaphragm. Next listen in the mitral area with the diaphragm of the stethoscope, which best reproduces higher pitched sounds, such as the systolic murmur of mitral regurgitation or a fourth heart sound. Then place the stethoscope in the tricuspid area (fifth left intercostal space) and listen. Next inch up the left sternal edge to the pulmonary (second left intercostal space) and aortic (second right intercostal space) areas, listening carefully in each position with the diaphragm.

For accurate auscultation, experience with what is normal is important. This can be obtained only through constant practice. Auscultation of the normal heart reveals two sounds called, not surprisingly, the first and second heart sounds. The explanation for the origin of these noises changes from year to year; the sounds are probably related to vibrations caused by the closing of the heart valves in combination with rapid changes in blood flow and tensing within cardiac structures that occur as the valves close.

The *first heart sound* (S1) has two components: mitral and tricuspid valve closure. Mitral closure occurs slightly before tricuspid, but usually only one sound is audible. The first heart sound indicates the beginning of ventricular systole.

The *second heart sound* (S2), which is at a slightly lower pitch than the first and marks the end of systole, is made up of aortic and pulmonary valve closures. In normal cases, because of lower pressure in the pulmonary circulation compared with the aorta, closure of the pulmonary valve is later than that of the aortic valve. These components are usually sufficiently separated in time so that splitting of the second heart sound is audible. Because the pulmonary component of the second heart sound (P2) may not be audible throughout the praecordium, splitting of the second heart sound may best be appreciated in the pulmonary area and along the left sternal edge. Pulmonary valve closure is further delayed with inspiration because of increased venous return to the right ventricle; thus splitting of the second heart sound is wider on inspiration. The second heart sound marks the beginning of diastole, which is usually longer than systole.

It can be difficult to decide which heart sound is which. Palpation of the carotid pulsation will indicate the timing of systole and enable the heart sounds to be more easily distinguished. It is obviously crucial to define systole and diastole during auscultation so that cardiac murmurs and abnormal sounds can be placed in the correct part of the cardiac cycle. Students are often asked to time a cardiac murmur; this is not a request to measure its length, but rather to say in which part of the cardiac cycle it occurs. Even the experts can mistake a murmur if they do not time it. An understanding of the cardiac cycle is helpful as one interprets the auscultatory findings (Figure 3.17).

Abnormalities of the Heart Sounds

Alterations in Intensity

The **first heart sound** (S1) is *loud* when the mitral or tricuspid valve cusps remain widely open at the end of diastole and shut forcefully with the onset of ventricular systole. This occurs in mitral stenosis and tricuspid stenosis because the narrowed valve orifice limits ventricular filling, so that there is no diminution in flow towards the end of diastole. The normal mitral valve cusps drift back towards the closed position at the end of diastole as ventricular filling slows down. Other causes of a loud S1 are related to reduced diastolic filling time, for example tachycardia or any cause of a short atrioventricular conduction time.

Soft first heart sounds can be due to a prolonged diastolic filling time (as with first degree heart block) or a delayed onset of left ventricular systole (as with left bundle branch block), or to failure of the leaflets to coapt normally (as in mitral regurgitation).

The **second heart sound** (S2) will have a *loud* aortic component (A2) in patients with systemic hypertension. This results in forceful aortic valve closure secondary to high aortic pressures. Congenital aortic stenosis is another cause because the valve is mobile but narrowed, and closes suddenly at the end of systole. The

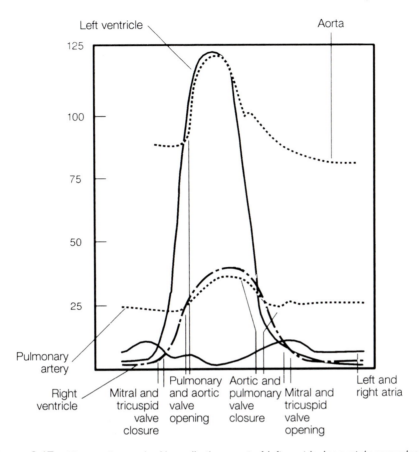

Figure 3.17 *The cardiac cycle. Normally the onset of left ventricular systole precedes the onset of pressure rise in the right ventricle. The mitral valve, therefore, closes before the tricuspid valve. Because the pulmonary artery diastolic pressure is lower than aortic diastolic pressure, the pulmonary valve opens before the aortic valve. Therefore, pulmonary ejection sounds occur closer to the first heart sound than do aortic ejection sounds. During systole the pressure in the ventricles slightly exceeds the pressure in the corresponding great arteries. Towards the end of systole, the ventricular pressure falls below the pressure in the great arteries, and when diastolic pressure is reached, the semilunar valves close. Normally, aortic valve closure precedes pulmonary valve closure. The mitral and tricuspid valves begin to open at the point at which the ventricular pressures fall below the corresponding atrial pressures.*

From Swash M, editor. Hutchison's clinical methods. 19th ed. London: Balliére Tindall, 1989, with permission.

pulmonary component of the second heart sound (P2) is *loud* in pulmonary hypertension, where the valve closure is forceful because of the high pulmonary pressure.

A *soft* A2 will be found when the aortic valve is calcified and leaflet movement is reduced, and in aortic regurgitation when the leaflets cannot coapt.

Splitting

Splitting of the **first heart sound** is usually not detectable clinically; however, when it occurs it is most often due to complete right bundle branch block.

Increased normal splitting (wider on inspiration) of the **second heart sound** occurs when there is any delay in right ventricular emptying, as in right bundle branch block (delayed right ventricular depolarisation), pulmonary stenosis (delayed right ventricular ejection), ventricular septal defect (increased right ventricular volume load), and mitral regurgitation (because of earlier aortic valve closure due to more rapid left ventricular emptying).

In the case of *fixed splitting* there is no respiratory variation (as is normal) and splitting tends to be wide. This is caused by an atrial septal defect where equalisation of volume loads between the two atria occurs through the defect. This results in the atria acting as a common chamber.

In the case of *reversed splitting* P2 occurs first and splitting occurs in expiration. This can be due to delayed left ventricular depolarisation (left bundle branch block), delayed left ventricular emptying (severe aortic stenosis, coarctation of the aorta) or increased left ventricular volume load (large patent ductus arteriosus). However, in the last-mentioned, the loud machinery murmur means that the second heart sound is usually not heard.

Extra Heart Sounds

The **third heart sound** (S3) is a low pitched mid-diastolic sound that is best appreciated by listening for a triple rhythm. It has been likened to the galloping of a horse and is often called a *gallop rhythm*. It is probably caused by tautening of the mitral or tricuspid papillary muscles at the end of rapid diastolic filling. A physiological left ventricular S3 occurs in children and young people and is due to very rapid diastolic filling. A pathological S3 is due to reduced ventricular compliance so that a filling sound is produced even when diastolic filling is not especially rapid.

A *left ventricular* S3 is louder at the apex than at the left sternal edge, and is louder on expiration. It can be physiological under the age of 40 years and in pregnancy. Otherwise, it is an important sign of left ventricular failure, but may also occur in aortic regurgitation, mitral regurgitation, ventricular septal defect and patent ductus arteriosus.

A *right ventricular* S3 is louder at the left sternal edge and with inspiration. It occurs in right ventricular failure or constrictive pericarditis.

The **fourth heart sound** (S4) is a late diastolic sound slightly more high pitched than the S3. Again, this is responsible for the impression of a triple (gallop) rhythm. It is never physiological and is due to a high pressure atrial wave reflected back from a poorly compliant ventricle. It does not occur if the patient is in atrial fibrillation because the sound depends on effective atrial contraction, which is lost when the atria fibrillate.

A *left ventricular* S4 occurs whenever left ventricular compliance is reduced due to aortic stenosis, acute mitral regurgitation, systemic hypertension, ischaemic heart disease or advanced age. It is often present during an episode of angina or with a myocardial infarction, and may be the only physical sign of that condition.

A *right ventricular* S4 occurs when right ventricular compliance is reduced in pulmonary hypertension or pulmonary stenosis.

If the heart rate is greater than 120 per minute, S3 and S4 may be superimposed, resulting in a **summation gallop**. In this case, two inaudible sounds may combine to produce an audible one. This does not necessarily imply ventricular stress unless one or both of the extra heart sounds persists when the heart rate slows or is slowed by carotid sinus massage. When both S3 and S4 are present the rhythm is described as a quadruple rhythm. It usually implies severe ventricular dysfunction.

Additional Sounds

An **opening snap** is a high pitched sound which occurs in mitral stenosis at a variable distance after S2. It is due to the sudden opening of the mitral valve and is followed by the diastolic murmur of mitral stenosis. It can be difficult to distinguish from a widely split S2, but normally occurs rather later in diastole than the pulmonary component of the second heart sound. It is more high pitched than a third heart sound and so is not usually confused with this. It is best heard at the lower left sternal edge with the diaphragm of the stethoscope. Use of the term 'opening snap' implies the diagnosis of mitral or tricuspid stenosis.

A **systolic ejection click** is an early systolic high pitched sound heard over the aortic or pulmonary and left sternal edge area which may occur in cases of congenital aortic or pulmonary stenosis where the valve remains mobile; it is followed by the systolic ejection murmur of aortic or pulmonary stenosis.

A **non-ejection systolic click** is a high pitched sound heard during systole and is best appreciated at the mitral area. It is a common finding. It may be followed by a systolic murmur. The click may be due to prolapse of one or more redundant mitral valve leaflets during systole. Non-ejection clicks may also be heard in atrial septal defects.

An atrial myxoma is a very rare tumour which may occur in either atrium. During atrial systole a loosely pedunculated tumour may be propelled into the mitral or tricuspid valve orifice causing a diastolic plopping sound, a **tumour plop**.

A **diastolic pericardial knock** may occur when there is sudden cessation of ventricular filling because of constrictive pericardial disease.

Prosthetic heart valves produce characteristic sounds (page 80). Rarely, a right ventricular pacemaker produces a late diastolic high pitched click due to contraction of the chest wall muscles (the **pacemaker sound**).

Murmurs of the Heart

In deciding the origin of a cardiac murmur one must consider a number of different features. These are: associated features (peripheral signs); timing; the area of greatest intensity; the loudness and pitch; and the effect of dynamic manoeuvres including respiration and the Valsalva manoeuvre (Figures 3.18a and 3.18b).

Associated Features

As already mentioned, the cause of a cardiac murmur can sometimes be elicited by careful analysis of the peripheral signs.

Timing (Table 3.9)

Systolic murmurs (which occur during ventricular systole) may be pansystolic, ejection systolic or late systolic.

The *pansystolic murmur* extends throughout systole beginning with the first heart sound then going right up to the second heart sound. Its loudness and pitch vary during systole. Pansystolic murmurs occur when a ventricle leaks to a lower pressure chamber or vessel. Since there is a pressure gradient from the moment the ventricle begins to contract (S1), blood flow and the murmur both begin at the first heart sound and continue until the pressures equalise (S2). Causes of pansystolic

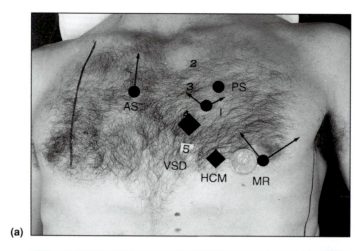

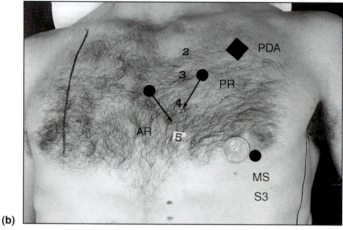

Figure 3.18 *Sites of maximum intensity and radiation of murmurs and heart sounds. (a) Systolic murmurs: AS = aortic stenosis; MR = mitral regurgitation; HCM = hypertrophic cardiomyopathy; PS = pulmonary stenosis; VSD = ventricular septal defect; I = innocent. (b) Diastolic murmurs and sounds: AR = aortic regurgitation; MS = mitral stenosis; S3 = third heart sound; PR = pulmonary regurgitation; PDA = patent ductus arteriosus (continuous murmur).*

murmurs include mitral regurgitation,* tricuspid regurgitation and ventricular septal defect.

With an *ejection (mid) systolic* murmur the murmur does not begin right at the first heart sound; its intensity is greatest in midsystole or later, and wanes again late in systole. This is described as a crescendo-decrescendo murmur. These murmurs are usually caused by turbulent flow through the aortic or pulmonary valve orifices or by greatly increased flow through a normal sized orifice or outflow tract.

---

* The term incompetence is synonymous with regurgitation, but the latter better describes the pathophysiology.

With a *late systolic* murmur one is able to distinguish an appreciable gap between the first heart sound and the murmur which then continues right up to the second heart sound. This is typical of mitral valve prolapse or papillary muscle dysfunction where mitral regurgitation begins in mid-systole.

Diastolic murmurs occur during ventricular diastole.

The *early diastolic* murmur begins immediately with the second heart sound and has a decrescendo quality (it is loudest at the beginning and extends for a variable distance into diastole). These early diastolic murmurs are typically high pitched and are due to regurgitation through leaking aortic or pulmonary valves. The murmur is loudest at the beginning because this is when aortic and pulmonary artery pressures are highest. Mid-diastolic murmurs begin later in diastole and may be short or extend right up to the first heart sound. They have a much lower pitched quality than early diastolic murmurs. They are due to impaired flow during ventricular filling and can be caused by mitral stenosis and tricuspid stenosis, where the valve is narrowed, or rarely by an atrial myxoma, where the tumour mass obstructs the valve orifice. In severe aortic regurgitation the regurgitant jet from the aortic valve may cause the anterior leaflet of the mitral valve to shudder, producing a diastolic murmur. Occasionally, normal mitral or tricuspid valves can produce flow murmurs, which are short and mid-diastolic and occur when there is torrential flow across the valve. Causes include a high cardiac output or intracardiac shunting (atrial or ventricular septal defects).

Presystolic murmurs may be heard when atrial systole increases blood flow across the valve just before the first heart sound. They are an extension of the mid-diastolic murmurs of mitral stenosis and tricuspid stenosis, and usually do not occur when atrial systole is lost in atrial fibrillation.

As the name implies, **continuous murmurs** extend throughout systole and diastole. They are produced when a communication exists between two parts of the circulation with a permanent pressure gradient so that blood flow occurs continuously. They can usually be distinguished from combined systolic and diastolic murmurs (due, for example, to aortic stenosis and aortic regurgitation), but this may sometimes be difficult. The causes are presented in Table 3.9.

A **pericardial friction rub** is a superficial scratching sound; there may be up to three distinct components occurring at any time during the cardiac cycle. They are not confined to systole or diastole. A rub is caused by movement of inflamed pericardial surfaces. It is a result of pericarditis. The sound can vary with respiration and posture; it is often louder when the patient is sitting up and breathing out. It tends to come and go and is often absent by the time students can be found to come and listen for it.

Area of Greatest Intensity

Although the place on the praecordium where a murmur is heard most easily is a guide to its origin, this is not a particularly reliable physical sign. For example, mitral regurgitation murmurs are usually loudest at the apex, over the mitral area, and tend to radiate towards the axillae, but they may be heard widely over the praecordium and even right up into the aortic area or over the back. Conduction of an ejection murmur up into the carotid arteries strongly suggests that this arises from the aortic valve.

Loudness and Pitch

Unfortunately, the *loudness* of the murmur is often not helpful in deciding the severity of the valve lesion. For example, in the severest forms of valve stenosis

Table 3.9 *Cardiac Murmurs*

Timing	Lesion
Pansystolic	Mitral regurgitation Tricuspid regurgitation Ventricular septal defect Aortopulmonary shunts
Mid-systolic	Aortic stenosis Pulmonary stenosis Hypertrophic cardiomyopathy Pulmonary flow murmur of an atrial septal defect
Late systolic	Mitral valve prolapse Papillary muscle dysfunction (due usually to ischaemia or hypertrophic cardiomyopathy)
Early diastolic	Aortic regurgitation Pulmonary regurgitation
Mid-diastolic	Mitral stenosis Tricuspid stenosis Atrial myxoma Austin Flint* murmur of aortic regurgitation Carey-Coombs† murmur of acute rheumatic fever
Presystolic	Mitral stenosis Tricuspid stenosis Atrial myxoma
Continuous	Patent ductus arteriosus Arteriovenous fistula (coronary artery, pulmonary, systemic) Aorto-pulmonary connection (e.g., congenital, Blalock‡ shunt) Venous hum (usually best heard over right supraclavicular fossa and abolished by ipsilateral internal jugular vein compression) Rupture of sinus of Valsalva into right ventricle or atrium 'Mammary souffle' (in late pregnancy or early postpartum period)

NB: The combined murmurs of aortic stenosis and aortic regurgitation, or mitral stenosis and mitral regurgitation, may sound as if they fill the entire cardiac cycle, but are not continuous murmurs by definition.

---

*   Austin Flint (1812–1886), New York physician.
†   Carey F Coombs (b. 1879), Bristol physician.
‡   Alfred Blalock (b. 1899), Baltimore physician.

murmurs may be soft or inaudible. However, murmurs are usually graded according to loudness. Cardiologists most often use a classification with six grades.

Grade 1/6: very soft and not heard at first (often audible only to consultants and to those students who have been told the murmur is present)
Grade 2/6: soft, but can be detected almost immediately by an experienced auscultator
Grade 3/6: moderate; there is no thrill
Grade 4/6: loud: thrill just palpable
Grade 5/6: very loud; thrill easily palpable
Grade 6/6: very, very loud; can be heard even without placing the stethoscope on the chest

Table 3.10 *Dynamic Manoeuvres and Systolic Cardiac Murmurs*

Manoeuvre	Lesion			
	Hypertrophic cardiomyopathy	Mitral valve prolapse	Aortic stenosis	Mitral regurgitation
Valsalva strain phase (decreases preload)	Louder	Longer	Softer	Softer
Squatting or leg raise (increases preload)	Softer	Shorter	Louder	Louder
Hand grip (increases afterload)	Softer	Shorter	Softer	Louder

This grading is useful, particularly because a change in the intensity of a murmur may be of great significance, for example, after a myocardial infarction.

It requires practice to appreciate the *pitch* of the murmur, but this may be of great use in identifying its type. In general, low pitched murmurs indicate turbulent flow under low pressure, as in mitral stenosis, and high pitched murmurs indicate a high velocity of flow, as in mitral regurgitation.

Dynamic Manoeuvres

All patients with a newly diagnosed murmur should undergo dynamic manoeuvre testing (Table 3.10).

Respiration: murmurs that arise on the right side of the heart tend to be louder during inspiration, as this increases venous return and therefore blood flow to the right side of the heart. Expiration has the opposite effect. This helps distinguish the site of a murmur. A routine part of the examination of the cardiovascular system involves leaning a patient forward in full expiration and listening to the base of the heart for aortic regurgitation, which may otherwise be missed. In this case the manoeuvre brings the base of the heart closer to the chest wall.

The Valsalva* manoeuvre: this is a forceful expiration against a closed glottis. One should ask the patient to hold the nose with his or her fingers, close the mouth, breathe out hard and completely so as to pop the eardrums, and hold this for as long as possible. Listen over the left sternal edge during this manoeuvre for changes in the systolic murmur of hypertrophic cardiomyopathy, and over the apex for changes when mitral valve prolapse is suspected.

The Valsalva manoeuvre has a number of phases. In phase 1 (beginning the manoeuvre) a rise in intrathoracic pressure and a transient increase in left ventricular output occur. In phase 2 (the straining phase) systemic venous return falls, filling of the right and then the left side of the heart is reduced, and stroke volume and blood pressure fall while the heart rate increases. As stroke volume and arterial blood pressure fall, most cardiac murmurs become softer; however, because the left ventricular volume is reduced, the systolic murmur of hypertrophic cardiomyopathy becomes louder and the systolic click and murmur of mitral valve prolapse begin earlier. In phase 3 (the release of the manoeuvre) first right-sided

---

*   Antonio Valsalva (1666–1723), Professor of Anatomy at Bologna, was noted for his studies of the ear.

and then left-sided cardiac murmurs become louder briefly before returning to normal.

Squatting increases venous return and systemic arterial resistance simultaneously causing a rise in stroke volume and arterial pressure. This makes most murmurs louder. However, left ventricular size is increased which reduces the obstruction to outflow and therefore reduces the intensity of the systolic murmur of hypertrophic cardiomyopathy, while the mid-systolic click and murmur of mitral valve prolapse are delayed.

Isometric exercise: sustained hand grip for 20 or 30 seconds increases systemic arterial resistance, blood pressure and heart size. The systolic murmur of aortic stenosis is softer because of a reduction in the pressure gradient across the valve. Most other murmurs become louder except the systolic murmur of hypertrophic cardiomyopathy, which is softer, and the mitral valve prolapse murmur, which is delayed because of an increased ventricular volume. This manoeuvre is only occasionally used.

The Back

It is now time to leave the praecordium. Percussion and auscultation of the *lung bases* (Chapter 4) are also part of the cardiovascular examination. Signs of cardiac failure may be detected in the lungs; in particular late or pan-inspiratory crackles or a pleural effusion may be present.

While the patient is sitting up, feel for pitting oedema of the sacrum which occurs in severe right heart failure, especially in patients who have been in bed. This is because the sacrum then becomes a dependent area and oedema fluid tends to settle under the influence of gravity.

The Abdomen

Lie the patient down flat (on one pillow) and examine the abdomen (Chapter 5). One is looking particularly for an enlarged tender *liver* which may be found when the hepatic veins are congested in the presence of right heart failure. Distension of the liver capsule is said to be the cause of liver tenderness in these patients. When tricuspid regurgitation is present the liver may be *pulsatile* as the right ventricular systolic pressure wave is transmitted to the hepatic veins. *Ascites* may occur with severe right heart failure. *Splenomegaly*, if present, may indicate infective endocarditis. An implanted cardioverter-defibrillator box may be palpable below the left costal margin. This feels like a very large pacemaker.

The Lower Limbs

Examine both *femoral arteries* by palpating and then auscultating them. A bruit may be heard if the artery is narrowed. Next palpate the following pulses (Figures 3.19 and 3.20): *popliteal* (behind the knee), *posterior tibial* (under the medial malleolus) and *dorsalis pedis* (on the forefoot) on both sides.

Palpate the distal shaft of the tibia for *oedema* by compressing the area for at least 15 seconds with the thumb. This area is often tender in normal people and gentleness in necessary. Oedema may be pitting (the skin is indented and only slowly refills (Figure 3.21)) or non-pitting. Pitting oedema occurs in cardiac failure unless the condition has been present for a long time and secondary changes in the

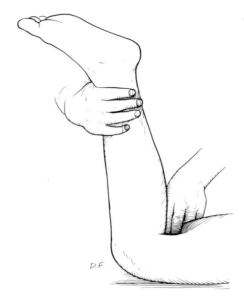

Figure 3.19 *Palpating the popliteal artery.*

Adapted from Dunphy JE, Botsford TW. Physical examination of the surgical patient. An introduction to clinical surgery. 4th ed. Philadelphia: WB Saunders, 1975. With permission.

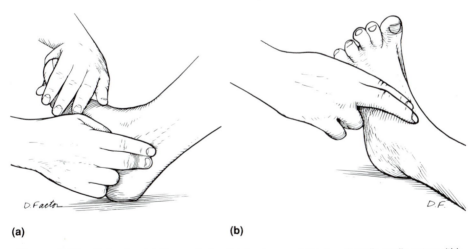

(a)   **(b)**

Figure 3.20 *Palpating (a) the posterior tibial artery and (b) the dorsalis pedis artery (this usually lies just lateral to the extensor hallucis longus tendon which can be seen when the patient dorsiflexes the big toe).*

Adapted from Dunphy JE, Botsford TW. Physical examination of the surgical patient. An introduction to clinical surgery. 4th ed. Philadelphia: WB Saunders, 1975. With permission.

Table 3.11   *Causes of Oedema*

Pitting Lower Limb Oedema

Cardiac: congestive cardiac failure, constrictive pericarditis
Drugs: calcium antagonists
Hepatic: cirrhosis (page 187) causing hypoalbuminaemia
Renal: nephrotic syndrome (page 214) causing hypoalbuminaemia
Gastrointestinal tract: malabsorption, starvation, protein-losing enteropathy causing
    hypoalbuminaemia
Beri beri (wet)
Cyclical oedema

Pitting Unilateral Lower Limb Oedema

Deep venous thrombosis
Compression of large veins by tumour or lymph nodes

Non-pitting Lower Limb Oedema

Hypothyroidism (page 302)
Lymphoedema
    Infectious (e.g., filariasis)
    Malignant (tumour invasion of lymphatics)
    Congenital (lymphatic development arrest)
    Allergy
    Milroy's* disease (unexplained lymphoedema which appears at puberty and is more
        common in females)

*   William Milroy (1855–1942), Professor of Medicine, University of Nebraska, described the disease in 1928.

lymphatic vessels have occurred. If oedema is present one should note its upper level. Severe oedema can involve the skin of the abdominal wall and the scrotum as well as the lower limbs. Causes of oedema are listed in Table 3.11.

Look for evidence of Achilles* tendon xanthomata due to hyperlipidaemia (Figure 3.22). Also look for cyanosis and clubbing of the toes (this may occur without finger clubbing in a patient with a patent ductus arteriosus because a rise in pulmonary artery pressures, sufficient to reverse the direction of flow in the shunt, has occurred).

Examine for signs of *peripheral vascular disease*: reduced or absent pulses, femoral systolic bruits, marked leg pallor, absence of hairs, cool skin and reduced capillary return (compress the toe nails—the return of the normal red colour is slow). In such cases, perform *Buerger's[†] test* to help confirm your diagnosis: elevate the legs to 45 degrees (pallor is rapid if there is a poor arterial supply) then place them dependent at 90 degrees over the edge of the bed (cyanosis occurs if the arterial supply is impaired).

Deep Venous Thrombosis

Deep venous thrombosis is a difficult clinical diagnosis. The patient may complain of calf pain. On examination one should look for swelling of the calf and the leg, and dilated superficial veins. Feel then for increased warmth and squeeze the calf

---

*   Achilles, mythical Greek hero, whose body was invulnerable except for his heels by which he was held when dipped in the River Styx as a baby.

†   Leo Buerger (1879–1943), New York physician, described thrombo-angiitis obliterans.

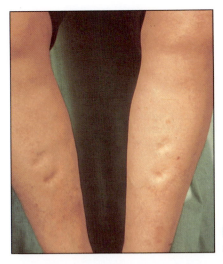

Figure 3.21
Severe pitting oedema of the legs.

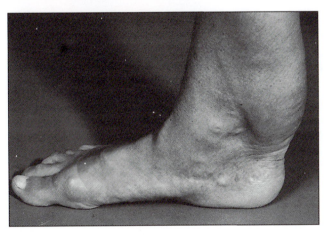

Figure 3.22
Achilles tendon xanthomata.

(gently) to determine if the area is tender. Homans'* sign, pain in the calf when the foot is sharply dorsiflexed, is of little diagnostic value and may theoretically be dangerous because of the possibility of dislodgment of loose clot. The causes of thrombosis were described by Virchow† in 1856 under three broad headings (his famous triad): (i) changes in the vessel wall; (ii) changes in blood flow; and (iii) changes in the constitution of the blood. Deep venous thrombosis is usually caused by prolonged immobilisation, cardiac failure (stasis) or trauma (vessel wall damage), but may also result from occult neoplasm, disseminated intravascular coagulation, the contraceptive pill and pregnancy (alterations in coagulability).

---

*   John Homans (1836–1903), Professor of Surgery, Harvard University, Boston.
†   Rudolph Virchow (1821–1902), brilliant German pathologist, and regarded as the founder of modern pathology.

Table 3.12 *Causes of Leg Ulcers*

1. Venous stasis ulcer—most common
   Site: around malleoli
   Associated pigmentation, stasis eczema
2. Ischaemic ulcer
   - large artery disease (atherosclerosis, thromboangiitis obliterans): usually lateral side of leg (pulses absent)
   - small vessel disease (e.g., leucocytoclastic vasculitis, palpable purpura)
3. Malignant ulcer, e.g., basal cell carcinoma (pearly translucent edge), squamous cell carcinoma (hard everted edge), melanoma, lymphoma, Kaposi's sarcoma
4. Infection, e.g., *Staphylococcus aureus*, syphilitic gumma, tuberculosis, atypical *Mycobacterium*, fungal
5. Neuropathic (painless penetrating ulcer on sole of foot: peripheral neuropathy, e.g., diabetes mellitus, tabes, leprosy)
6. Underlying systemic disease
   - Diabetes mellitus: vascular disease, neuropathy, or necrobiosis lipoidica (front of leg)
   - Pyoderma gangrenosum
   - Rheumatoid arthritis
   - Lymphoma
   - Haemolytic anaemia (small ulcers over malleoli), e.g., sickle cell anaemia

Acute Arterial Occlusion

This can be the result of embolism, thrombosis or injury. Peripheral arterial embolism usually arises from thrombus in the heart, where it is often secondary to (i) myocardial infarction or dilated cardiomyopathy; (ii) atrial fibrillation; or (iii) infective endocarditis. Acute arterial occlusion of a major peripheral limb artery results in a painful, pale, pulseless and 'paralysed' limb (the four Ps).

Varicose Veins

If a patient complains of 'varicose veins', ask him or her to *stand* with the legs fully exposed. *Inspect* the front of the whole leg for tortuous, dilated branches of the long saphenous vein (below the femoral vein in the groin to the medial side of the lower leg). Then inspect the back of the calf for varicosities of the short saphenous vein (from the popliteal fossa to the back of the calf and lateral malleolus). Look to see if the leg is inflamed, swollen or pigmented (venous stasis).

Palpate the veins. Hard leg veins suggest thrombosis, while tenderness indicates thrombophlebitis. Perform the *cough impulse test*. Put the fingers over the long saphenous vein opening in the groin, medial to the femoral vein (NB: Don't forget the anatomy—femoral vein (medial), artery (your landmark), nerve (lateral)). Ask the patient to cough: a fluid thrill is felt if the saphenofemoral valve is incompetent.

The following supplementary tests are occasionally helpful (and surgeons like to quiz students on them in exams).

Trendelenburg* test: with the patient lying down, the leg is elevated. Firm pressure is placed on the saphenous opening in the groin, and the patient is

---

*   Friedrich Trendelenburg (1844–1924), Professor of Surgery, Leipzig.

instructed to stand. The sign is positive if the veins stay empty until the groin pressure is released (incompetence at the saphenofemoral valve). If the veins fill despite groin pressure, the incompetent valves are in the thigh or calf, and Perthes'* test is performed.

Perthes' test: repeat Trendelenburg's test, but when the patient stands allow some blood to be released and then get him or her to stand up and down on the toes a few times. The veins will become less tense if the perforating calf veins are patent and have competent valves (the muscle pump is functioning).

If the pattern of affected veins is unusual (e.g., pubic varices), one should try to exclude secondary varicose veins. These may be due to an intrapelvic neoplasm which has obstructed deep venous return. A rectal (page 178) and pelvic (page 219) examination should be performed to look for these.

Finally, chronic venous stasis is one cause of ulceration of the lower leg. This is often associated with pigmentation and eczema, which are due to venous stasis. The differential diagnosis of leg ulcers is shown in Table 3.12.

Correlation of Physical Signs and Cardiovascular Disease

When a disease is named after some author, it is very likely that we don't know much about it.

August Bier (1861–1949)

Cardiac Failure

This is one of the commonest syndromes: the signs of cardiac failure should be sought in all patients admitted to hospital. Cardiac failure has been defined as a reduction in cardiac function such that cardiac output is reduced relative to the metabolic demands of the body and compensating mechanisms have occurred. The specific signs depend on whether the left, right or both ventricles are involved.

Left Ventricular Failure (LVF)

Symptoms: exertional dyspnoea, orthopnoea, paroxysmal nocturnal dyspnoea.

General signs: tachypnoea, due to raised pulmonary pressures; central cyanosis, due to pulmonary oedema; Cheyne-Stokes breathing, especially in sedated elderly patients; peripheral cyanosis, due to low cardiac output; hypotension, due to low cardiac output. Cardiac cachexia.

Arterial pulse: sinus tachycardia, due to increased sympathetic tone; pulsus alternans (alternate strong and weak beats)—rare, mechanism unknown.

Apex beat: displaced, with dilatation of the left ventricle; dyskinetic in anterior myocardial infarction or dilated cardiomyopathy; palpable gallop rhythm.

Auscultation: left ventricular S3; functional mitral regurgitation (secondary to valve ring dilatation).

Lung fields: signs of pulmonary congestion or pulmonary oedema, due to raised venous pressures (increased preload).

Signs of the underlying cause.

---

*   Georg Clemens Perthes (1869–1927), German surgeon.

Causes of LVF: (i) myocardial disease (ischaemic heart disease, cardio-myopathy); (ii) volume overload (aortic regurgitation, mitral regurgitation, patent ductus arteriosus); (iii) pressure overload (systolic hypertension, aortic stenosis).

Right Ventricular Failure (RVF)

Symptoms: ankle or abdominal swelling, anorexia, nausea.

General signs: peripheral cyanosis, due to low cardiac output.

Arterial pulse: low volume, due to low cardiac output.

Jugular venous pulse: raised, due to the raised venous pressure (right heart preload); Kussmaul's sign, due to poor right ventricular compliance (e.g., right ventricular myocardial infarction); large *v* waves (functional tricuspid regurgitation secondary to valve ring dilatation).

Apex beat: right ventricular heave.

Auscultation: right ventricular S3; pansystolic murmur of functional tricuspid regurgitation (absence of a murmur does not exclude tricuspid regurgitation).

Abdomen: *tender hepatomegaly*, due to increased venous pressure transmitted via the hepatic veins; pulsatile liver, if tricuspid regurgitation is present.

Oedema, due to sodium and water retention plus raised venous pressure may be manifested by pitting ankle and sacral oedema, ascites, or pleural effusions (small).

Signs of the underlying cause.

Causes of RVF: (i) left ventricular failure (severe chronic LVF causes raised pulmonary pressures resulting in secondary right ventricular failure); (ii) volume overload (atrial septal defect, primary tricuspid regurgitation); (iii) pressure overload (pulmonary stenosis, pulmonary hypertension); (iv) myocardial disease (right ventricular myocardial infarction, cardiomyopathy).

Myocardial Infarction

There may be very few signs in *uncomplicated* cases.

General signs: anxiety and restlessness (from the chest pain); pallor, diaphoresis (sweating) and cool limbs; mild fever (usually not exceeding 38°C).

Pulse and blood pressure: tachycardia and/or hypotension (25% with anterior infarction from sympathetic hyperactivity), bradycardia and/or hypotension (up to 50% with inferior infarction from parasympathetic hyperactivity). Other arrhythmias including atrial fibrillation, ventricular tachycardia and heart block may be present.

The JVP: increased with right ventricular infarction; Kussmaul's sign may be present.

Apex beat: dyskinetic in patients with large anterior infarction.

Auscultation: S4, S3, decreased intensity of heart sounds, transient apical mid-systolic or late-systolic murmur (in 25% from mitral regurgitation secondary to papillary muscle dysfunction), or a pericardial friction rub (with transmural infarction).

Complications: arrhythmias, heart failure, cardiogenic shock, rupture of a papillary muscle, perforation of the ventricular septum, ventricular aneurysm, thromboembolism or cardiac rupture. Signs of these complications include the development of a new murmur, recurrent chest pain, dyspnoea or sudden hypotension.

Pericardial Disease

Acute Pericarditis

Signs: fever, pericardial friction rub.

Causes of acute pericarditis: (i) viral infection (Coxsackie A or B virus, influenza); (ii) after myocardial infarction: early, or late (10 to 14 days, termed Dressler's* syndrome); (iii) after pericardiotomy (cardiac surgery); (iv) uraemia; (v) neoplasia—tumour invasion (e.g., bronchus, breast, lymphoma) or after irradiation for tumour; (vi) connective tissue disease (e.g., systemic lupus erythematosus, rheumatoid arthritis); (vii) hypothyroidism; (viii) other infections (e.g., tuberculosis, pyogenic pneumonia or septicaemia); (ix) acute rheumatic fever.

Chronic Constrictive Pericarditis

General signs: cachexia.

Pulse and blood pressure: pulsus paradoxus (more than the normal 10 mmHg fall in the arterial pulse pressure on inspiration, because increased right ventricular filling compresses the left ventricle); low blood pressure.

The JVP: raised; Kussmaul's sign (uncommon); prominent x and y descents.

Apex beat: impalpable.

Auscultation: heart sounds distant, early S3; early pericardial knock (rapid ventricular filling abruptly halted).

Abdomen: hepatomegaly, due to raised venous pressure; splenomegaly, due to raised venous pressure; ascites.

Peripheral oedema.

Causes of chronic constrictive pericarditis: (i) cardiac operation or trauma; (ii) tuberculosis, histoplasmosis or pyogenic infection; (iii) neoplastic disease; (iv) mediastinal irradiation; (v) connective tissue disease (especially rheumatoid arthritis); (vi) chronic renal failure.

Acute Cardiac Tamponade

General signs: tachypnoea; anxiety; syncope.

Pulse and blood pressure: rapid pulse rate; pulsus paradoxus; hypotension.

The JVP: raised; Kussmaul's sign; prominent x but an absent y descent.

Apex beat: impalpable.

Auscultation: reduced heart sounds.

Lungs: dullness and bronchial breathing at the left base, due to lung compression by the distended pericardial sac.

Chronic pericardial tamponade causes signs similar to constrictive pericarditis, except that there is no prominent x descent (which is not an easy sign to pick clinically).

Infective Endocarditis

General signs: fever; arthropathy (especially metacarpophalangeal joints, wrists, elbows, knees, ankles).

---

* William Dressler (1890–1969), New York cardiologist, described this syndrome in 1956.

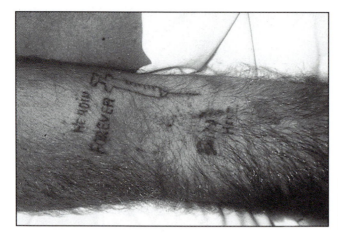

Figure 3.23

Example of an intravenous drug addict's forearm.

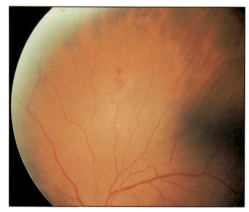

Figure 3.24

A Roth's spot.

Hands: splinter haemorrhages; clubbing (within six weeks of onset); Osler's nodes (rare); Janeway lesions (very rare).

Arms: evidence of intravenous drug use (Figure 3.23)—right (and left) heart endocarditis can result from this.

Eyes: pale conjunctivae (anaemia); retinal or conjunctival haemorrhages—Roth's* spots are fundal vasculitic lesions with a yellow centre surrounded by a red ring (Figure 3.24).

Heart—signs of *underlying heart disease*: (i) acquired (mitral regurgitation, mitral stenosis, aortic stenosis, aortic regurgitation); (ii) congenital (patent ductus arteriosus, ventricular septal defect, coarctation of the aorta); (iii) prosthetic valves.

Abdomen: splenomegaly.

Urine analysis: blood.

Peripheral evidence of embolisation to limbs or central nervous system.

---

*   Moriz von Roth (1839–1914), Swiss physician and pathologist, described these changes in 1872.

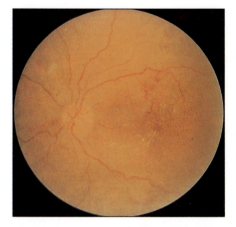

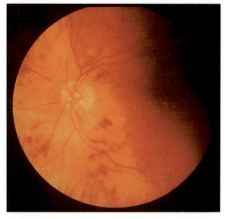

Figure 3.25 *Hypertensive retinopathy grade 3. Note flame-shaped haemorrhages and cotton wool spots.*

Figure 3.26 *Hypertensive retinopathy grade 4. Note A-V nipping, silver wiring and papilloedema.*

Systemic Hypertension

It is important to have in mind a method for the examination of a patient with systemic hypertension. The examination aims to measure the blood pressure level, determine if there is an underlying cause present, and assess the severity as determined by signs of end-organ damage. It is a common clinical problem.

On general inspection the signs of associated diseases must be sought: for example, Cushing's* syndrome (page 310), acromegaly (page 308), polycythaemia (page 241) or chronic renal failure (page 206).

Take the blood pressure, with the patient lying and standing, using an appropriately sized cuff (page 41). A rise in diastolic pressure on standing occurs typically in essential hypertension; a fall on standing may suggest a secondary cause, but is usually an effect of antihypertensive medications. Palpate for radiofemoral delay, and check the blood pressure in the legs if coarctation of the aorta is suspected or if severe hypertension is discovered before 30 years of age (page 83).

Next examine the fundi for hypertensive changes (Figures 3.25 and 3.26) which can be classified from grades 1 to 4: grade 1—'silver wiring' of the arteries only (sclerosis of the vessel wall reduces its transparency so that the central light streak becomes broader and shinier); grade 2—silver wiring of arteries plus arteriovenous nipping or nicking (indentation or deflection of the veins where they are crossed by the arteries); grade 3—grade 2 plus haemorrhages (flame shaped) and exudates (soft—cottonwool spots due to ischaemia, or hard—lipid residues from leaking vessels); grade 4—grade 3 changes plus papilloedema (page 346). It is important to describe the changes present rather than just give a grade.

Now examine the rest of the cardiovascular system for signs of left ventricular failure, secondary to hypertension, and for coarctation of the aorta. A fourth heart sound is almost always detectable if the blood pressure is greater than 180/110 mmHg.

---

* Harvey Cushing (1869–1939), Professor of Surgery, Harvard University, and a renowned neurosurgeon.

Then go to the abdomen to palpate for renal or adrenal masses (possible causes), and for the presence of an abdominal aortic aneurysm (page 170, a possible complication). Auscultate for a renal bruit (page 210) due to renal artery stenosis. Remember that most left-sided abdominal bruits arise from the splenic artery and are of no significance.

Examine the central nervous system for signs of previous cerebrovascular accidents (page 391), and palpate and auscultate the carotid arteries for bruits (stenosis may be a manifestation of vascular disease, and may be associated with renal artery stenosis). Urinalysis should also be performed to look for evidence of renal disease (page 212).

Causes of Systemic Hypertension

Hypertension may be essential or idiopathic (more than 95% of cases), or secondary (less than 5%). Immoderate alcohol and salt consumption and obesity are associated with hypertension. Obstructive sleep apnoea may also be an association.

Secondary causes include: (i) renal disease—renal artery stenosis, chronic pyelonephritis, analgesic nephropathy, connective tissue disease, glomerulonephritis, polycystic disease, diabetic nephropathy, reflux nephropathy; (ii) endocrine disorders—Cushing's syndrome, Conn's syndrome (primary aldosteronism), phaeochromocytoma, acromegaly; (iii) coarctation of the aorta; and (iv) other, such as the contraceptive pill, polycythaemia rubra vera, toxaemia of pregnancy, neurogenic causes (increased intracranial pressure, lead poisoning, acute porphyria), or hypercalcaemia.

Complications of Hypertension

These include left ventricular failure, cerebrovascular ischaemic events, renal failure, and eye disease (blindness). Hypertension is also a risk factor for ischaemic heart disease and peripheral vascular disease.

Malignant Hypertension

This can be defined as papilloedema as a result of severe hypertension.

Pulmonary Hypertension

Systolic pulmonary artery pressures higher than 30 mmHg are abnormal and constitute pulmonary hypertension. It is important to know what signs to look for in a patient who may have pulmonary hypertension.

General signs: (usually only in patients with severe hypertension) tachypnoea; peripheral cyanosis and cold extremities, due to low cardiac output; hoarseness (very rare, due to pulmonary artery compression of the left recurrent laryngeal nerve).

The pulse: usually of small volume, due to the low cardiac output (only in severe disease).

The JVP: prominent *a* wave, due to forceful right atrial contraction.

The apex beat: right ventricular heave; palpable P2.

Auscultation: systolic ejection click, due to dilatation of the pulmonary artery; loud P2, due to forceful valve closure because of high pulmonary artery pressures; S4; pulmonary ejection murmur, due to dilatation of the pulmonary artery resulting in turbulent blood flow; murmur of pulmonary regurgitation if dilatation of the pulmonary artery occurs.

Signs of right ventricular failure (late: termed cor pulmonale—page 115).

Causes of Pulmonary Hypertension

Pulmonary hypertension may be primary (idiopathic), or secondary.

Secondary causes include: (i) pulmonary emboli—e.g., blood clots, tumour particles, fat globules; (ii) lung disease—chronic airflow limitation (page 122), obstructive sleep apnoea, interstitial lung disease (e.g., pulmonary fibrosis); (iii) congenital heart disease causing a left to right shunt—atrial septal defect, ventricular septal defect, patent ductus arteriosus; and (iv) severe kyphoscoliosis.

Innocent Murmurs

The detection of a systolic murmur on routine examination is a common problem. It can cause considerable alarm to both the patient and the examining clinician. These murmurs in asymptomatic people are often the result of normal turbulence within the heart and great vessels. When no structural abnormality of the heart or great vessels is present these are called innocent, functional or organic murmurs. They probably arise from vibrations within the aortic arch near the origins of the head and neck vessels or from the right ventricular outflow tract. They are more common in children and young adults .

Innocent murmurs are always systolic. (A venous hum, which is not really a murmur, has both systolic and diastolic components.) They are usually soft and ejection-systolic in character. Those arising from the aortic arch may radiate to the carotids and be heard in the neck. Those arising from the right ventricular outflow tract are loudest in the pulmonary area.

These outflow tract murmurs must be distinguished from the pulmonary flow murmur of an atrial septal defect (page 82). Therefore it is important to listen carefully for wide or fixed splitting of the second heart sound before pronouncing a murmur innocent.

Valve Diseases of the Left Heart

Mitral Stenosis

The normal area of the mitral valve is 4 to 6 cm². Reduction of the valve area to half normal or less causes significant obstruction to left ventricular filling and blood will only flow from the left atrium to the left ventricle if the left atrial pressure is raised.

Symptoms: dyspnoea, orthopnoea, paroxysmal nocturnal dyspnoea (increased left atrial pressure); haemoptysis (ruptured bronchial veins); ascites, oedema, fatigue (pulmonary hypertension).

General signs: tachypnoea; 'mitral facies' (page 43); and peripheral cyanosis (severe mitral stenosis).

The pulse and blood pressure: normal or reduced in volume, due to a reduced cardiac output; atrial fibrillation may be present because of left atrial enlargement.

The JVP: normal; prominent *a* wave if pulmonary hypertension is present; loss of the *a* wave if the patient is in atrial fibrillation.

Palpation: tapping quality of the apex beat (palpable S1); right ventricular heave and palpable P2 if pulmonary hypertension is present; diastolic thrill rarely (lie patient on the left side).

Auscultation (Figure 3.27): loud S1 (valve cusps widely apart at the onset of systole)—this also indicates that the valve cusps remain mobile; loud P2 if pulmonary hypertension is present; opening snap (high left atrial pressure forces the valve cusps apart, but the valve cone is halted abruptly); low pitched rumbling diastolic murmur (best heard with the bell of the stethoscope with the patient in the left lateral position, and quite different in quality and timing from the murmur of aortic regurgitation); a late diastolic accentuation of the diastolic murmur may occur if the patient is in sinus rhythm, but is usually absent if atrial fibrillation has supervened—this is best heard in the left lateral position; exercise accentuates the murmur (ask the patient to sit up and down quickly in bed several times).

Signs indicating severe mitral stenosis (valve area less than 1cm^2): small pulse pressure; soft first heart sound (immobile valve cusps); early opening snap (due to increased left atrial pressure); long diastolic murmur (persists as long as there is a gradient); diastolic thrill at the apex; signs of pulmonary hypertension.

Causes of mitral stenosis: (i) rheumatic (following acute rheumatic fever); (ii) congenital parachute valve (all chordae insert into one papillary muscle—rare).

Mitral Regurgitation (Chronic)

A regurgitant mitral valve allows part of the left ventricular stroke volume to regurgitate into the left atrium, imposing a volume load on both the left atrium and the left ventricle.

Symptoms: dyspnoea (increased left atrial pressure); fatigue (decreased cardiac output).

General signs: tachypnoea; mitral facies (rare, as pulmonary hypertension is unusual).

The pulse: normal, or sharp upstroke due to rapid left ventricular decompression; atrial fibrillation is relatively common.

The JVP: normal unless right ventricular failure has occurred; the *a* wave is lost in atrial fibrillation.

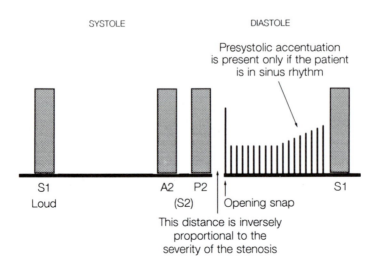

Figure 3.27 *Mitral stenosis (MS) (at the apex).*

Palpation: the apex beat is displaced, diffuse and hyperdynamic; a pansystolic thrill may be present at the apex; a parasternal impulse (due to left atrial enlargement behind the right ventricle—the left atrium is often larger in mitral regurgitation than in mitral stenosis and can be enormous).

Auscultation (Figure 3.28): soft or absent S1 (by the end of diastole, atrial and ventricular pressures have equalised and the valve cusps have drifted back together); left ventricular S3, due to rapid left ventricular filling in early diastole; pansystolic murmur maximal at the apex and usually radiating towards the axilla.

Signs indicating severe chronic mitral regurgitation: small volume pulse; enlarged left ventricle; S3; soft S1; A2 is early, because rapid left ventricular decompression into the left atrium causes the aortic valve to close early; early diastolic rumble; signs of pulmonary hypertension; signs of left ventricular failure.

Causes of chronic mitral regurgitation: (i) rheumatic; (ii) mitral valve prolapse; (iii) papillary muscle dysfunction, due to left ventricular failure or ischaemia; (iv) connective tissue disease—e.g., Marfan's syndrome, rheumatoid arthritis, ankylosing spondylitis; (v) congenital parachute valve; (vi) cardiomyopathy—hypertrophic, dilated or restrictive cardiomyopathy.

Acute Mitral Regurgitation

In this case patients can present with pulmonary oedema and cardiovascular collapse. There is usually a loud apical ejection murmur present (it is short because atrial pressure is increased). With anterior leaflet chordae rupture the murmur radiates to the axilla and back; with posterior leaflet rupture the murmur radiates to the cardiac base and carotids.

Causes: (i) myocardial infarction (dysfunction or rupture of papillary muscles); (ii) infective endocarditis; (iii) trauma or surgery; (iv) spontaneous rupture of a chord.

Mitral Valve Prolapse (Systolic-Click Murmur Syndrome)

This syndrome can cause a systolic murmur or click or both at the apex. The presence of the murmur indicates that there is some mitral regurgitation present.

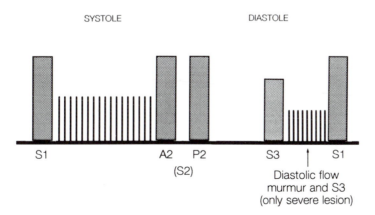

Figure 3.28   *Mitral regurgitation (at the apex).*

Auscultation (Figure 3.29): systolic click or clicks at a variable time (usually mid-systolic) may be the only abnormality audible, but a click is not always audible; systolic murmur—high pitched late-systolic murmur, commencing with the click and extending throughout the rest of systole.

Dynamic auscultation: murmur and click occur earlier and may become louder with the Valsalva manoeuvre and with standing, but both occur later and may become softer with squatting and isometric exercise.

Causes of mitral valve prolapse: (i) myxomatous degeneration of the mitral valve tissue—this is very common and the severity may increase with age so that significant mitral regurgitation may supervene; (ii) may be associated with atrial septal defect (secundum) (page 82), hypertrophic cardiomyopathy (page 79), or Marfan's syndrome (page 33).

Aortic Stenosis

The normal area of the aortic valve is more than $2\,cm^2$. Significant narrowing of the aortic valve restricts left ventricular outflow and imposes a pressure load on the left ventricle.

Symptoms: exertional angina (50% do not have coronary artery disease), exertional dyspnoea and exertional syncope.

General signs: usually there is nothing remarkable about the general appearance.

The pulse: there may be a plateau or anacrotic pulse, or the pulse may be late peaking (tardus). This is of small volume (parvus) and the pulse pressure is also reduced.

Palpation: the apex beat is hyperdynamic and may be slightly displaced; systolic thrill at the base of the heart (aortic area).

Auscultation (Figure 3.30): a narrowly split or reversed S2 because of delayed left ventricular ejection; a harsh mid-systolic ejection murmur, maximal over the aortic area and extending into the carotid arteries is characteristic and may be heard quite well at the apex too—the murmur is loudest with the patient sitting up and in full expiration; associated aortic regurgitation is common; in congenital aortic stenosis where the valve cusps remain mobile and the dome of the valve comes to a sudden halt, an ejection click may precede the murmur—the ejection

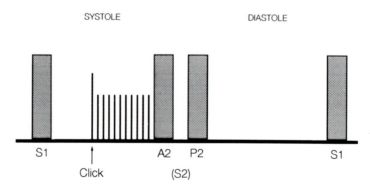

Figure 3.29 *Mitral valve prolapse (MVP) (at the apex).*

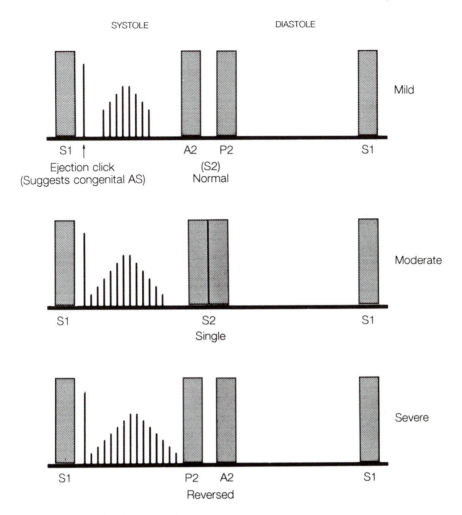

SYSTOLE   DIASTOLE

S1 ↑
Ejection click
(Suggests congenital AS)

A2   P2
(S2)
Normal

S1

Mild

S1

S2
Single

S1

Moderate

S1

P2   A2
Reversed

S1

Severe

Figure 3.30   *Aortic stenosis (AS) (at the aortic area).*

click is absent if the valve is calcified or if the stenosis is not at the valve level but above or below it.

Signs indicating severe aortic stenosis (valve area less than 1 cm², or valve gradient greater than 50–70 mmHg: plateau pulse; thrill in the aortic area; length of the murmur and lateness of the peak of the systolic murmur; S4; paradoxical splitting of S2, due to greatly delayed aortic valve closure; absent A2; left ventricular failure (very late sign; right ventricular failure is preterminal).

Causes of aortic stenosis: (i) degenerative calcific aortic stenosis, particularly in elderly patients; (ii) calcific in younger patients, usually on a congenital bicuspid valve; (iii) rheumatic.

Two other sorts of aortic outflow obstruction are possible: (i) with supravalvular obstruction there is narrowing of the ascending aorta or a fibrous diaphragm just above the aortic valve—this is rare and may be associated with a characteristic

Table 3.13 *Eponymous Signs of Aortic Regurgitation*

1. Quincke's sign: capillary pulsation in the nail beds—it is of no value, as this sign occurs normally
2. Corrigan's sign: prominent carotid pulsations
3. De Musset's sign: head nodding in time with the heart beat
4. Hill's sign: increased blood pressure in the legs compared with the arms
5. Mueller's sign: pulsation of the uvula in time with the heart beat
6. Duroziez's sign: systolic and diastolic murmurs over the femoral artery on gradual compression of the vessel
7. Traube's sign: a double sound heard over the femoral artery on compressing the vessel distally; this is *not* a 'pistol shot' sound that may be heard over the femoral artery with very severe aortic regurgitation

NB: These signs are uncommon and usually unhelpful

1. Heinrich Quincke (1842–1922), German neurologist.
2. Dominic Corrigan (1802–1880), Edinburgh graduate who worked in Dublin and is credited with discovering aortic regurgitation.
3. Alfred de Musset, nineteenth Century French poet who suffered from aortic regurgitation. The sign was noticed by his brother, a physician.
4. Leonard Hill (b. 1866), English physiologist who also described the physiology of the cerebral circulation.
5. Frederick Von Mueller (1858–1941), German physician who also noted an increase in metabolism in exophthalmic goitre.
6. Paul Duroziez (1826–1897), French physician.
7. Ludwig Traube (1818–1876), Hungarian physician who worked in Germany.

facies (a broad forehead, widely set eyes and a pointed chin); there is a loud A2 and often a thrill in the sternal notch area; (ii) with subvalvular obstruction there is a membranous diaphragm or fibrous ridge just below the aortic valve; aortic regurgitation is associated and is due to a jet lesion on the coronary cusp.

Dynamic left ventricular outflow tract obstruction may occur in hypertrophic cardiomyopathy. Here there may be a double apical impulse. Atrial contraction into a stiff left ventricle may be palpable before the left ventricular impulse (only in the presence of sinus rhythm of course).

Aortic sclerosis presents in the elderly; there are no peripheral signs of aortic sclerosis. The diagnosis implies the absence of a gradient across the aortic valve despite some thickening and a murmur.

Aortic Regurgitation

The incompetent aortic valve allows regurgitation of blood from the aorta to the left ventricle during diastole for as long as the aortic diastolic pressure exceeds the left ventricular diastolic pressure.

Symptoms: occur in the late stages of disease and include exertional dyspnoea, fatigue, palpitations (hyperdynamic circulation) and exertional angina.

General signs: Marfan's syndrome, ankylosing spondylitis or one of the other seronegative arthropathies (page 274) or, rarely, Argyll–Robertson pupils (page 323) may be obvious.

The pulse and blood pressure: the pulse is characteristically collapsing, a 'water hammer'* pulse (Table 3.13); there may be a wide pulse pressure.

---

* This Victorian children's toy consisted of a sealed tube half-filled with fluid with the other half being a vacuum. Inversion of the tube caused the fluid to fall rapidly without air resistance and strike the other end with a noise like a hammer blow. It is not easy to imagine a child today being entertained by this for very long.

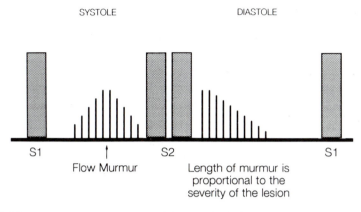

Figure 3.31 *Aortic regurgitation (at the left sternal edge).*

The neck: prominent carotid pulsations (Corrigan's sign).

Palpation: the apex beat is characteristically displaced and hyperkinetic. A diastolic thrill may be felt at the left sternal edge when the patient sits up and breathes out.

Auscultation (Figure 3.31): A2 (the aortic component of the second heart sound) may be soft; a decrescendo high pitched diastolic murmur beginning immediately after the second heart sound and extending for a variable time into diastole—it is loudest at the third and fourth left intercostal spaces; a systolic ejection murmur is usually present (due to associated aortic stenosis or to torrential flow across a normal diameter aortic valve). Aortic stenosis is distinguished from an aortic flow murmur by the presence of the peripheral signs of significant aortic stenosis, such as a plateau pulse.

An *Austin Flint* murmur* should also be listened for. This is a low pitched rumbling mid-diastolic and presystolic murmur audible at the apex (the regurgitant jet from the aortic valve causes the anterior mitral valve leaflet to shudder). It can be distinguished from mitral stenosis because S1 (the first heart sound) is not loud and there is no opening snap.

Many other signs have been described, but they are generally not helpful (Table 3.13).

Signs indicating severe chronic aortic regurgitation: collapsing pulse; wide pulse pressure; long decrescendo diastolic murmur; left ventricular S3 (third heart sound); soft A2; Austin Flint murmur; signs of left ventricular failure.

Causes of aortic regurgitation: disease may affect the valvular area or aortic root, and may be acute or chronic.

Causes of chronic aortic regurgitation: (i) valvular—rheumatic (rarely the only murmur in this case), congenital (e.g., bicuspid valve; ventricular septal defect—an associated prolapse of the aortic cusp is not uncommon), seronegative arthropathy, especially ankylosing spondylitis; (ii) aortic root dilatation (murmur may be maximal at the right sternal border)—Marfan's syndrome, aortitis (e.g., seronegative arthropathies, rheumatoid arthritis, tertiary syphilis), dissecting aneurysm.

---

*   Austin Flint (1812–1886), New York physician.

Causes of acute aortic regurgitation (Note: murmur may be soft because of increased left ventricular end-diastolic pressure): (i) valvular—infective endocarditis; (ii) aortic root—Marfan's syndrome, hypertension, dissecting aneurysm.

Valve Diseases of the Right Heart

Tricuspid Stenosis

This is very rare.

The JVP: raised; giant *a* waves with a slow *y* descent may be seen.

Auscultation: a diastolic murmur audible at the left sternal edge, accentuated by inspiration, very similar to the murmur of mitral stenosis except for the site of maximal intensity and the effect of respiration (louder on inspiration); tricuspid regurgitation and mitral stenosis are often present as well; no signs of pulmonary hypertension.

Abdomen: presystolic pulsation of the liver, caused by forceful atrial systole.

Cause of tricuspid stenosis: rheumatic heart disease.

Tricuspid Regurgitation

The JVP: large *v* waves; the JVP is elevated if right ventricular failure has occurred.

Palpation: right ventricular heave.

Auscultation: there may be a pansystolic murmur maximal at the lower end of the sternum that increases on inspiration, but the diagnosis can be made on the basis of the peripheral signs alone.

Abdomen: a pulsatile, large and tender liver is usually present and may cause the right nipple to dance in time with the heart beat; ascites, oedema and pleural effusions may also be present.

Legs: dilated, pulsatile veins.

Causes of tricuspid regurgitation:[*] (i) functional (no disease of the valve leaflets)—right ventricular failure; (ii) rheumatic—only very rarely does rheumatic tricuspid regurgitation occur alone, usually mitral valve disease is also present; (iii) infective endocarditis (right-sided endocarditis in intravenous drug addicts); (iv) tricuspid valve prolapse; (v) right ventricular papillary muscle infarction; (vi) trauma (usually a steering wheel injury to the sternum); (vii) congenital— Ebstein's[†] anomaly (page 83).

Pulmonary Stenosis (in adults)

General signs: peripheral cyanosis, due to a low cardiac output, but only in severe cases.

The pulse: normal or reduced if cardiac output is low.

The JVP: giant *a* waves because of right atrial hypertrophy; the JVP may be elevated.

Palpation: right ventricular heave; thrill over the pulmonary area.

---

[*] Doppler echocardiography has shown that trivial tricuspid regurgitation is very common and is then considered physiological.

[†] Wilhelm Ebstein, Professor of Medicine at Göttingen in Germany, who invented and developed palpation.

Auscultation: the murmur may be preceded by an ejection click; a harsh ejection systolic murmur heard best in the pulmonary area and with inspiration is typically present; right ventricular S4 may be present (due to right atrial hypertrophy).

Abdomen: presystolic pulsation of the liver may be present.

Signs of severe pulmonary stenosis: an ejection systolic murmur peaking late in systole; absence of an ejection click (also absent when the pulmonary stenosis is infundibular—i.e., below the valve level); presence of S4; signs of right ventricular failure.

Causes of pulmonary stenosis: (i) congenital; (ii) carcinoid syndrome (rare).

Pulmonary Regurgitation

This is an uncommon pathological condition; trivial pulmonary regurgitation is often found at echocardiography and is considered physiological.

Auscultation: a decrescendo diastolic murmur which is high pitched and audible at the left sternal edge is characteristic—this increases on inspiration (unlike the murmur of aortic regurgitation) and is called the Graham-Steell* murmur; signs of pulmonary hypertension may also be present.

NB: If there are no signs of pulmonary hypertension a decrescendo diastolic murmur at the left sternal edge is more likely to be due to aortic regurgitation than to pulmonary regurgitation.

Causes of pulmonary regurgitation: (i) pulmonary hypertension; (ii) infective endocarditis; (iii) congenital absence of the pulmonary valve.

Prosthetic Heart Valves

The physical signs with common types of valves are presented in Table 3.14.

Cardiomyopathy

Hypertrophic Cardiomyopathy

This is abnormal hypertrophy of the muscle in the left ventricular or right ventricular outflow tract, or both. It can obstruct outflow from the left ventricle late in systole when the hypertrophied area contracts. Systolic displacement of the mitral valve apparatus into the left ventricular outflow tract also occurs causing mitral regurgitation and contributing to the outflow obstruction. Although the outflow tract is narrowed by the hypertrophied septum, the major contribution to the dynamic increase in obstruction comes from the systolic movement of the mitral valve. Variants of hypertrophic cardiomyopathy may involve the mid-ventricle or apex with varying degrees of obstruction.

Symptoms: dyspnoea (increased left ventricular end-diastolic pressure due to abnormal diastolic compliance), angina, syncope or sudden death (secondary to ventricular fibrillation or a sudden increase in outflow obstruction).

The pulse: sharp, rising and jerky. Rapid ejection by the hypertrophied ventricle early in systole is followed by obstruction caused by the displacement of the mitral valve into the outflow tract. This is quite different from the pulse of aortic stenosis.

The JVP: there is usually a prominent *a* wave, due to forceful atrial contraction against a non-compliant right ventricle.

---

* Graham Steell (1851–1942), Birmingham physician, described this murmur in 1888.

Table 3.14 *Prosthetic Heart Valves: Physical Signs*

Type	Mitral	Aortic
Ball valve (e.g., Starr-Edwards)*	Sharp mitral opening sound after S2, sharp closing sound at S1 Systolic ejection murmur, no diastolic murmur	Sharp aortic opening sound after S1, sharp closing sound at S2 Systolic ejection murmur (harsh), no diastolic murmur
Disc valve (e.g., Bjork-Shiley)*	Sharp closing sound at S1, soft systolic ejection murmur and diastolic rumble	Sharp closing sound at S2, soft systolic ejection murmur (diastolic murmur occasionally) (NB an early diastolic murmur indicates AR usually due to a paravalvular leak
Porcine valve†	Diastolic rumble (50%), systolic ejection murmur (soft) (50%), mitral opening sound (50%)	Closing sound usually heard, systolic ejection murmur (soft), no diastolic murmur
Bileaflet valve	—	Aortic valve opening and closing sounds common, soft systolic ejection murmur common

Modified with permission from Smith ND, Raizada V, Abrams J. Auscultation of the normally functioning prosthetic valve. *Ann Intern Med* 1981; 95: 594.
NB: An aortic regurgitation murmur present after aortic valve replacement suggests regurgitation of the valve ring. It is not uncommon. Less often a mitral regurgitation murmur suggests the same problem with a prosthetic mitral valve.
* Severe prosthetic dysfunction causes absence of the opening or closing sounds. Ball and cage valves cause more haemolysis than other types, while disc valves are more thrombogenic.
† Bioprosthetic obstruction or patient–prosthetic mismatch cause diastolic rumbling.

Palpation: double or triple apical impulse, due to presystolic expansion of the ventricle caused by atrial contraction.

Auscultation: late systolic murmur at the lower left sternal edge and apex (due to the obstruction) and a pansystolic murmur at the apex (due to mitral regurgitation); S4.

Dynamic manoeuvres: the outflow murmur is increased by the Valsalva manoeuvre, by standing and by isotonic exercise; it is decreased by squatting and isometric exercise.

Causes of hypertrophic cardiomyopathy: (i) autosomal dominant with variable expressivity; (ii) idiopathic; (iii) Friedreich's* ataxia (page 410).

Dilated Cardiomyopathy

This heart muscle abnormality results in a global reduction in cardiac function. Coronary artery disease is excluded as a cause by definition. The signs are those of congestive cardiac failure including those of mitral and tricuspid regurgitation. The heart sounds themselves may be very quiet. Ventricular arrhythmias are common. It is a common indication for cardiac transplantation.

---

* Nikolaus Friedreich (1825–1882), German physician, described this disease in 1863.

Causes of dilated cardiomyopathy: (i) idiopathic; (ii) alcohol; (iii) post-viral; (iv) postpartum; (v) drugs (e.g., doxorubicin); (vi) connective tissue disease (e.g., systemic lupus erythematosus); (vii) dystrophia myotonica; (viii) haemochromatosis.

Restrictive Cardiomyopathy

This causes similar signs to constrictive pericarditis (page 67), but Kussmaul's sign is more common and the apex beat is usually easily palpable.

Causes of restrictive cardiomyopathy: (i) idiopathic; (ii) eosinophilic endomyocardial disease; (iii) endomyocardial fibrosis; (iv) infiltrative disease (e.g., amyloid); (v) granulomas (e.g., sarcoid).

Aortic Dissection

A tear in the intima leads to blood surging into the aortic media, separating the intima and adventitia; this may present acutely or chronically. There are three different types: *type I* begins in the ascending aorta and extends proximally and distally; *type II* is limited to the ascending aorta and aortic arch (this is particularly associated with Marfan's syndrome); *type III* begins distal to the left subclavian artery and has the best prognosis.

Symptoms: chest pain (typically very severe, maximum in intensity at the time of onset due to either the aortic tear or associated myocardial infarction); stroke; syncope (associated with tamponade); symptoms of LVF; and, rarely, limb pain (ischaemia), paraplegia (spinal cord ischaemia), or abdominal pain (mesenteric ischaemia).

Signs: hypertension, decreased or absent pulses, signs of acute aortic regurgitation or acute cardiac tamponade.

Acyanotic Congenital Heart Disease

Ventricular Septal Defect

In this condition one or more holes are present in the membranous or muscular ventricular septum.

Palpation: hyperkinetic displaced apex if the defect is large; and a thrill at the left sternal edge.

Auscultation (Figure 3.32): a harsh pansystolic murmur maximal at, and almost confined to, the lower left sternal edge with a third or fourth heart sound—the

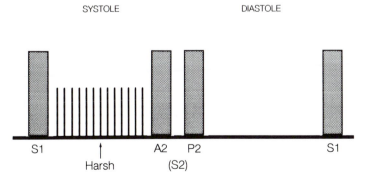

Figure 3.32 *Ventricular septal defect (VSD) (at the left sternal edge).*

murmur is louder on expiration; sometimes a mitral regurgitation murmur is associated. The murmur is often louder and harsher when the defect is small.

Causes of ventricular septal defect: (i) congenital; (ii) acquired—e.g., myocardial infarction involving the septum.

Atrial Septal Defect

There are two main types: *ostium secundum* (90%), where there is a defect in the part of the septum which does not involve the atrioventricular valves, and *ostium primum*, where the defect does involve the atrioventricular valves.

Palpation: normal or right ventricular enlargement.

Auscultation (Figure 3.33): fixed splitting of S2; the defect produces no murmur directly, but increased flow through the right side of the heart can produce a low pitched diastolic tricuspid flow murmur and more often a pulmonary systolic ejection murmur—these are both louder on inspiration.

The signs of an ostium primum defect are the same as for an ostium secundum defect, but associated mitral regurgitation, tricuspid regurgitation or a ventricular septal defect may be present. The left ventricular impulse is often impalpable.

Patent Ductus Arteriosus

This is a persistent embryonic vessel which connects the pulmonary artery and the aorta. The shunt is from the aorta to the pulmonary artery unless pulmonary hypertension has supervened.

Pulse and blood pressure: a collapsing pulse with a sharp upstroke (due to ejection of a large volume of blood into the empty aorta with systole); low diastolic blood pressure (due to rapid decompression of the aorta).

Palpation: often there is a hyperkinetic apex beat.

Auscultation: if the shunt is of moderate size a single second heart sound is heard, but if the shunt is of significant size reversed splitting of the second heart sound occurs (due to a delayed A2 because of an increased volume load in the left ventricle); a continuous loud 'machinery' murmur maximal at the first left intercostal space is usually present; flow murmurs through the left side of the heart, including a mitral mid-diastolic murmur, may be heard.

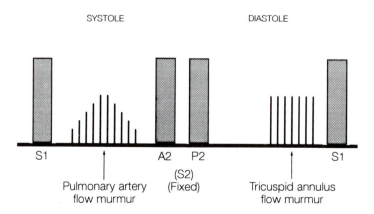

Figure 3.33 *Atrial septal defect (ASD): ostium secundum (at the left sternal edge).*

Table 3.15 *Classification of Congenital Heart Disease*

Acyanotic

With Left to Right Shunt

Ventricular septal defect
Atrial septal defect
Patent ductus arteriosus

With No Shunt

Bicuspid aortic valve, congenital aortic stenosis
Coarctation of aorta
Dextrocardia
Pulmonary stenosis, tricuspid stenosis
Ebstein's anomaly

Cyanotic

Eisenmenger's syndrome (pulmonary hypertension and a right to left shunt)
Tetralogy of Fallot
Ebstein's anomaly (if an atrial septal defect and right to left shunt are also present)
Truncus arteriosus
Transposition of the great vessels
Tricuspid atresia
Total anomalous pulmonary venous drainage

Coarctation of the Aorta

This is congenital narrowing of the aorta usually just distal to the origin of the left subclavian artery. It is more common in males. The underlying cause is uncertain but seems related to abnormal placement of tissue involved in the closing of the ductus arteriosus. There is an association with bicuspid aortic valve and Turner's syndrome.

Signs: the upper body may be better developed than the lower; radiofemoral delay is present, and the femoral pulses are weak; hypertension occurs in the arms but not in the legs; a mid-systolic murmur is usually audible over the praecordium and the back, due to blood flow through collateral chest vessels and across the coarct itself.

Ebstein's Anomaly

This is a very rare lesion. The abnormality is a downward displacement of the tricuspid valve apparatus into the right ventricle so that the right atrium becomes very large and consists partly of ventricular muscle, while the right ventricle becomes small. An atrial septal defect is commonly associated. Characteristically, multiple clicks occur due to asynchronous closure of the tricuspid valve. Tricuspid regurgitation is usually present.

Cyanotic Congenital Heart Disease

This is a difficult area. The causes are listed in Table 3.15. The important point to determine is whether or not signs of pulmonary hypertension are present (page 70). Congenital heart disease in which a shunt from the left to the right side of the circulation occurs leads to an increase in pulmonary blood flow. This can cause reactive pulmonary hypertension so that pulmonary pressures eventually exceed systemic pressures. When that happens the systemic to pulmonary (left to right) shunt will reverse. This right to left shunt leads to deoxygenated blood being mixed in the systemic circulation, resulting in cyanosis. This is called Eisenmenger's* syndrome.

Eisenmenger's Syndrome (right to left shunt)

Signs: central cyanosis; clubbing; polycythaemia; signs of pulmonary hypertension.

It may be possible to decide at what level the shunt occurs by listening to the second heart sound (S2). If there is wide fixed splitting this suggests an atrial septal defect. If a single second heart sound is present this suggests truncus arteriosus or a ventricular septal defect. A normal or reversed S2 suggests a patent ductus arteriosus.

Tetralogy of Fallot†

There are four features which are due to a single developmental abnormality: (i) ventricular septal defect (VSD); (ii) right ventricular outflow obstruction, which determines the severity of the condition, and can be at the pulmonary valve or infundibular level; (iii) an aorta which over-rides the VSD and is responsible for the cyanosis; and (iv) right ventricular hypertrophy secondary to outflow obstruction.

Signs: central cyanosis—this occurs without pulmonary hypertension because venous mixing is possible at the ventricular level, where pressures are balanced The aorta over-rides both ventricles and so receives right and left ventricular blood. Clubbing and polycythaemia are usually present. There may be evidence of right ventricular enlargement—a parasternal impulse at the left sternal edge. A systolic thrill caused by pulmonary valve or right ventricular outflow obstruction may be present. There is no overall cardiomegaly. On auscultation the second heart sound is single and there are no signs of pulmonary hypertension; a pulmonary systolic ejection murmur is present.

The Chest X-Ray: A Systematic Approach

Analysis of the chest X-ray is complementary to the patient's physical examination. It provides much information about the heart and lungs.

The interpretation of the chest X-ray is not easy. It requires knowledge of anatomy and pathology, and appreciation of the whole range of normal appearances (Figure 3.34), and knowledge of the likely X-ray changes occurring with pathological processes. One should feel personally responsible for viewing a patient's radiographs.

Most medical students faced with giving their interpretation of a chest X-ray either opt for a 'spot diagnosis' (usually wrong) or raise their eyes to heaven, hoping for divine inspiration. However, a systematic approach is necessary. More is missed by not looking than by not knowing.

---

*   Victor Eisenmenger (1864–1932), German physician.

†   Etienne-Louis Fallot (1850–1911), Professor of Hygiene, Marseilles, described this in 1888.

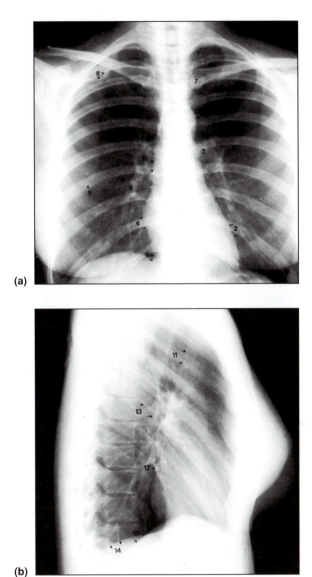

Figure 3.34 *Normal chest X-ray showing, in the posteroanterior view (top): (1) aortic knuckle; (2) left heart border formed by the lateral border of the left ventricle; (3) left hilum formed mostly by the left main pulmonary artery and partly by the left upper pulmonary veins; (4) right heart border formed by the right atrium; (5) inferior angle of the scapula; (6) right basal pulmonary artery; (7) medial aspect of the left clavicle; (8) spine of the scapula; (9) right cardiophrenic angle; (10) superimposition of right lateral margins of the superior vena cava and the ascending aorta. Lateral view (bottom) shows: (11) anterior border of trachea; (12) pulmonary vein, entering left atrium; (13) oblique fissure; (14) left hemidiaphragm; (15) right hemidiaphragm.*

Frontal Film

Name, Date and Projection

First, it is important to check the name and date, to be sure that it is the correct patient's film. Checking the left or right marker prevents missing dextrocardia. The film markings will also indicate the projection and patient position. The standard frontal film is taken by a posteroanterior (PA) projection of an erect patient. Anteroposterior and supine films are only second-best. On a supine film there is distension of all the posterior (gravity-dependent) vessels and thus the lung fields appear more plethoric. A small pleural effusion may not be visible if it is lying posteriorly and the heart often appears large on a supine film.

Centring

The medial ends of the clavicles should be equidistant from the midline spinous processes. If the patient is rotated, this will accentuate the hilum that is turned forward.

Exposure

The quality of the film is important. There should be enough X-ray penetration for the spine to be just seen through the mediastinum, otherwise the film will be too white. With good radiographic technique, the scapulae are projected outside the lung fields.

The film needs to be exposed on full inspiration so that there is no basal crowding of the pulmonary vessels and so that estimation of the cardiothoracic ratio is accurate.

On full inspiration, the diaphragm lies at the level of the tenth or eleventh rib posteriorly or at the level of the sixth costal cartilage anteriorly. The right hemi-diaphragm usually lies about 2cm higher than the left.

Correct Orientation

Do not miss dextrocardia—the heart apex will be to the right and the stomach gas to the left. Do not be misled by left or right markers wrongly placed by a radiographer.

Systematic Film Interpretation

Mediastinum: the trachea should lie in the midline. It may be deviated by a goitre or mediastinal mass. It is normally deviated a little to the left as it passes the aortic knuckle. (The aortic arch becomes wider and unfolded with age because of loss of elasticity.)

The mediastinum, including the trachea, can be deviated by a large pleural effusion, a tension pneumothorax, or pulmonary collapse.

Rotation of the patient may make the mediastinum appear distorted.

Hila: the hila are mostly formed by the pulmonary arteries with the upper lobe veins superimposed. The left hilum is higher than the right. The left has a squarish shape whereas the right has a V shape.

A hilum can be more prominent if the patient is rotated. Lymphadenopathy or a large pulmonary artery will cause hilar enlargement.

Heart: the heart shape is ovoid with the apex pointing to the left. Characteristically, about two-thirds of the heart projects to the left of the spine.

The right heart border is formed by the outer border of the right atrium, and the left heart border by the left ventricle. The left margin of the right ventricle lies about a thumb's breadth in from the left heart border. (On the surface of the heart this is marked by the left anterior descending coronary artery.)

The cardiothoracic diameter is a good way of determining whether the heart is enlarged. If the heart size is more than 50% of the transthoracic diameter, enlargement is present.

Valve calcification, if present, is better seen on the lateral view. On the frontal view, the valve calcification cannot be visualised over the spine.

Diaphragm: the hemidiaphragms visualised on the frontal films are the top of the domes seen tangentially. Much lung in the posterior costophrenic angles is not seen on the frontal film.

If the hemidiaphragms are low and flat, emphysema may be present. A critical look must be made beneath the diaphragm to see if there is free peritoneal gas (Figure 5.23, page 194).

Lung fields: on the frontal field, it is convenient to divide the lung fields into zones. It is easy then to compare one zone with another for density differences and the distribution of the vascular 'markings'.

The apices lie above the level of the clavicles. The upper zones include the apices and pass down to the level of the second costal cartilages. The mid-zones lie between the second and fourth costal cartilage levels. The lower zones lie between the fourth and sixth costal cartilages.

The radiolucency of the lung fields is due to the air filling the lung. The 'greyness' is due to blood in the pulmonary vessels.

The upper zones of the lungs are normally less well perfused, resulting in smaller blood vessels. With raised left atrial pressure, there is upper zone blood diversion and the vessels are congested.

An increase in lung radiolucency occurs with pulmonary vessel loss, as with emphysema. Lung radiolucency is lost with an effusion or consolidation.

Terms such as opacity, consolidation, and patchy shadowing are used to describe the lung fields. It is usually unwise to attempt to make too precise a diagnosis of the underlying pathology.

The lungs are divided into lobes by reflections of the visceral pleura. The right lung is composed of the upper, middle and lower lobes. On the left, there are only the upper and lower lobes.

The right upper lobe has three segments: anterior, posterior and apical. The right middle lobe has a lateral and medial segment. Apical, medial basal, lateral basal, anterior basal and posterior basal segments compose the lower lobe.

There are three differences in the segmental anatomy of the left lung (Figure 4.10, page 127). The left upper lobe has four segments: an apicoposterior, anterior, and two lingular segments. The superior and inferior lingular segments are the equivalent of the right middle lobe. The left lower lobe has four segments: it does not contain a medial basal segment.

The fissures are seen as hairline shadows. The horizontal fissure is at the level of the right fourth costal cartilage. The oblique fissures are not seen on the frontal view.

Bones and soft tissue: nipple shadows are often seen over the lower zones and are about 5mm in diameter. They can be confused with a 'coin' lesion. In such a case, nipple markers may be helpful.

Look carefully for a missing breast shadow in a female patient. A mastectomy may provide a diagnostic clue to explain bony or pulmonary metastases, or upper zone postradiation fibrosis.

Soft tissue gas may accompany a pneumothorax or be present after a thoracotomy.

Calcified tuberculous glands in the neck should be looked for in patients with lung scarring or calcified hilar lymph nodes.

Check that there are no rib fractures or space occupying lesions. Look for rib notching, due to increased blood flow through intercostal vessels (e.g., coarctation of the aorta). Cervical ribs or a thoracic scoliosis should be noted. Erosions or arthritis around the shoulder joints should be looked for.

Review: certain parts of the film should be double-checked if the radiograph appears normal.

The retrocardiac region should be looked at again. A collapsed left lower lobe will reveal itself as a triangular opacity behind the heart shadow.

Both apices should be re-checked for lesions, especially Pancoast tumours or tuberculosis.

Has the patient a pneumothorax? There will be a difference between the translucency of the two lungs.

Lateral Film

The lateral view is used largely for localisation of an already visible lesion on the frontal film. Examine it just as carefully. Sometimes a lesion is seen only on the lateral view. If there is clinical evidence of heart or lung disease, frontal and lateral views should always be obtained.

Points to remember: (i) the retrosternal and retrocardiac triangles are normally of a similar radiodensity; (ii) the thoracic vertebrae become less opaque lower down the spine, unless there is pulmonary or pleural disease; and (iii) the posterior costophrenic angle is sharp unless there is fluid or adjacent consolidation.

The hemidiaphragms are well defined unless there is pleural or pulmonary disease.

The oblique fissure placement is '4 to 4'. It passes from approximately 4cm behind the anterior costophrenic angle, through the hilum to the T4 vertebral body level.

Heart

The right ventricle forms the anterior heart border on the lateral film. The left atrium forms the upper posterior border.

Mitral valve calcification is seen below an imaginary line drawn from the anterior costophrenic angle to the hilum, whereas aortic valve calcification lies above this line.

Examples of Chest X-Rays in Cardiac Disease

The radiological changes seen in pulmonary venous congestion, interstitial pulmonary oedema, and alveolar pulmonary oedema are shown in Figures 3.35 to 3.37, respectively. Mitral valve disease is shown in Figure 3.38, while a ventricular aneurysm is seen in Figure 3.39. The characteristic notching of the inferior aspects of the ribs, due to hypertrophy of the intercostal arteries, appears in Figure 3.40,

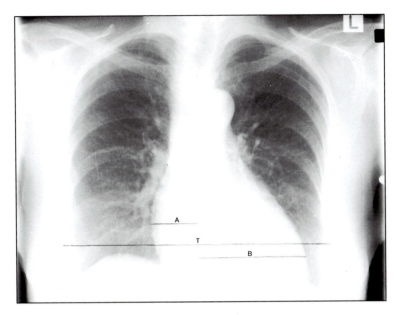

Figure 3.35 *Pulmonary venous congestion. The heart is enlarged due to failure. This failure is not severe enough to cause pulmonary oedema. However, the increased pulmonary venous pressure has caused upper zone blood diversion so the vessels above the hilum appear wider than those below. (The mechanism of the blood diversion is not fully understood.) These changes are seen when the pulmonary venous pressure is about 15 to 20 mmHg.*

The cardiothoracic ratio $\frac{A+B}{T}$ is a useful indicator of cardiac enlargement if it is greater than 50%. The thoracic measurement (T) is the widest diameter above the costophrenic angles, usually at the level of the right hemidiaphragm. The cardiac diameter is the addition of the two widths A and B.

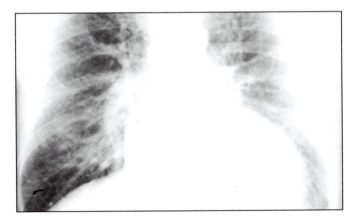

Figure 3.36 *Interstitial pulmonary oedema. The heart is moderately enlarged. The interstitial oedema causes fine diffuse shadowing in the lung fields with blurring of the vessel margins. The escape of fluid into the interstitial tissue occurs when the capillary pressure exceeds the plasma osmotic pressure of 25 mmHg .*

The interstitial oedema is characterised by Kerley 'B' lines which are oedematous interlobular septa. They are best seen peripherally in the right costophrenic angle (arrow), where they lie horizontally, and are about 1cm long. They contain the engorged lymphatics which were originally thought by Kerley to be the sole cause of the 'B' lines.

Sternal sutures are present from previous cardiac surgery.

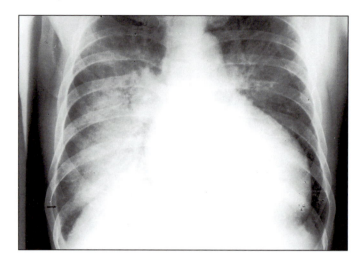

Figure 3.37 *Alveolar pulmonary oedema. When the pulmonary venous pressure reaches 30 mmHg, oedema fluid will pass into the alveoli. This causes shadowing (patchy to confluent depending on the extent) in the lung fields. This usually occurs first around the hila and gives a bat's wing appearance. These changes are usually superimposed on the interstitial oedema.*
     A lamellar pleural effusion (arrow) is seen at the right costophrenic angle where Kerley 'B' lines are also evident.

while the pulmonary plethora which is characteristic of a left to right shunt is obvious in Figure 3.41. A prosthetic aortic valve, which was inserted when a regurgitant valve was replaced in a patient with Marfan's syndrome, is illustrated in Figure 3.42.

Summary

The Cardiovascular Examination: A Suggested Method (Figure 3.43)

Position the patient at 45 degrees and make sure his or her chest and neck are fully exposed. Cover the breasts of a female patient with a towel or loose garment.

Inspect while standing back for the appearance of Marfan's, Turner's or Down's syndromes. Also look for dyspnoea, cyanosis, jaundice and cachexia.

Pick up the patient's hand. Feel the radial pulse. Inspect the hands then for clubbing. Also look for the peripheral stigmata of infective endocarditis: splinter haemorrhages are common (and are also caused by trauma), while Osler's nodes and Janeway lesions are rare. Look quickly, but carefully, at each nail bed, otherwise it is easy to miss these signs. Note any tendon xanthoma (Type II hyperlipidaemia).

The pulse at the wrist should be timed for rate and rhythm. Feel for radiofemoral delay (which occurs in coarctation of the aorta) and radioradial inequality. Pulse character is best assessed at the carotids.

Take the blood pressure.

Next inspect the face. Look at the eyes briefly for jaundice (e.g., valve haemolysis), xanthelasma (Type II or III hyperlipidaemia), or the rare Argyll-

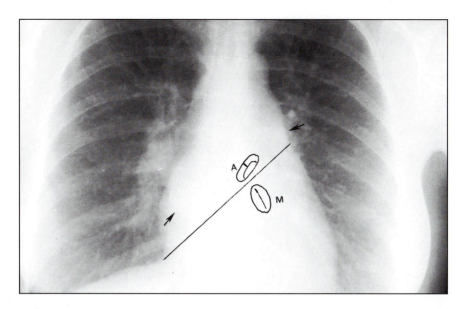

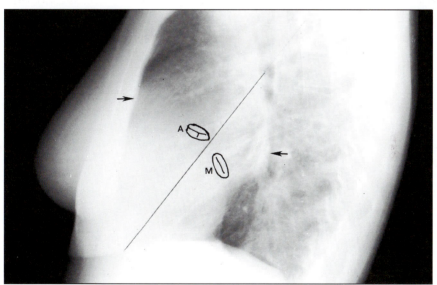

Figure 3.38 *Mitral valve disease. The left atrium enlarges because of the pressure and volume load. It bulges posteriorly and to both sides (arrows). The atrial appendage bulges out below the left hilum. The prominent right border of the atrium causes the 'double right heart border' appearance.*

To distinguish the valves if calcification is present, draw imaginary lines. On the PA view, the line passes from the right cardiophrenic angle to the inferior aspect of the left hilum. The line on the lateral view passes from the anteroinferior angle through the midpoint of the hilum. The aortic valve lies above this line whereas the mitral valve lies below it.

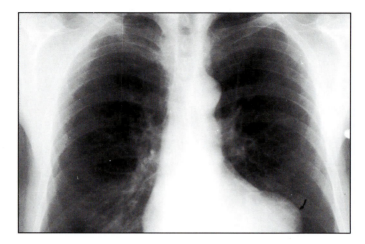

Figure 3.39   *Ventricular aneurysm. There is a bulge of the left cardiac border (arrow) which indicates an aneurysm of the left ventricular wall. The most common cause is weakness following myocardial infarction.*

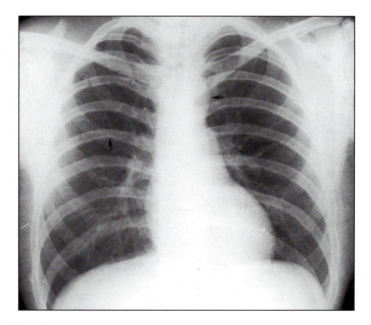

Figure 3.40   *Aortic coarctation. The classical sign in aortic coarctation is notching of the inferior aspects of the ribs. This is due to hypertrophy of the intercostal arteries in which retrograde flow from the axillary collaterals is taking blood back to the descending aorta.*

    Because of the increased resistance to the left heart flow, left ventricular hypertrophy and then failure can occur. Failure causing cardiac enlargement has not yet occurred in this patient.

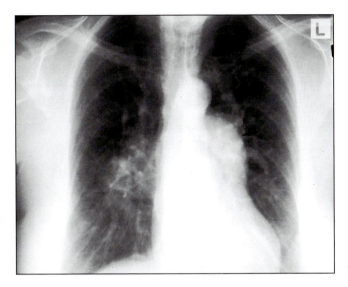

Figure 3.41   *Atrial septal defect (ASD). The most important thing to recognise is that there is pulmonary plethora indicating a left to right shunt. Left to right shunts occur in ASD, ventricular septal defect (VSD), and patent ductus arteriosus (PDA).*

The shunted flow causes enlargement of the main pulmonary artery and its branches. The right hilum is enlarged because of the very dilated right pulmonary artery. The left hilum is hidden by the very dilated main pulmonary artery (arrow).

The ascending aorta is small (in contrast with its enlargement in PDA). The left atrium and ventricle are not enlarged, as they are in VSD and PDA.

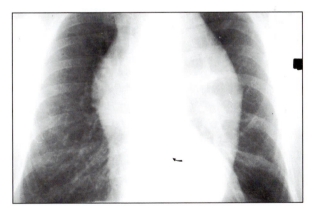

Figure 3.42   *Marfan's syndrome. The mediastinum is widened by uniform dilatation of the ascending aorta, the aortic arch, and the descending aorta. This patient had Marfan's syndrome. Dissecting aneurysms can also occur and have a similar appearance.*

There is a prosthetic aortic valve (arrow) from repair of previous regurgitation. Sternal sutures should be noted as well. No left ventricular enlargement is evident at this stage.

Figure 3.43 *Cardiovascular System*

Lying at 45°

GENERAL INSPECTION
  Marfan's, Turner's, Down's syndrome
  Rheumatological disorders, e.g.,
      ankylosing spondylitis (aortic
      regurgitation)
  Acromegaly, etc.
  Dyspnoea

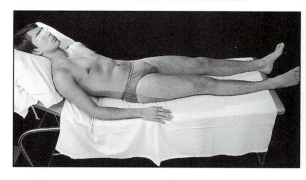

HANDS
  Radial pulses—right and left
  Radiofemoral delay
  Clubbing
  Signs of infective endocarditis—splinter
      haemorrhages, Osler's nodes etc.
  Peripheral cyanosis
  Xanthomata

BLOOD PRESSURE

FACE
  Eyes
    Sclerae—pallor, jaundice
    Pupils—Argyll Robertson (aortic
        regurgitation)
    Xanthelasma
  Malar flush (mitral stenosis, pulmonary
      stenosis)
  Mouth
    Cyanosis
    Palate (high arched—Marfan's)
    Dentition

NECK
  Jugular venous pressure
    Central venous pressure height
    Wave form (especially large v waves)
  Carotids—pulse character

PRAECORDIUM
  Inspect
    Scars—whole chest, back
    Deformity
    Apex beat—position, character
    Abnormal pulsations
  Palpate
    Apex beat—position, character
    Thrills
    Abnormal impulses
  NB: Beware of dextrocardia

AUSCULTATE
  Heart sounds
  Murmurs
  Position patient
    Left lateral position
    Sitting forward (forced expiratory
        apnoea)
  NB: Palpate for thrills again after
      positioning
  Dynamic auscultation
    Respiratory phases
    Valsalva
    Exercise (isometric, e.g., hand grip)
    Standing
    Squatting

BACK (sitting forward)
  Scars, deformity
  Sacral oedema
  Pleural effusion (percuss)
  Left ventricular failure (auscultate)

ABDOMEN (lying flat—1 pillow only)
  Palpate liver (pulsatile etc.), spleen, aorta
  Percuss for ascites (right heart failure)
  Femoral arteries—palpate, auscultate

LEGS
  Peripheral pulses
  Cyanosis, cold limbs, trophic changes,
      ulceration (peripheral vascular
      disease)
  Oedema
  Xanthomata
  Calf tenderness
  Clubbing of toes

OTHER
  Urine analysis (infective endocarditis)
  Fundi (endocarditis)
  Temperature chart (endocarditis)

Robertson pupils (suggesting one should be on guard for aortic regurgitation from syphilis). You may also notice the classical mitral facies. Then inspect the mouth using a torch for a high arched palate (Marfan's syndrome), petechiae and state of dentition (endocarditis). Look at the tongue or lips for central cyanosis and for tongue enlargement (e.g., amyloidosis).

The neck is very important. The jugular venous pressure (JVP) must be assessed for height and character. Use the right internal jugular vein for this. Look for a change with inspiration (Kussmaul's sign).

Now feel each carotid pulse separately (never together!). Assess the pulse character.

Proceed to the praecordium. Always begin by inspecting for scars, deformity, site of the apex beat and visible pulsations. Do not forget about pacemaker boxes. Mitral valvotomy scars (usually under the left breast) can be quite lateral and very easily missed.

Palpate for the position of the apex beat. Count down the correct number of interspaces. The normal position is the fifth left intercostal space, one centimetre medial to the midclavicular line. The character of the apex beat is important. There are a number of types. A *pressure-loaded* (hyperdynamic, systolic over-loaded) apex beat is a forceful and sustained impulse which is not displaced (e.g., aortic stenosis, hypertension). A *volume-loaded* (hyperkinetic, diastolic over-loaded) apex beat is a forceful but unsustained impulse which is displaced down and laterally (e.g., aortic regurgitation, mitral regurgitation). Do not miss the tapping apex beat of mitral stenosis (a palpable first heart sound). The double or triple apical impulse of hypertrophic obstructive cardiomyopathy is very important too. Feel also for an apical thrill, and time it.

Then palpate with the heel of your hand for a left parasternal impulse (which indicates right ventricular enlargement or left atrial enlargement) and for thrills. Now feel at the base of the heart for a palpable pulmonary component of the second heart sound (P2) and aortic thrills. Percussion is usually unnecessary.

Auscultation begins with listening in the mitral area with both the bell and the diaphragm. Listen for each component of the cardiac cycle separately. Identify the first and second heart sounds and decide if they are of normal intensity and whether the second heart sound is normally split. Now listen for extra heart sounds and for murmurs. Do not be satisfied at having identified one abnormality.

Repeat the approach at the left sternal edge and then the base of the heart (aortic and pulmonary areas). Time each part of the cycle with the carotid pulse.

It is now time to reposition the patient. First put him or her in the left lateral position. Again feel the apex beat for character (particularly tapping) and auscultate. Sit the patient up and palpate for thrills (with the patient in full expiration) at the left sternal edge and base. Then listen in those areas, particularly for aortic regurgitation.

Dynamic auscultation should always be done if there is any doubt about the diagnosis. The Valsalva manoeuvre should be performed whenever there is a pure systolic murmur. Hypertrophic cardiomyopathy is easily missed otherwise.

The patient is now sitting up. Percuss the back quickly to exclude a pleural effusion (e.g., due to left ventricular failure), and auscultate for inspiratory crackles (left ventricular failure). If there is a radiofemoral delay, also listen for a coarctation murmur over the back. Feel for sacral oedema and note any back deformity (e.g., ankylosing spondylitis with aortic regurgitation).

Next lie the patient flat and examine the abdomen properly for hepatomegaly (right ventricular failure) and a pulsatile liver (tricuspid regurgitation). Feel for splenomegaly (endocarditis) and an aortic aneurysm. Palpate both femoral arteries and auscultate here for bruits. Go on and examine all the peripheral pulses. Look for signs of peripheral vascular disease, peripheral oedema, clubbing of the toes, Achilles tendon xanthomata and stigmata of infective endocarditis.

Finally, examine the fundi (for hypertensive changes, and Roth's spots in endocarditis) and the urine (haematuria in endocarditis). Take the temperature.

Suggested Reading

Original and Review Articles

Anonymous. Is clubbing a growth disorder? *Lancet* 1990; 336: 848–849.

Brugada P, Gursoy S, Brugada J, Ardries E. Investigation of palpitations *Lancet* 1993; 341: 1254–1258.

Butie A, Clinical examination of varicose veins. *Dermat Surg* 1995; 21: 52–6.

Calkins H, Shyr Y, Frumin H, Schork A, Morady F, The value of the clinical history of the differentiation of syncope due to ventricular tachycardia, atrioventricular block, and neurocardiogenic syncope. *Am J Med* 1995; 98: 365–73.

Evan AT, Sensitivity and specificity of the history and physical examination for coronary artery disease. *Ann Intern Med* 1994; 120: 344–5.

Folland ED, Kriegel BJ, Henderson WG, et al. Implications of third heart sounds in patients with valvular heart disease. The Veterans Affairs Cooperative Study on Valvular Heart Disease. *N Engl J Med* 1992; 327: 458–462.

Harvey WP, Cardiac pearls. *Disease-A-Month* 1994; 40: 41–113.

Heckerling PS, Wiener SL, Wolfkiel CJ, et al. Accuracy and reproducibility of precordial percussion and palpation for detecting increased left ventricular end-diastolic volume and mass. A comparison of physical findings and ultrafast computed tomography of the heart. *JAMA* 1993; 270: 1943–1948.

Hurst JW, Hopkins LC, Smith RB III. Noises in the neck. *N Engl J Med* 1980; 302: 862–863.

O'Keeffe ST, Woods BO, Breslin DJ, Tsapatsaris NP. Blue toe syndrome. Causes and management. *Arch Intern Med* 1992; 152: 2197–2202.

Rothman A, Goldberger AL. Aids to cardiac auscultation. *Ann Intern Med* 1983; 99: 346–353.

Smith ND, Raizada V, Abrams J. Auscultation of the normally functioning prosthetic valve. *Ann Intern Med* 1981; 95: 594–598.

Special Writing Group of the Committee on Rheumatic Fever, Endocarditis and Kawasaki Disease of the Council on Cardiovascular Disease in the Young of the American Heart Association. Guidelines for the diagnosis of rheumatic fever. Jones Criteria, 1992 Update. *JAMA* 1992; 268: 2069–2073.

Timmis AJ. The third heart sound. *BMJ* 1987; 294: 326–327.

Tsapatsaris NP, Napolitana GT, Rothchild J. Osler's maneuver in an outpatient clinic setting. *Arch Intern Med* 1991; 151: 2209–2211.

Tyberg TI, Goodyer AVN, Langou RA. Genesis of pericardial knock in constrictive pericarditis. *Am J Cardiol* 1980; 46: 570–575.

Whitworth JA. The management of hypertension: a consensus statement. *Med J Aust* 1994; 160(Suppl 21 March): S1–S16.

Textbooks

Abrams J. Essentials of cardiac physical diagnosis. Philadelphia: Lea & Febiger, 1987.

Braunwald E, editor. Heart disease. A textbook of cardiovascular medicine. 4th ed. Philadelphia: WB Saunders, 1993.

Julian DG, Cowan JC. Cardiology. 6th ed. London: Baillière Tindall, 1992.

Chapter 4

THE RESPIRATORY SYSTEM AND BREAST EXAMINATION

A medical chest specialist is long-winded about the short-winded.

Kenneth T Bird (b. 1917)

This chapter deals with common respiratory symptoms, and the examination of the respiratory system and the breasts.

The Respiratory History

Presenting Symptoms (Table 4.1)

Cough and Sputum

Cough is a common presenting respiratory symptom. It occurs when deep inspiration is followed by explosive expiration. Flow rates of air in the trachea approach the speed of sound during a forceful cough. Coughing enables the airways to be cleared of secretions and foreign bodies. The duration of a cough is important. A cough of recent origin, particularly if associated with fever and other symptoms of respiratory tract infection, may be due to acute bronchitis or pneumonia. A chronic cough associated with wheezing may be due to asthma; sometimes asthma can present with just cough alone. An irritating chronic dry cough can result from oesophageal reflux and acid irritation of the lungs. A similar cough is not uncommonly associated with the use of the angiotensin-converting enzyme (ACE) inhibitors. These are drugs used in the treatment of hypertension and cardiac failure. A chronic cough which is productive of large volumes of purulent sputum may be due to bronchiectasis. A change in the character of a chronic cough may indicate the development of a new and serious underlying problem (e.g., infection or lung cancer).

The patient's description of his or her cough may be helpful. A cough associated with inflammation of the epiglottis may have a barking quality. Cough caused by tracheal compression by a tumour may be loud and brassy. Cough associated with recurrent laryngeal nerve palsy has a hollow sound because the vocal cords are unable to close completely; this has been described as a bovine cough. A cough that is worse at night is suggestive of asthma or heart failure, while coughing that comes on immediately after eating or drinking may be due to a tracheo-oesophageal fistula or oesophageal reflux.

Table 4.1   *Respiratory History*

Major Symptoms
Cough
Sputum
Haemoptysis
Dyspnoea (acute, progressive or paroxysmal)
Wheeze
Chest pain
Fever
Hoarseness
Night sweats

Table 4.2   *Causes of Haemoptysis*

Respiratory
Bronchitis
Bronchial carcinoma
Pulmonary infarction
Bronchiectasis
Cystic fibrosis
Lung abscess
Pneumonia
Tuberculosis
Foreign body
Goodpasture's* syndrome: pulmonary haemorrhage, glomerulonephritis, antibody to basement membrane antigens
Rupture of a mucosal blood vessel after vigorous coughing
Cardiovascular
Mitral stenosis (severe)
Acute left ventricular failure
Bleeding Diatheses
NB: Exclude spurious causes, such as nasal bleeding or haematemesis.

*   Ernest W Goodpasture (1886–1960), pathologist at Johns Hopkins, Baltimore.

It is an important, though perhaps a somewhat unpleasant task, to inquire about the type of sputum produced. Be warned that some patients have more interest in their sputum than others and may go into more detail than you really want. A large volume of purulent (yellow or green) sputum suggests the diagnosis of bronchiectasis or lobar pneumonia. Foul-smelling dark coloured sputum may indicate the presence of a lung abscess with anaerobic organisms. Pink frothy secretions from the trachea, which occur in pulmonary oedema, should not be confused with sputum. Haemoptysis (coughing up of blood) can be a sinister sign of lung disease (Table 4.2) and must always be investigated. It is best to rely on the patient's assessment of the taste of the sputum which is, not unexpectedly, foul in conditions like bronchiectasis or lung abscess.

Breathlessness (Dyspnoea) (Table 4.3)

The awareness that an abnormal amount of work is required for breathing is called dyspnoea. It can be due to respiratory or cardiac disease (page 28). Careful questioning about the timing of onset, severity and pattern of dyspnoea is helpful in making the diagnosis. The patient may be aware of this only on heavy exertion or have much more limited exercise tolerance. Dyspnoea can be graded from I to IV based on the New York Heart Association classification:

Table 4.3 *Causes of Dyspnoea*

Respiratory	
1. Airways Disease	Chronic bronchitis and emphysema
	Asthma
	Bronchiectasis
	Cystic fibrosis
	Laryngeal or pharyngeal tumour
	Bilateral cord palsy
	Tracheal obstruction or stenosis
	Tracheomalacia
	Crico-arytenoid rheumatoid arthritis
2. Parenchymal Disease	Pneumonia
	Allergic alveolitis
	Sarcoidosis
	Fibrosis and diffuse alveolitis
	Obliterative bronchiolitis
	Diffuse infections
	Respiratory distress syndrome
	Infiltrative and metastatic tumour
	Pneumothorax
	Pneumoconiosis
3. Pulmonary Circulation	Pulmonary embolism
	Chronic thromboembolic pulmonary hypertension
	Pulmonary arteriovenous malformation
	Pulmonary arteritis
4. Chest Wall and Pleura	Effusion or massive ascites
	Pleural tumour
	Fractured ribs
	Ankylosing spondylitis
	Kyphoscoliosis
	Neuromuscular diseases
	Bilateral diaphragmatic paralysis
Cardiac	Left ventricular failure
	Mitral valve disease
	Cardiomyopathy
	Pericardial effusion or constrictive pericarditis
	Intracardiac shunt
Anaemia	
Non-cardiorespiratory	Psychogenic
	Acidosis (compensatory respiratory alkalosis)
	Hypothalamic lesions

- Class I—dyspnoea on heavy exertion
- Class II—dyspnoea on moderate exertion
- Class III—dyspnoea on minimal exertion
- Class IV—dyspnoea at rest

It is more useful, however, to determine the amount of exertion that actually causes dyspnoea, i.e., the distance walked, or the number of steps climbed. The association of dyspnoea with wheeze suggests airways disease, which may be due to asthma or chronic airflow limitation. The duration and variability of the dyspnoea are important. Dyspnoea that worsens progressively over a period of weeks, months or years may be due to pulmonary fibrosis. Dyspnoea of more rapid onset may be due to an acute respiratory infection (including bronchopneumonia or lobar pneumonia) or to pneumonitis (which may be infective or secondary to a hypersensitivity reaction). Dyspnoea that varies from day to day or even from hour to hour suggests a diagnosis of asthma. Dyspnoea on moderate exertion is not uncommonly due to the combination of obesity and a lack of physical fitness.

Wheeze

A number of conditions can cause a continuous whistling noise during breathing. These include asthma or chronic airflow limitation, and airways obstruction by a foreign body or tumour. Wheeze is usually maximal during expiration and is accompanied by prolonged expiration.

Chest Pain

Chest pain due to respiratory disease is usually different from that associated with myocardial ischaemia (page 25). It is characteristically pleuritic in nature, i.e., sharp and made worse by deep inspiration and coughing. It is typically localised to one area of the chest. It may be of sudden onset in patients with lobar pneumonia, pulmonary infarction or pneumothorax and is often associated with dyspnoea.

Other Presenting Symptoms

Patients may occasionally present with episodes of *fever at night*. Tuberculosis, pneumonia and mesothelioma should always be considered in these cases. *Hoarseness* may sometimes be considered a respiratory system symptom. It can be due to transient inflammation of the vocal cords (laryngitis), vocal cord tumour or recurrent laryngeal nerve palsy. Occasionally patients with tuberculosis present with episodes of *drenching sweating* at night.

Sleep apnoea is an abnormal increase in the periodic cessation of breathing during sleep. Patients with *obstructive sleep apnoea* (where airflow stops despite persistent respiratory efforts) typically present with daytime somnolence, chronic fatigue, morning headaches and personality disturbances. Very loud snoring may be reported by anyone within earshot. Patients with *central sleep apnoea* (where there is cessation of inspiratory muscle activity) may also present with somnolence but do not snore excessively (Table 4.4).

Some patients respond to anxiety by increasing the rate and depth of their breathing. This is called hyperventilation. The result is an increase in CO_2 excretion and the development of alkalosis—a rise in the pH of the blood. These patients may complain of variable dyspnoea; they have more difficulty breathing in than out. The alkalosis results in paraesthesiae of the fingers and around the

Table 4.4 *Abnormal Patterns of Breathing*

Type of Breathing	Cause(s)
1. Sleep apnoea—cessation of airflow for more than 10 seconds more than 10 times a night during sleep	Obstructive (e.g., obesity with upper airway narrowing, enlarged tonsils, pharyngeal soft tissue changes in acromegaly or hypothyroidism)
2. Cheyne-Stokes* breathing—periods of apnoea alternate with periods of hyperpnoea. This is due to a delay in the medullary chemoreceptor response to blood gas changes	Left ventricular failure Brain damage (e.g., trauma, cerebral haemorrhage) High altitude
3. Kussmaul's breathing (air hunger)— deep rapid respiration due to stimulation of the respiratory centre	Metabolic acidosis (e.g., diabetes mellitus, chronic renal failure)
4. Hyperventilation, which results in alkalosis and tetany	Anxiety
5. Ataxic (Biot†) breathing—irregular in timing and depth	Brainstem damage
6. Apneustic breathing—a post-inspiratory pause in breathing	Brain (pontine) damage
7. Paradoxical respiration—the abdomen sucks inward with inspiration (it normally pouches outward due to diaphragmatic descent)	Diaphragmatic paralysis

* John Cheyne (1777–1836), Scottish physician who worked in Dublin, described this in 1818. William Stokes (1804–1878), French physician.
† Camille Biot (b. 1878), French physician.

mouth, lightheadedness, chest pain and a feeling of impending collapse. Anxiety can also make patients aware of the need to take an occasional large breath. This is not really dyspnoea, but it can be what patients mean when they complain of shortness of breath.

Past History

One should always ask about previous respiratory illness including pneumonia, tuberculosis or chronic bronchitis, or abnormalities of the chest X-ray which have been previously reported to the patient. Patients with the acquired immuno-deficiency syndrome (AIDS) have a high risk of developing *Pneumocystis carinii* pneumonia and indeed other chest infections including tuberculosis.

Treatment

It is important to find out what drugs the patient is using, how often they are taken and whether they are inhaled or swallowed. The patient's previous and current medications may give a clue to the current diagnosis. Bronchodilators are pre-scribed for chronic airflow limitation, asthma and bronchiectasis. Chronic respira-tory disease including sarcoidosis, hypersensitivity pneumonias and asthma may have been treated with steroids. Steroid use may predispose to tuberculosis. Patients with chronic lung conditions like cystic fibrosis or bronchiectasis will often be very knowledgeable about their treatment and can describe the various forms of physiotherapy that are essential for keeping their airways clear.

Almost every class of drug can produce lung toxicity. Examples include pulmonary embolism from use of the oral contraceptive pill, interstitial lung disease from cytotoxic agents (e.g., methotrexate, cyclophosphamide, bleomycin), bronchospasm from beta-blockers or non-steroidal anti-inflammatory drugs and cough from ACE inhibitors. Some medications known to cause lung disease may not be mentioned by the patient because they are illegal (e.g., cocaine), are used sporadically (e.g., hydrochlorothiazide), can be obtained over the counter (e.g., tryptophan) or are not taken orally (e.g., timolol eye drops). The clinician therefore needs to ask about these types of drug specifically.

Occupational History

In no system are the patient's present and previous occupations of more importance. A detailed occupational history is essential. One must ask about exposure to dusts in mining industries and factories (e.g., asbestos, coal, silica, iron oxide, tin oxide, cotton, beryllium, titanium oxide, silver, nitrogen dioxide, anhydrides). Working or household exposure to animals, including birds, is also relevant (e.g., Q fever or psittacosis). Exposure to mouldy hay, humidifiers or air conditioners may also result in lung disease (e.g., allergic alveolitis). The patient may be unaware that his or her occupation involved exposure to dangerous substances; for example, factories making insulating cables and boards very often used asbestos until 20 years ago. Asbestos exposure can result in the development of asbestosis, mesothelioma or carcinoma of the lung up to 30 years later.

It is most important to find out what the patient actually does when at work, the duration of any exposure, use of protective devices and whether other workers have become ill. An improvement in symptoms over the weekend is a valuable clue to the presence of occupational lung disease, particularly occupational asthma. This can occur as a result of exposure to spray paints or plastic or soldering fumes.

Social History

A smoking history should be routine, as it is the major cause of chronic airflow limitation and lung cancer (Table 1.2). It is necessary to ask how many packets of cigarettes a day a patient has smoked and how many years the patient has smoked. An estimate should be made of the number of packet years of smoking. Remember that this is based on 20-cigarette packets and that packets of cigarettes are getting larger; curiously, most manufacturers now make packets of 30 or 35. More recently giant packets of 50 have appeared. These are too large to fit into pockets and must be carried in the hands as a constant reminder to the patient of his or her addiction. Occupation may further affect cigarette smokers; for example, asbestos workers who smoke are at an especially high risk of lung cancer. Passive smoking is now regarded as a significant risk, and exposure to other people's cigarette smoke at home and at work should be asked about.

Many respiratory conditions are chronic and may interfere with the ability to work. Housing conditions may be inappropriate for a person with a limited exercise tolerance or an infectious disease. An inquiry about the patient's alcohol consumption is important. The drinking of large amounts of alcohol in binges can sometimes result in aspiration pneumonia, and alcoholics are more likely to develop pneumococcal or *Klebsiella* pneumonia. Intravenous drug users are at risk of lung abscess and drug-related pulmonary oedema. Such information may influence the decision about whether to advise treatment at home or in hospital.

Family History

A family history of asthma, cystic fibrosis or emphysema should be sought. $Alpha_1$-antitrypsin deficiency, for example, is an inherited disease, and carriers are extremely susceptible to the development of emphysema. A family history of infection with tuberculosis is also important.

The Respiratory Examination

Positioning the Patient

The patient should be undressed to the waist. If he or she is not acutely ill the examination is easiest to perform with the patient sitting over the edge of the bed or even on a chair.

General Appearance

It is important to look for the following signs before beginning the detailed examination.

Dyspnoea

Watch the patient for signs of dyspnoea at rest (page 28). Count the respiratory rate; the normal rate at rest should not exceed 14 breaths per minute. Tachypnoea refers to a rapid respiratory rate. Look to see whether the accessory muscles of respiration are being used. These muscles include the sternomastoids, the platysma and the strap muscles of the neck. Characteristically the accessory muscles cause elevation of the shoulders with inspiration and aid respiration by increasing chest expansion. In some cases, the pattern of breathing is diagnostically helpful (Table 4.4).

Cyanosis

Look for evidence of cyanosis (page 18). Central cyanosis is best detected by inspecting the tongue. Examination of the tongue differentiates central from peripheral cyanosis. Lung disease severe enough to result in significant ventilation-perfusion imbalance, such as pneumonia, chronic airflow limitation and pulmonary embolism, may cause reduced arterial oxygen saturation and central cyanosis. Cyanosis becomes evident when the absolute concentration of deoxygenated haemoglobin is 5g/100mL of blood. Cyanosis is usually obvious when the arterial oxygen saturation falls below 90% in a person with a normal haemoglobin level. Central cyanosis is therefore a relatively late sign of hypoxaemia. In patients with anaemia cyanosis does not occur until even greater levels of arterial desaturation are reached. The detection of cyanosis is much easier in good lighting conditions and is said to be more difficult if the patient's bed is surrounded by cheerful pink curtains.

Character of the Cough

Coughing is a protective response to irritation of sensory receptors in the submucosa of the upper airways or bronchi. Ask the patient to cough several times. Lack of the usual explosive beginning may indicate vocal cord paralysis (the 'bovine' cough). A muffled, wheezy ineffective cough suggests airflow limitation. A very loose productive cough suggests excessive bronchial secretions due to chronic bronchitis, pneumonia or bronchiectasis. A dry irritating cough may occur with chest infection, asthma or carcinoma of the bronchus and sometimes with left ventricular failure or interstitial lung disease. It is also typical of the cough produced by the ACE inhibitors. These drugs are used commonly in the treatment of hypertension and cardiac failure.

Sputum

Sputum should be inspected. Careful study of the sputum is an essential part of the physical examination. The volume and type (purulent, mucoid or mucopurulent), and the presence or absence of blood, should be recorded.

Stridor

Obstruction of the larynx, trachea or large airways may cause stridor, a rasping or croaking noise loudest on inspiration. This can be due to a foreign body, a tumour, infection (e.g., epiglottitis) or inflammation (Table 4.5). It is a sign that requires urgent attention.

Hoarseness

Listen to the voice for hoarseness, as this may indicate recurrent laryngeal nerve palsy associated with carcinoma of the lung (usually left sided), or laryngeal carcinoma. However, the commonest cause is laryngitis.

The Hands

As usual, examination in detail begins with the hands.

Clubbing

Look for clubbing (Figure 4.1) which is commonly due to respiratory disease (Table 3.3, page 34). An uncommon association with clubbing is hypertrophic

Table 4.5 *Some Causes of Stridor in Adults*

Sudden Onset (minutes)	Anaphylaxis
	Toxic gas inhalation
	Acute epiglottitis
	Inhaled foreign body
Gradual Onset (days, weeks)	Laryngeal and pharyngeal tumours
	Crico-arytenoid rheumatoid arthritis
	Bilateral vocal cord palsy
	Tracheal carcinoma
	Paratracheal compression by lymph nodes
	Post-tracheostomy or intubation granulomata

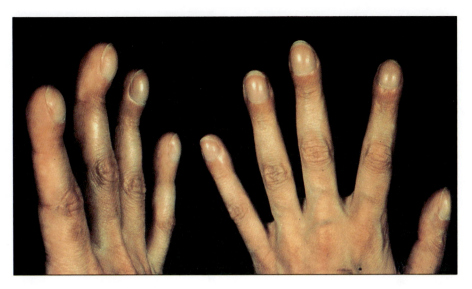

Figure 4.1   *Finger clubbing.*

pulmonary osteoarthropathy (HPO). HPO is characterised by the presence of periosteal inflammation at the distal ends of long bones, the wrists, the ankles, the metacarpal and the metatarsal bones. There is swelling and tenderness over the wrists and other involved areas. Rarely HPO may occur without clubbing. The causes of HPO include primary lung carcinoma and pleural mesothelioma. Remember chronic bronchitis and emphysema do not cause clubbing.

Staining

Look for staining of the fingers (actually caused by tar, as nicotine is colourless), a sign of cigarette smoking. The density of staining does not indicate the number of cigarettes smoked, but depends rather on the way the cigarette is held in the hand.

Wasting and Weakness

Compression and infiltration by a peripheral lung tumour of a lower trunk of the brachial plexus results in wasting of the small muscles of the hand and weakness of finger abduction (page 385).

Pulse Rate

Tachycardia and pulsus paradoxus are important signs of severe asthma (page 122).

Flapping Tremor (Asterixis)

Ask the patient to dorsiflex the wrists with the arms outstretched and to spread out the fingers. A flapping tremor may occur with severe carbon dioxide retention, usually due to severe chronic airflow limitation. However, this is a late and unreliable sign.

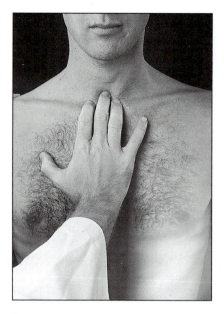 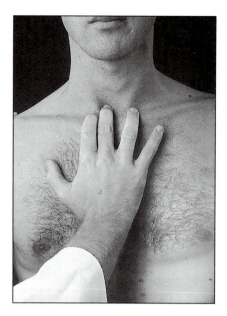

Figure 4.2   *Feeling for the position of the trachea—a similar gap should be palpable on each side.*

The Face

Inspect the *eyes* for evidence of Horner's* syndrome (a constricted pupil, partial ptosis and loss of sweating) which can be due to an apical lung tumour compressing the sympathetic nerves in the neck (page 369).

The *nose* is sited conveniently in the centre of the face. In this position it may readily be inspected inside and out. Look for polyps (associated with asthma), engorged turbinates (various allergic conditions) and a deviated septum (nasal obstruction).

As already discussed, look at the *tongue* for central cyanosis. Look in the *mouth* for evidence of an upper respiratory tract infection (a reddened pharynx and tonsillar enlargement with or without a coating of pus). A broken tooth or a rotten tooth stump may predispose to lung abscess or pneumonia.

Sinusitis is indicated by tenderness over the *sinuses* on palpation. There may be facial plethora or cyanosis if superior vena caval obstruction is present (page 125). Some patients with obstructive sleep apnoea will be obese with a receding chin, a small pharynx and a short thick neck.

The Trachea

The position of the trachea is most important and time should be spent establishing it accurately. From in front of the patient the forefinger of the right hand is pushed up and backwards from the suprasternal notch until the trachea is felt (Figure 4.2). If the trachea is displaced to one side its edge rather than its middle

---

* Johann Horner (1831–1886), Professor of Ophthalmology in Zurich.

Table 4.6 *Causes of Tracheal Displacement*

1. Towards the side of the lung lesion
    Upper lobe collapse
    Upper lobe fibrosis
    Pneumonectomy

2. Away from the side of the lung lesion (uncommon)
    Massive pleural effusion
    Tension pneumothorax

3. Upper mediastinal masses, such as retrosternal goitre

will be felt and a larger space will be present on one side than the other. Slight displacement to the right is fairly common in normal people. This examination is uncomfortable for the patient so one must be gentle.

Significant displacement of the trachea suggests, but is not specific for, disease of the upper lobes of the lung (Table 4.6).

Tracheal tug is demonstrated when the finger resting on the trachea feels it move inferiorly with each inspiration. This is a sign of gross overexpansion of the chest because of airflow obstruction.

The Chest

The chest should be examined anteriorly and posteriorly by inspection, palpation, percussion and auscultation. Compare the right and left sides during each part of the examination.

Inspection

Shape and Symmetry of the Chest

When the anteroposterior (AP) diameter is increased compared with the lateral diameter, the chest is described as barrel-shaped. An increase in the AP diameter indicates hyperinflation and is seen frequently in patients with severe asthma or emphysema. It is not always a reliable guide to the severity of the underlying lung disease.

A **pigeon chest (pectus carinatum)** is a localised prominence (an outward bowing of the sternum and costal cartilages). It may be a manifestation of chronic childhood respiratory illness, in which case it is thought to result from repeated strong contractions of the diaphragm while the thorax is still pliable. It also occurs in rickets (page 317).

A **funnel chest (pectus excavatum)** is a developmental defect involving a localised depression of the lower end of the sternum (Figure 4.3). In severe cases lung capacity may be restricted.

Harrison's* sulcus is a linear depression of the lower ribs just above the costal margins at the site of attachment of the diaphragm. It can result from severe asthma in childhood, or rickets.

Kyphosis refers to an exaggerated forward curvature of the spine, while scoliosis is lateral bowing. **Kyphoscoliosis** may be idiopathic (80%), secondary to poliomy-

---

*   Edward Harrison (1766–1838), British general practitioner, described this deformity in rickets in 1798.

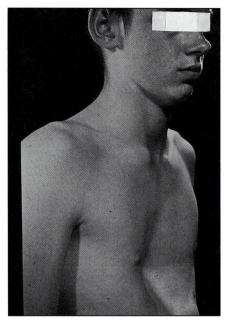

Figure 4.3
Pectus excavatum.

elitis, or associated with Marfan's syndrome. Severe thoracic kyphoscoliosis may reduce the lung capacity and increase the work of breathing.

Lesions of the chest wall may be obvious. Look for *scars* from previous thoracic operations, or from chest drains for a previous pneumothorax or pleural effusion. Thoracoplasty causes severe chest deformity; this operation was performed for tuberculosis and involved removal of a large number of ribs on one side of the chest to achieve permanent collapse of the affected lung. It is no longer performed because of the availability of effective antituberculosis chemotherapy. *Radiotherapy* may cause erythema and thickening of the skin over the irradiated area. There is sharp demarcation between abnormal and normal skin. There may be small tattoo marks indicating the limits of the irradiated area. Signs of radiotherapy usually indicate that the patient has been treated for carcinoma of the lung or, less often, for lymphoma.

Subcutaneous emphysema is a crackling sensation felt on palpating the skin of the chest or neck. On inspection, there is often diffuse swelling of the chest wall and neck. It is caused by air tracking from the lungs and is usually due to a pneumothorax; less commonly it can follow rupture of the oesophagus or a pneumo-mediastinum (air in the mediastinal space).

Prominent veins may be seen in patients with superior vena caval obstruction. It is important to determine the direction of blood flow (page 162).

Movement of the chest wall should be noted. Look for asymmetry of chest wall movement anteriorly and posteriorly. Assessment of expansion of the upper lobes is best achieved by inspection from behind the patient, looking down at the clavicles during moderate respiration (Figure 4.4). Diminished movement indicates underlying lung disease. The affected side will show delayed or decreased movement. For assessment of lower lobe expansion, the chest should be inspected posteriorly.

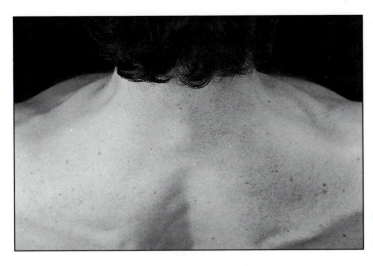

Figure 4.4

Inspecting upper lobe expansion.

Reduced chest wall movement on one side may be due to localised pulmonary fibrosis, consolidation, collapse, pleural effusion or pneumothorax. Bilateral reduction of chest wall movement indicates a diffuse abnormality such as chronic airflow limitation or diffuse pulmonary fibrosis.

Palpation

Chest Expansion

Place the hands firmly on the chest wall with the fingers extending around the sides of the chest. The thumbs should almost meet in the middle line and should be lifted slightly off the chest so that they are free to move with respiration (Figure 4.5). As the patient takes a big breath in, the thumbs should move symmetrically apart at least 5cm. Reduced expansion on one side indicates a lesion on that side. The causes have been discussed above.

Lower lobe expansion is assessed from the back by palpation. Some idea of upper and middle lobe expansion is possible when the manoeuvre is repeated on the front of the chest, but this is better gauged by inspection.

Apex Beat

When the patient is lying down, establishing the position of the apex beat may be helpful (page 49) since displacement towards the side of the lesion can be caused by collapse of the lower lobe or by localised pulmonary fibrosis. Movement of the apex beat away from the side of the lung lesion can be caused by pleural effusion or tension pneumothorax. The apex beat is often impalpable in a chest which is hyperexpanded secondary to chronic airflow limitation.

Vocal Fremitus

Palpate the chest wall with the palm of the hand while the patient repeats 'ninety-nine'. The front and back of the chest are each palpated in two comparable positions with the palm of one hand on each side of the chest. In this way differences in vibration on the chest wall can be detected. This can be a difficult sign to interpret. The causes of change in vocal fremitus are the same as those for vocal resonance (page 115).

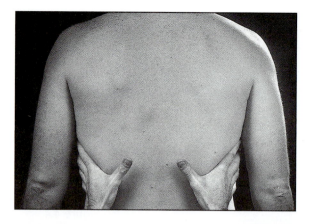

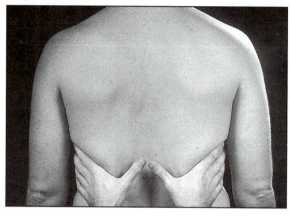

Figure 4.5

Palpation for lower lobe expansion. Inspiration (top) and expiration (bottom).

Ribs

Gently compress the chest wall anteroposteriorly and laterally. Localised pain suggests a rib fracture, which may be secondary to trauma, or may be spontaneous as a result of tumour deposition or bone disease.

Percussion

With the left hand on the chest wall and the fingers slightly separated and aligned with the ribs, the middle finger is pressed firmly against the chest. Then the pad of the right middle finger is used to strike firmly the middle phalanx of the middle finger of the left hand. The percussing finger is quickly removed so that the note generated is not dampened. The percussing finger must be held partly flexed and a loose swinging movement should come from the wrist and not from the forearm. Medical students will soon learn to keep the right middle fingernail short. Percussion of symmetrical areas of the anterior, posterior and axillary regions is necessary (Figure 4.6). Percussion in the supraclavicular fossa over the apex of the lung should not be forgotten. Percuss the clavicle directly with the percussing finger. On percussion posteriorly, the scapulae should be moved out of the way by asking the

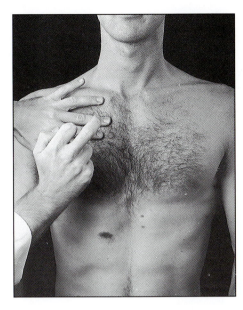

Figure 4.6
Percussion of the chest.

patient to move the elbows forward across the front of the chest; this rotates the scapulae anteriorly.

The feel of the percussion note is as important as its sound. The note is affected by the thickness of the chest wall, as well as by underlying structures. Percussion over a solid structure, such as the liver or a consolidated area of lung, produces a dull note. Percussion over a fluid-filled area, such as a pleural effusion, produces an extremely dull (stony dull) note. Percussion over the normal lung produces a resonant note and percussion over hollow structures, such as the bowel or a pneumothorax, produces a hyperresonant note.

Considerable practice is required before expert percussion can be performed, particularly in front of an audience. The ability to percuss well is usually obvious in clinical examinations and counts strongly in a student's favour, as it indicates a reasonable amount of experience in the wards.

Liver Dullness

The upper level of liver dullness is determined by percussing down the anterior chest in the mid-clavicular line. Normally, the upper level of the liver dullness is the sixth rib in the right mid-clavicular line. If the chest is resonant below this level it is a sign of hyperinflation, usually due to emphysema or asthma.

Cardiac Dullness

An area of cardiac dullness is usually present on the left side of the chest, but this may be decreased in emphysema or asthma.

Auscultation

Breath Sounds

Using the diaphragm of the stethoscope one should listen to the breath sounds in the areas shown in Figure 4.7. It is important to compare each side with the other.

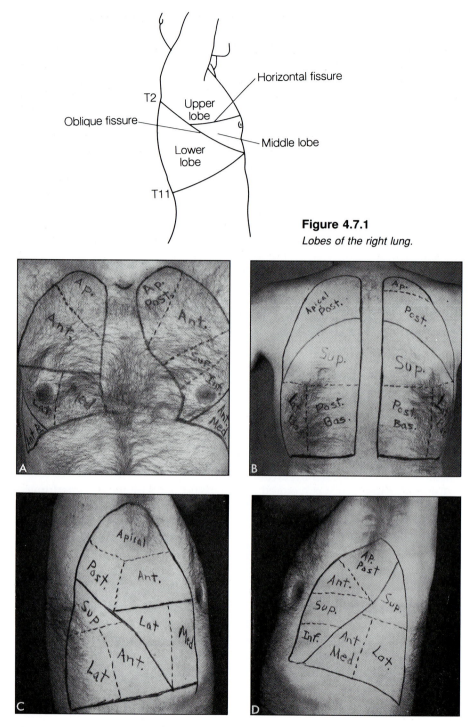

Figure 4.7.1

Lobes of the right lung.

Figure 4.7.2 *Outlines of the lung segments projected on the thoracic wall: (A) anterior view; (B) posterior view; (C) right lateral view; (D) left lateral view. Refer to Figure 4.10, page 127, for a list of the segments in each lobe.*

From Delp MH, Manning RT. Major's physical diagnosis. An introduction to the clinical process. 9th ed. Philadelphia: WB Saunders, 1981, with permission.

Remember to listen high up into the axillae and, using the bell of the stethoscope applied above the clavicles, to listen to the lung apices. A number of observations must be made while auscultating and, as with auscultation of the heart, different parts of the cycle must be considered. Listen for the quality of the breath sounds; the intensity of the breath sounds; and the presence of additional (adventitious) sounds.

Quality of breath sounds: *normal breath sounds* are heard with the stethoscope over all parts of the chest. These sounds are produced in the airways rather than the alveoli. They had once been thought to arise in the alveoli (vesicles) of the lungs and are therefore called vesicular sounds. They have rather fancifully been compared to the sound of wind rustling in leaves. Their intensity is related to total airflow at the mouth and to regional airflow. Normal (vesicular) breath sounds are louder and longer on inspiration than on expiration and there is no gap between the inspiratory and expiratory sounds. They are due to the transmission of air turbulence in the large airways filtered through the normal lung to the chest wall.

Bronchial breath sounds: here turbulence in the large airways is heard without being filtered by the alveoli, producing a different quality. Bronchial breath sounds have a hollow, blowing quality. They are audible throughout expiration and there is often a gap between inspiration and expiration. The expiratory sound has a higher intensity and pitch than the inspiratory sound. Bronchial breath sounds are more easily remembered than described. They are heard over areas of consolidation since solid lung conducts the sound of turbulence in main airways to peripheral areas without filtering. Causes of bronchial breath sounds are shown in Table 4.7.

Occasionally breath sounds over a large cavity have an exaggerated bronchial quality. This very hollow or *amphoric* sound has been likened to that heard when air passes over the top of a hollow jar (Greek *amphoreus*).

Intensity of the breath sounds: it is better to describe breath sounds as being of normal or reduced intensity than to speak about air entry. The entry of air into parts of the lung cannot be directly gauged from the breath sounds.

Causes of reduced breath sounds include chronic airflow limitation (especially emphysema), pleural effusion, pneumothorax, pneumonia, a large neoplasm, and pulmonary collapse.

Added (adventitious) sounds: there are two types of added sounds: continuous (wheezes) and interrupted (crackles).

Continuous sounds are called *wheezes*. They are abnormal findings and have a musical quality. The wheezes must be timed in relation to the respiratory cycle. They may be heard in expiration or inspiration or both. Wheezes are due to

Table 4.7 *Causes of Bronchial Breath Sounds*

NB: The large airways must be patent
Common
Lung consolidation (lobar pneumonia)
Uncommon
Localised pulmonary fibrosis
Pleural effusion (above the fluid)
Collapsed lung (e.g., adjacent to a pleural effusion)

continuous oscillation of opposing airway walls and imply significant airway narrowing. Wheezes tend to be louder on expiration. This is because the airways normally dilate during inspiration and are narrower during expiration. An inspiratory wheeze implies severe airway narrowing.

The pitch (frequency) of wheezes varies. It is determined only by the velocity of the air jet and is not related to the length of the airway. High pitched wheezes are produced in the smaller bronchi and have a whistling quality, whereas low pitched wheezes arise from the larger bronchi.

Wheezes are usually the result of acute or chronic airflow obstruction due to asthma (often high pitched) or chronic airflow limitation (often low pitched). Here a combination of bronchial muscle spasm, mucosal oedema and excessive secretions results in airflow limitation. Wheezes are a poor guide to the severity of airflow obstruction. In severe airways obstruction wheeze can be absent because ventilation is so reduced that the velocity of the air jet is reduced below a critical level necessary to produce the sound.

A fixed bronchial obstruction, usually due to a carcinoma of the lung, tends to cause a localised wheeze which has a single musical note (monophonic) and does not clear with coughing.

Interrupted non-musical sounds are best called *crackles*. There is a lot of confusion about the naming of these sounds, perhaps as a result of mistranslations of Laënnec. Some authors describe low pitched crackles as râles and high pitched ones as crepitations, but others do not make this distinction. The simplest approach is to call all these sounds crackles, but also to describe their timing and pitch.

Crackles are probably the result of loss of stability of peripheral airways which collapse on expiration. With high inspiratory pressures, there is rapid air entry into the distal airways. This causes the abrupt opening of alveoli and of small or medium sized bronchi containing secretions in regions of the lung deflated to residual volume. More compliant (distensible) areas open up first followed by the increasingly stiff areas.

The timing of crackles is of great importance. *Early inspiratory crackles* suggest disease of the small airways, and are characteristic of chronic airflow limitation. The crackles are only heard in early inspiration and are of medium coarseness. They are different from those heard in left ventricular failure, which occur later in the respiratory cycle.

Late or paninspiratory crackles suggest disease confined to the alveoli. They may be fine, medium or coarse in quality. Fine crackles have been likened to the sound of hair rubbed between the fingers or to the sound Velcro makes when being unstrapped—they are typically caused by pulmonary fibrosis. Medium crackles are usually due to left ventricular failure. Here the presence of alveolar fluid disrupts the function of the normally secreted surfactant. Coarse crackles are characteristic of pools of retained secretions and have an unpleasant gurgling quality. They tend to change with coughing, which also has an unpleasant gurgling quality. Bronchiectasis is a common cause, but any disease that leads to retention of secretions may produce these features.

Pleural friction rub: when thickened, roughened pleural surfaces rub together as the lungs expand and contract a continuous or intermittent grating sound may be audible. A pleural rub indicates pleurisy, which may be secondary to pulmonary infarction or pneumonia. Rarely, malignant involvement of the pleura, a spontaneous pneumothorax or pleurodynia may cause a rub.

Vocal Resonance

Auscultation over the chest while a patient speaks gives further information about the lungs' ability to transmit sounds. Over normal lung the low pitched components of speech are heard with a booming quality and high pitched components are attenuated. Consolidated lung, however, tends to transmit high frequencies so that speech heard through the stethoscope takes on a bleating quality (called aegophony: Greek *aix* goat, *phone* voice). When a patient with aegophony says 'e' as in 'bee' it sounds like 'a' as in 'bay'.

Ask the patient to say 'ninety-nine' while you listen over each part of the chest. Over consolidated lung the numbers will become clearly audible while over normal lung the sound is muffled. If vocal resonance is present, bronchial breathing is likely to be heard (Table 4.7). Sometimes vocal resonance is increased to such an extent that whispered speech is distinctly heard; this is called whispering pectoriloquy.

If a very localised abnormality is found at auscultation, try to determine the lobe and approximately which segment or segments are involved (Figure 4.7).

The Heart

Lie the patient at 45 degrees and measure the jugular venous pressure for evidence of right heart failure (page 66). Next examine the praecordium. It is important to pay close attention to the pulmonary component of the second heart sound (P2). This is best heard at the second intercostal space on the left. It should not be louder than the aortic component, best heard at the right second intercostal space. If the P2 is louder, pulmonary hypertension should be strongly suspected. There may be signs of right ventricular failure or hypertension. A right ventricular fourth heart sound is said to be audible in the epigastium in some of these patients. Pulmonary hypertensive heart disease (cor pulmonale) may be due to chronic airflow limitation, pulmonary fibrosis, pulmonary thromboembolism, marked obesity, sleep apnoea or severe kyphoscoliosis.

The Abdomen

Palpate the liver for ptosis* (page 165), due to emphysema, or for enlargement from secondary deposits of tumour in cases of lung carcinoma.

Other

Pemberton's[†] Sign

Ask the patient to lift the arms over the head. Look for the development of facial plethora, inspiratory stridor and non-pulsatile elevation of the jugular venous pressure. This occurs in superior vena caval obstruction (page 125).

Feet

Inspect for swelling (oedema) or cyanosis which may be clues to cor pulmonale, and look for evidence of deep venous thrombosis.

---

*   From the Greek word for falling, this was once mostly applied to the eyelid but now seems accepted as a description of the position of any organ.

[†]   John de Jarnett Pemberton (1887–1968), Mayo Clinic surgeon.

Respiratory Rate on Exercise and Positioning

Patients complaining of dyspnoea should have their respiratory rate measured at rest, at maximal tolerated exertion (e.g., after climbing one or two flights of stairs), and supine. If dyspnoea is not accompanied by tachypnoea when a patient climbs stairs one should consider the possibility of malingering.

Look for paradoxical inward motion of the abdomen during inspiration when the patient is supine (indicating diaphragmatic paralysis).

Temperature

Fever may occur with any acute or chronic chest infection.

Bedside Assessment of Lung Function

Forced Expiratory Time

Physical examination should always include an estimate of the forced expiratory time (FET). Here one measures the time taken by a patient to exhale forcefully and completely through the open mouth after taking a maximum inspiration. The normal forced expiratory time is three seconds or less. Note any audible wheeze or cough. An increased FET indicates airways obstruction. A peak flow meter or spirometer, however, will provide a much more accurate measurement.

Peak Flow Meter

A peak flow meter is a simple gauge which is used to measure the maximum flow rate of expired air. Again the patient is asked to take a full breath in, but rather than a prolonged expiration a rapid forced maximal expiratory puff is made through the mouth. The value obtained (the peak expiratory flow rate (PEFR)) depends largely on airways diameter. Normal values for young men are approximately 600 litres a minute and for women 400 litres a minute. The value depends on age, sex and height, so tables of normal values should be consulted. Airways obstruction, such as that caused by asthma or chronic airflow limitation, results in a reduced and variable PEFR. It is a simple way of assessing and following patients with airways obstruction.

Spirometry (Figure 4.8)

The spirometer records graphically or numerically the forced expiratory volume and the forced vital capacity. The forced expiratory volume (FEV) is the volume of air expelled from the lungs after maximum inspiration using maximum forced effort, and is measured in a given time. Usually this is one second (FEV_1). The forced vital capacity (FVC) is the total volume of air expelled from the lungs after maximum inspiratory effort followed by maximum forced expiration. The FVC is often nearly the same as the vital capacity, but in airways obstruction it may be less because of premature airways closure. It is usual to record the best of three attempts and calculate the FEV_1/FVC ratio as a percentage. In healthy youths, the normal value is 80%, but this may decline to as little as 60% in old age. Normal values also vary with sex and race.

Obstructive Ventilatory Defect

When the FEV_1/FVC ratio is reduced this is referred to as an obstructive defect. Both values tend to be reduced, but the FEV_1 is disproportionately low. The

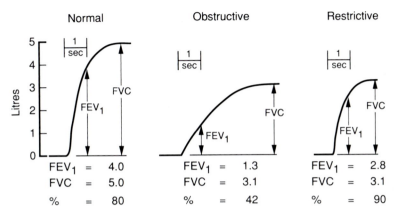

Figure 4.8   *Spirometry tracings.*

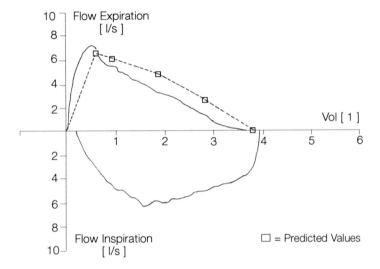

Figure 4.9   *Flow volume curve.*

causes are loss of elastic recoil or airways narrowing, as in asthma or chronic airflow limitation.

Restrictive Ventilatory Defect

When the FEV$_1$/FVC ratio is normal or higher than normal, but both values are reduced, the pattern is described as a restrictive defect. This occurs in parenchymal lung disease, such as pulmonary fibrosis, sarcoidosis, or when lung expansion is reduced by pneumonia or chest wall abnormalities.

Flow Volume Curve

As an alternative to spirometry the flow volume curve may be measured using a portable electronic device. This measures expiratory and inspiratory flow as a function of exhaled volume. It is a simple and reproducible test easily performed in the respiratory laboratory or at the bedside. The FVC, FEV_1 and various flow measurements (e.g., peak flow) can be calculated from the curve (Figure 4.9).

Correlation of Physical Signs and Respiratory Disease
(Table 4.8)

Consolidation (Lobar Pneumonia)

Pneumonia is defined as inflammation of the lung which is characterised by exudation into the alveoli. Pneumonia may be classified on an anatomical basis into lobar, segmental or lobular pneumonia. The signs of lobar pneumonia are characteristic and are referred to clinically as consolidation.

Signs

Expansion: reduced on the affected side.
Vocal fremitus: increased on the affected side (in other chest disease this sign is of very little use!).
Percussion: dull, but not stony dull.
Breath sounds: bronchial.
Additional sounds: medium, late or paninspiratory crackles as the pneumonia resolves.
Vocal resonance: increased.
Pleural rub: may be present.

Causes

Lobar pneumonia: pneumococcal (90% of cases), staphylococcal.
Bronchopneumonia (lobular): bacteria (commonest), viruses such as influenza virus, adenovirus, measles virus, cytomegalovirus. In bronchopneumonia, crackles are often the only chest sign.
Primary atypical pneumonia: *Mycoplasma pneumoniae* (majority), psittacosis, Legionnaires' disease, Q fever, chlamydial pneumonia.

Collapse

If a bronchus is obstructed by a tumour mass, retained secretions or a foreign body, the air in the part of the lung supplied by the bronchus is absorbed and the affected part of the lung collapses.

Signs

Trachea: displaced towards the collapsed side.
Expansion: reduced on the affected side with flattening of the chest wall on the same side.
Percussion: dull over the collapsed area.
Breath sounds: reduced, with or without bronchial breathing above the area of collapse.

N.B. 1. There may be no signs with complete lobar collapse.
    2. The early changes after the inhalation of a foreign body may be over-inflation of the affected side,

Table 4.8 Comparison of the Chest Signs in Common Respiratory Disorders

Disorder	Mediastinal Displacement	Chest Wall Movement	Percussion Note	Breath Sounds	Added Sounds	Vocal Resonance
Consolidation	None	Reduced over affected area	Dull	Bronchial	Crackles	Increased
Collapse	Ipsilateral shift	Decreased over affected area	Dull	Absent or reduced	Absent	Absent
Pleural Effusion	Heart displaced to opposite side (trachea displaced only if massive)	Reduced over affected area	Stony dull	Absent over fluid; may be bronchial at upper border	Absent; pleural rub may be found above effusion	Absent over effusion
Pneumothorax	Tracheal deviation to opposite side if under tension	Decreased over affected area	Resonant	Absent or greatly reduced	Absent	Absent
Bronchial Asthma	None	Decreased symmetrically	Normal or decreased	Normal or reduced	Wheeze	Normal or decreased
Interstitial Pulmonary Fibrosis	None	Decreased symmetrically (minimal)	Normal	Normal	Fine inspiratory crackles over affected lobes unaffected by cough or posture	Normal

Causes

Intraluminal: mucus (e.g., postoperative, asthma, cystic fibrosis), foreign body, aspiration.
Mural: bronchial carcinoma.
Extramural: peribronchial lymphadenopathy, aortic aneurysm.

Pleural Effusion

This is a collection of fluid in the pleural space. Note that pleural collections consisting of blood (haemothorax), chyle (chylothorax) or pus (empyema) have specific names, and are not called pleural effusions, although the physical signs are similar.

Signs

Trachea and apex beat: displaced away from a massive effusion.
Expansion: reduced on the affected side.
Percussion: stony dullness over the fluid.
Breath sounds: reduced or absent. There may be an area of bronchial breathing audible above the effusion due to compression of overlying lung.
Vocal resonance: reduced.

Causes

Transudate (less than 30g of protein per litre of fluid): (i) cardiac failure; (ii) hypoalbuminaemia from the nephrotic syndrome or chronic liver disease; (iii) hypothyroidism; (iv) Meigs'* syndrome (ovarian fibroma causing pleural effusion and ascites).
   Exudate (more than 30g of protein per litre of fluid): (i) pneumonia; (ii) neoplasm—bronchial carcinoma, metastatic carcinoma, mesothelioma; (iii) tuberculosis; (iv) pulmonary infarction; (v) subphrenic abscess; (vi) acute pancreatitis; (vii) connective tissue disease such as rheumatoid arthritis, systemic lupus erythematosus; (viii) drugs, e.g., methysergide, cytotoxics; (ix) irradiation; (x) trauma.
   Haemothorax (blood in the pleural space): (i) severe trauma to the chest; (ii) rupture of a pleural adhesion containing a blood vessel.
   Chylothorax (milky appearing pleural fluid due to leakage of lymph): (i) trauma or surgery to the thoracic duct; (ii) carcinoma or lymphoma involving the thoracic duct.
   Empyema (pus in the pleural space): (i) pneumonia; (ii) lung abscess; (iii) bronchiectasis; (iv) tuberculosis; (v) penetrating chest wound.

Yellow Nail Syndrome

This is a rare condition in which the nails are thickened and yellow and there is separation of the distal nail plate from the nail bed (onycholysis). It may be associated with a pleural effusion and bronchiectasis, and usually with lymphoedema of the legs.

---

* Joe Vincent Meigs (b. 1892), Boston gynaecologist, described this in 1934.

Pneumothorax

Leakage of air from the lung or a chest wall puncture into the pleural space causes a pneumothorax.

Signs

Expansion: reduced on the affected side.
Percussion: hyper-resonance if the pneumothorax is large.
Breath sounds: greatly reduced or absent.
There may be subcutaneous emphysema.
There may be no signs if the pneumothorax is small (less than 30%).

Causes

'**Spontaneous':** (i) subpleural bullae rupture, usually in tall, healthy young males; (ii) emphysema with rupture of bullae, usually in middle-aged or elderly patients with generalised emphysema; (iii) rarely in asthma, lung abscess, bronchial carcinoma, eosinophilic granuloma, end-stage fibrosis or Marfan's syndrome.

  Traumatic: rib fracture, penetrating chest wall injury, or during pleural or pericardial aspiration.

Tension Pneumothorax

This occurs when there is a communication between the lung and the pleural space, with a flap of tissue acting as a valve, allowing air to enter the pleural space during inspiration and preventing it from leaving during expiration. A tension pneumothorax results from air accumulating under increasing pressure in the pleural space; it causes considerable displacement of the mediastinum with obstruction and kinking of the great vessels, and represents a medical emergency.

Signs

The patient is often tachypnoeic and cyanosed, and may be hypotensive.
Trachea and apex beat: displaced away from the affected side.
Expansion: reduced or absent on affected side.
Percussion: hyper-resonant over the affected side.
Breath sounds: absent.
Vocal resonance: absent.

Causes

Trauma.
Mechanical ventilation at high pressure.
Spontaneous (rare cause of tension pneumothorax).

Bronchiectasis

This is a pathological dilatation of the bronchi resulting in impaired clearance of mucus, and chronic infection.

Signs

Systemic signs: fever, cachexia; sinusitis (70%).
Clubbing and cyanosis (if disease is severe).

Sputum: voluminous, purulent, foul smelling, sometimes bloodstained.

NB: History of chronic cough and purulent sputum since childhood is virtually diagnostic.

Coarse pan-inspiratory or late inspiratory crackles over the affected lobe.

Signs of severe bronchiectasis: very copious sputum and haemoptysis, clubbing, widespread crackles, signs of airways obstruction, signs of respiratory failure and cor pulmonale, signs of secondary amyloidosis.

Causes of Bronchiectasis

Congenital: (i) immotile cilia syndrome; (ii) cystic fibrosis; (iii) congenital hypogammaglobulinaemia.

Acquired: (i) infections in childhood, such as whooping cough, pneumonia, or measles; (ii) localised disease such as a foreign body, a bronchial adenoma, or tuberculosis; (iii) allergic bronchopulmonary aspergillosis—this causes proximal bronchiectasis.

Bronchial Asthma

This may be defined as paroxysmal recurrent attacks of wheezing (or in childhood of cough) due to airways narrowing which changes in severity over short periods of time.

Signs

Wheezing.
Tachypnoea.
Tachycardia.
Prolonged expiration.
Prolonged forced expiratory time (decreased peak flow, decreased FEV_1).
Use of accessory muscles of respiration.
Hyperinflated chest (increased anteroposterior diameter with high shoulders and, on percussion, decreased liver dullness).
Inspiratory and expiratory wheezes.

Signs of severe asthma: appearance of exhaustion and fear, inability to speak because of breathlessness, drowsiness due to hypercapnia (preterminal), cyanosis (a very sinister sign), tachycardia (pulse above 130/min correlates with significant hypoxaemia), pulsus paradoxus (more than 20 mmHg), reduced breath sounds or a 'silent' chest.

Chronic Airflow Limitation (Chronic Obstructive Pulmonary Disease)

This represents a spectrum of abnormalities from predominantly emphysema, where there is pathologically an increase beyond normal in the size of the air spaces distal to the terminal bronchioles, to chronic bronchitis, where there is mucous gland hypertrophy, increased numbers of goblet cells and hypersecretion of mucus in the bronchial tree resulting in a chronic cough and sputum. Chronic airflow limitation does not cause clubbing or haemoptysis. Fifty per cent of patients with chronic bronchitis have emphysema, so there is often considerable overlapping of signs.

Signs of Emphysema

The patients are usually not cyanosed but are dyspnoeic and are sometimes called 'pink puffers'. The signs result from hyperinflation.

Barrel-shaped chest with increased anteroposterior diameter.

Pursed lip breathing (this occurs in emphysema and not in chronic bronchitis): expiration through partly closed lips increases the end-expiratory pressure and keeps airways open, helping to minimise air trapping.

Use of accessory muscles of respiration and drawing in of the lower intercostal muscles with inspiration.

Palpation: reduced expansion and a hyperinflated chest.

Percussion: hyper-resonant with decreased liver dullness.

Breath sounds: decreased.

Wheeze is often absent.

Signs of right heart failure may occur, but only late in the course of the disease, when they usually indicate a preterminal state.

Causes of Generalised Emphysema

Emphysema associated with chronic bronchitis and smoking.

Alpha$_1$-antitrypsin deficiency.

Chronic Bronchitis

This is defined as the daily production of sputum for three months a year for at least two consecutive years

Signs of Chronic Bronchitis

The signs are the result of bronchial hypersecretion and airways obstruction.

Loose cough and sputum (mucoid or mucopurulent).

Cyanosis: these patients are sometimes called 'blue bloaters' because of cyanosis present in the latter stages, and because of associated oedema from right ventricular failure.

Palpation: hyperinflated chest with reduced expansion.

Percussion: increased resonance.

Breath sounds: reduced with end-expiratory high or low pitched wheezes and early inspiratory crackles.

Signs of right ventricular failure.

Causes of Chronic Bronchitis

Smoking is the major cause, but recurrent bronchial infection may cause progression of the disease.

Pulmonary Fibrosis

Diffuse fibrosis of the lung parenchyma impairs gas transfer and causes ventilation-perfusion mismatching. It can result from inhalation of mineral dusts (focal fibrosis), replacement of lung tissue following disease which damages the lungs (e.g., tuberculosis) or interstitial disease (e.g., fibrosing alveolitis).

Signs

General: dyspnoea, cyanosis and clubbing may be present.
Palpation: expansion is slightly reduced.
Auscultation: fine (Velcro-like) late-inspiratory or pan-inspiratory crackles heard over the affected lobes.
Signs of associated connective tissue disease: rheumatoid arthritis (page 271), systemic lupus erythematosus (page 277), scleroderma (page 281), Sjögren's* syndrome (page 250), polymyositis and dermatomyositis (page 405).

Causes

Upper lobe: SCHART— S = silicosis (progressive massive fibrosis), sarcoidosis; C = coal workers' pneumoconiosis (progressive massive fibrosis); H = histiocytosis; A = ankylosing spondylitis, allergic bronchopulmonary aspergillosis; R = radiation; T = tuberculosis.
Lower lobe: RASCO— R = rheumatoid arthritis; A = asbestosis; S = scleroderma; C = cryptogenic fibrosing alveolitis; O = other (drugs, e.g., busulphan, bleomycin, nitrofurantoin, hydralazine, methotrexate, amiodarone).

Tuberculosis

Primary Tuberculosis

A Ghon⁺ focus with hilar lymphadenopathy occurs usually in children.

Usually no abnormal chest signs are found, but segmental collapse, due to bronchial obstruction by the hilar lymph nodes, occasionally occurs. Erythema nodosum (page 192) is an important associated sign, but is rare.

Post-primary Tuberculosis

Reactivation of a primary lesion or occasionally reinfection are the causes of post-primary or adult tuberculosis. Immune suppression and malnutrition predispose to reactivation of tuberculosis.

There are often no chest signs. The clues to the diagnosis are the classical symptoms of cough, haemoptysis, weight loss, night sweats and malaise.

Miliary Tuberculosis

Widespread haematogenous dissemination of tubercle bacilli causes multiple millet-seed tuberculous nodules in various organs—spleen, liver, lymph nodes, kidneys, brain, joints. Miliary tuberculosis may complicate both childhood and adult tuberculosis.

Fever, anaemia and cachexia are the general signs. The patient may also be dyspnoeic, and pleural effusions, lymphadenopathy, hepatosplenomegaly or signs of meningitis may be present.

Mediastinal Compression

Mediastinal structures may be compressed by a variety of pathological masses including carcinoma of the lung (90%), other tumours (lymphoma, thymoma, dermoid cyst), a large retrosternal goitre or rarely an aortic aneurysm.

---

*   Henrik Samuel Conrad Sjögren (b. 1899), Stockholm ophthalmologist.
⁺   Anton Ghon (1866–1936), Austrian pathologist.

Signs

Superior vena caval obstruction:* the face is plethoric and cyanosed with periorbital oedema; the eyes may show exophthalmos, conjunctival injection, and venous dilatation in the fundi; in the neck the jugular venous pressure is raised but not pulsatile, the thyroid may be enlarged, there may be supraclavicular lymphadenopathy and a positive Pemberton's sign; the chest may show dilated collateral vessels, or signs of lung carcinoma.

Tracheal compression: stridor, usually accompanied by respiratory distress.

Recurrent laryngeal nerve involvement: hoarseness of the voice.

Horner's syndrome (page 369).

Paralysis of the phrenic nerve: dullness to percussion at the affected base, which does not change with deep inspiration (abnormal tidal percussion), and absent breath sounds suggest a paralysed diaphragm due to phrenic nerve involvement.

Carcinoma of the Lung

Many patients have no signs.

Respiratory Signs

Haemoptysis.
Clubbing, sometimes with hypertrophic pulmonary osteoarthropathy (usually not small cell carcinoma).
Lobar collapse or volume loss.
Pneumonia.
Pleural effusion.
Fixed inspiratory wheeze.
Tender ribs (secondary deposits of tumour in the ribs).
Mediastinal compression including signs of nerve involvement.
Supraclavicular or axillary lymphadenopathy.

Distant Metastases

Brain, liver and bone are the most commonly affected organs.

Non-metastatic Extrapulmonary Manifestations

Anorexia, weight loss, cachexia, fever.

Endocrine changes: (i) hypercalcaemia, due to secretion of parathyroid hormone-like substances, occurs in squamous cell carcinoma; (ii) hyponatraemia—antidiuretic hormone is released by small (oat) cell carcinomas; (iii) ectopic ACTH syndrome (small cell carcinoma); (iv) carcinoid syndrome (small cell carcinoma); (v) gynaecomastia (gonadotrophins); (vi) hypoglycaemia (insulin-like peptide from squamous cell carcinoma).

Neurological manifestations: Eaton-Lambert[†] syndrome (small cell carcinoma); peripheral neuropathy; subacute cerebellar degeneration; polymyositis; cortical degeneration.

Haematological features: migrating venous thrombophlebitis; disseminated intravascular coagulation; anaemia.

---

* First described by William Hunter in a patient with a syphilitic aortic aneurysm.

† M L Eaton, 20th Century American physician, and E H Lambert (b. 1915), American neurologist.

Skin: acanthosis nigricans; dermatomyositis (rare).
Renal: nephrotic syndrome due to membranous glomerulonephritis (rare).

Sarcoidosis

This is a systemic disease, characterised by the presence of non-caseating granulomas which commonly affect the lungs, skin, eyes, lymph nodes, liver and spleen, and nervous system. The aetiology is unknown.

Pulmonary Signs

Lungs: no signs usually, although 80% of patients have lung involvement. In severe disease there may be signs of pulmonary fibrosis.

Extrapulmonary Signs

Skin: lupus pernio (violaceous patches on the face, especially the nose, fingers or toes), pink nodules and plaques (granulomata) in old scars, erythema nodosum on the shins.
Eyes: ciliary injection, anterior uveitis.
Lymph nodes: generalised lymphadenopathy.
Liver and spleen: enlarged (uncommon).
Parotids: gland enlargement (uncommon) (page 156).
Central nervous system: cranial nerve lesions, peripheral neuropathy (uncommon).
Musculoskeletal system: arthralgia, swollen fingers, bone cysts (rare).
Heart: heart block presenting as syncope, cor pulmonale (both rare).
Signs of hypercalcaemia (page 314).

Pulmonary Embolism

Embolism to the lungs often occurs without symptoms. One should always entertain this diagnosis if there has been sudden and unexplained dyspnoea. Pleuritic chest pain and haemoptysis only occur when there is infarction. Syncope or the sudden onset of severe substernal pain can occur with massive embolism.

General signs: tachycardia; tachypnoea; fever (with infarction).

Lungs: pleural friction rub if infarction has occurred.

Massive embolism: elevated jugular venous pressure; right ventricular gallop; right ventricular heave; tricuspid regurgitation murmur; increased pulmonary component of the second heart sound.

Signs of deep venous thrombosis: fewer than 50% of patients have clinical evidence of a source.

NB: A firm diagnosis cannot be made on the symptoms and signs alone.

The Chest X-ray

The radiological appearance of a normal lung, with the lung segments labelled, is shown in Figure 4.10.

The radiological changes of consolidation, pleural effusion, pneumothorax and hydropneumothorax, are shown in Figures 4.11 to 4.14.

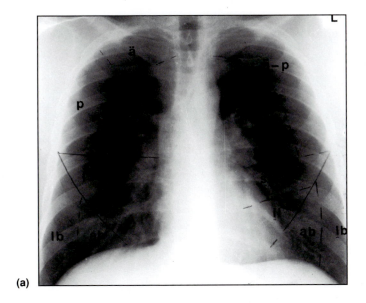

(a)

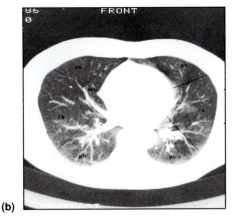

(b)

Figure 4.10 *Lung segments. (a) Postero-anterior view; (b) CT scan through lung bases; (c) left lateral view; (d) right lateral view.*

Right upper lobe: ä = *apical segment; a = anterior segment, p = posterior segment.*
Left upper lobe: ä-p = *apico-posterior segment, s = anterior segment, sl = superior lingular segment, il = inferior lingular segment. **Right middle lobe (rml):** m = medial segment, l = lateral segment. **Right lower lobe:** äl = apical segment, mb = medial basal segment, lb = lateral basal segment, ab = anterior basal segment, pb = posterior basal segment. **Left lower lobe:** äl = apical segment, lb = lateral basal segment, ab = anterior basal segment, pb = posterior basal segment.*

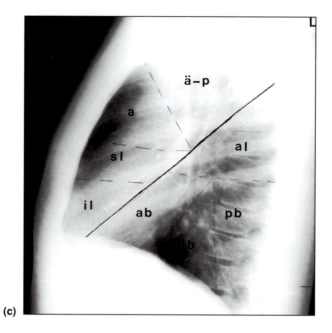

(c)

(d)

Figure 4.10 *Continued*

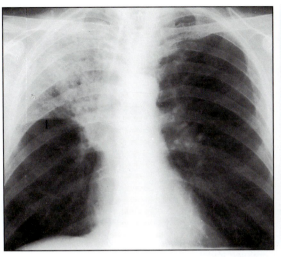
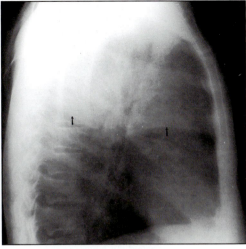

Figure 4.11 *Right upper lobe consolidation. The right upper lobe is opacified and is limited inferiorly by the horizontal fissure (arrow). There must be some collapse as well, as the fissure shows some elevation. These changes could be due to a bacterial lobar pneumonia per se, but a central bronchostenotic lesion should be considered. If the pneumonia persists a bronchoscopy is indicated to search for a central carcinoma.*

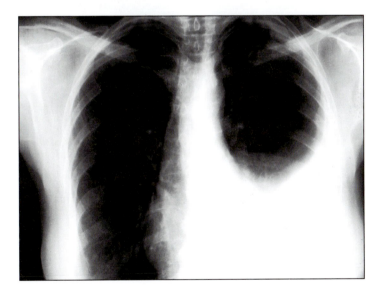

Figure 4.12 *Pleural effusion. The upper margin of the effusion is curved ('meniscus sign'). The left hemidiaphragm is not seen because there is no adjacent aerated lung for contrast.*
The heart shows some deviation to the right. It is unlikely that this is caused by an effusion of this size. It is probably related to the lower thoracic scoliosis.

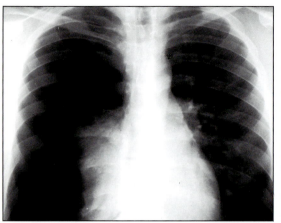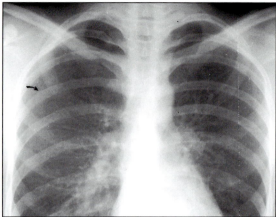

Figure 4.13 *Pneumothorax. (Left) There is a massive right pneumothorax with collapsed lung seen against the hilum (arrow). There is increased translucency because of the absence of vascular shadows. (Right) Different patient with a smaller pneumothorax. Small pneumothoraces are easier to see on an expiratory film as the pneumothorax volume remains constant surrounding the partly deflated lung. The visceral pleural surface is marked (arrow).*

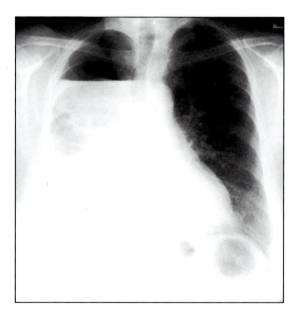

Figure 4.14 *Hydropneumothorax. An air-fluid level is seen in the upper portion of the right hemithorax. When air and fluid are present in the pleural space, the fluid no longer forms a meniscus at its upper margin. Some aerated lung is seen deep to the fluid.*

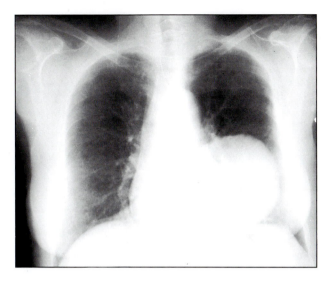

Figure 4.15   *A pulmonary mass. There is a large solitary mass lesion in the left lower zone. The differential diagnosis is primary or secondary neoplasm, hydatid cyst or large abscess. No air-fluid level is seen within it to indicate cavitation.*

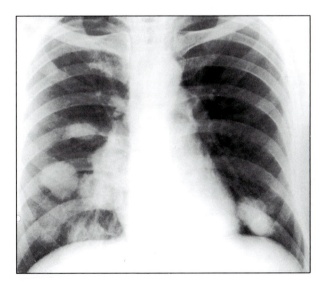

Figure 4.16   *Pulmonary metastases. Multiple rounded opacities are seen in both lung fields, mainly at the left base and around the right hilum.*
   The most likely cause is multiple pulmonary metastases. Other rare possibilities are hydatid cysts, large sarcoid nodules, or large rheumatoid nodules. Multiple abscesses are extremely unlikely in the absence of cavitation.

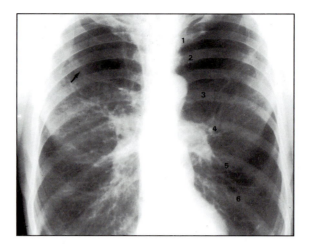

Figure 4.17   *Emphysema. The lungs are overinflated with low, flat hemidiaphragms. The level of the hemidiaphragms is well below the anterior aspects of the sixth ribs. The diaphragm normally projects over the sixth rib anteriorly and the tenth intercostal space posteriorly. Count the ribs anteriorly (1–6).*

There is increased translucency of both upper zones with loss of the vascular markings due to bulla formation (arrow). This increased translucency is not due to overexposure.

The hila are prominent because of the enlarged central pulmonary arteries. In contrast, the smaller peripheral pulmonary arteries (the lung markings) are decreased in size and number. This is due to actual destruction, displacement around bullae, and decreased perfusion through emphysematous areas.

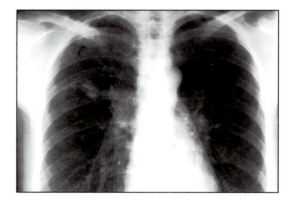

Figure 4.18   *Primary tuberculosis. Two small rounded areas of shadowing are seen in the right upper zone (black arrows).*

The right hilum is enlarged by the enlarged draining lymph nodes (open arrow). This combination of focal shadowing and enlarged lymph nodes is the primary (Ghon) complex of tuberculosis. With healing, calcification may occur in the parenchymal and nodal lesions.

In contrast, in tuberculosis reactivation or reinfection, cavitation may occur and there is no lymphadenopathy.

A pulmonary mass is obvious in Figure 4.15, while multiple metastases are seen in Figure 4.16. Figure 4.17 illustrates the features of emphysema, and primary tuberculosis is shown in Figure 4.18.

Chest X-Ray Checklist

A—airway (midline, no obvious deformities, no paratracheal masses).

B—bones and soft tissue (no fractures, subcutaneous emphysema).

C—cardiac size, silhouette, and retrocardiac density normal.

D—diaphragms (right above left by 1cm to 3cm, costophrenic angles sharp, diaphragmatic contrast with lung sharp).

E—equal volume (count ribs, look for mediastinal shift).

F—fine detail (pleura and lung parenchyma).

G—gastric bubble (above the air bubble one shouldn't see an opacity of any more than 0.5cm width).

H—hilum (left normally above right by up to 3cm, no larger than a thumb), hardware (in the intensive care unit: endotracheal tube, central venous catheters).

Examination of the Breasts

Breast examination is a vitally important part of the general physical examination.

Inspection

Ask the patient to sit up with her chest fully exposed. Look at the *nipples* for retraction (due to cancer or fibrosis; in some patients retraction may be normal) and Paget's disease of the nipple (where underlying breast cancer causes a unilateral red, bleeding area).

Next inspect the rest of the *skin*. Look for visible veins (which if unilateral suggest a cancer), skin dimpling, and for peau d'orange skin (where advanced breast cancer causes oedematous skin pitted by the sweat glands).

Ask the patient to *raise her arms above her head* and then lower them slowly. Look for tethering of the nipples or skin, a shift in the relative position of the nipples or a fixed mass distorting the breast (Figure 4.19). Also note if there are any masses in the axillae. Next ask her to rest her hands on her hips and then press her hands against her hips (the pectoral contraction manoeuvre). This accentuates areas of dimpling or fixation.

Palpation

Examine both the supraclavicular and axillary regions for lymphadenopathy (page 227). Then ask the patient to lie down. It can be helpful to have the patient place her hand behind her head. Palpation is performed gently with the palmar surface of the middle three fingers parallel to the contour of the breast. Feel the four quadrants of each breast systematically. Start at the areola and roll the fingers over the breast tissue pressing towards the chest wall. Examine in a concentric circular pattern moving away from the nipple (Figure 4.20). Then ask her to rest both arms above her head. Feel the axillary tail of the breast between your thumb and fingers.

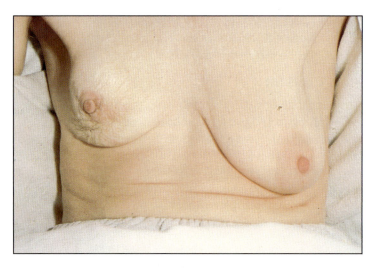

Figure 4.19 *Carcinoma of the right breast showing elevation of the breast, dimpling of skin, and retraction of the nipple.*

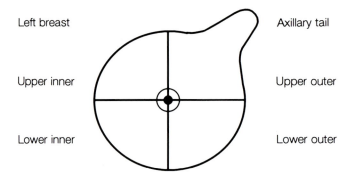

Figure 4.20 *Quadrants of the breast.*

Next feel behind the nipple for lumps and note if any fluid can be expressed: bright blood (from a duct papilloma, fibroadenosis or carcinoma), yellow serous (fibroadenosis) or serous fluid (early pregnancy), milky (lactation) or green fluid (mammary duct ectasia).

Evaluation of a Breast Lump

The following points need to be carefully elucidated if a lump is detected.

1. Position—the breast quadrant involved and proximity to the nipple.
2. Size, shape and consistency—a hard, irregular nodule is characteristic of carcinoma.
3. Tenderness—suggests an inflammatory or cystic lesion; breast cancer is usually not tender.

Table 4.9 *Causes of a Breast Lump*

Non-tender	Tender
Carcinoma	Breast abscess
Fibroadenosis (chronic mastitis)	Fibroadenosis
Fibroadenoma (benign highly mobile 'breast mouse')	Costal cartilage chondritis
Uncommon causes	Inflammatory breast cancer
Trauma, fat necrosis	
Other cysts—e.g., galactocele	
Other neoplasms—e.g., duct papilloma	
Chest wall—e.g., lipoma, costal cartilage, chondritis	
(Tietze's* disease)	

*   Alexander Tietze (1864–1927), German surgeon.

4. Fixation—mobility is determined by taking the breast between the hands and moving it over the chest wall; in advanced carcinoma the lump may be fixed to the chest wall.

5. Single or multiple lesions present—multiple nodules suggest benign cystic disease or fibroadenosis.

Causes of a lump in the breast are listed in Table 4.9. Causes of breast enlargement in males are presented on page 319. In men with true gynaecomastia a disc of breast tissue can be palpated under the areola. This is not present in men who are merely obese.

Summary

The Respiratory Examination: A Suggested Method (Figure 4.21)

Undress the patient to the waist and sit him or her over the side of the bed. While standing back to make your usual inspection, ask if sputum is available for inspection. Purulent sputum always indicates respiratory infection, and a large volume of purulent sputum is an important clue to bronchiectasis. Haemoptysis is also an important sign. Look for dyspnoea at rest and count the respiratory rate. Note any paradoxical inward motion of the abdomen during inspiration (diaphragmatic paralysis). Look for use of the accessory muscles of respiration, and any intercostal indrawing of the lower ribs anteriorly (an important sign of emphysema). General cachexia should also be noted.

Pick up the hands. Look for clubbing, peripheral cyanosis, nicotine staining and anaemia. Note any wasting of the small muscles of the hands and weakness of finger abduction (lung cancer involving the brachial plexus). Palpate the wrists for tenderness (hypertrophic pulmonary osteoarthropathy). While holding the hand, palpate the radial pulse for obvious pulsus paradoxus. Take the blood pressure if indicated.

Go on to the face. Look closely at the eyes for constriction of the pupils and ptosis (Horner's syndrome from an apical lung cancer). Inspect the tongue for central cyanosis.

Palpate the position of the trachea. This is a most important sign, so spend time on it. If the trachea is displaced, you must concentrate on the upper lobes for physical signs. Also note the presence of a tracheal tug, which indicates severe airflow obstruction. Now ask the patient to speak (hoarseness) and then cough and note whether this is a loose cough, a dry cough, or a bovine cough. Next measure the forced expiratory time (FET). Tell the patient to take a maximal inspiration and blow out as rapidly and forcefully as possible while you listen. Note audible wheeze and prolongation of the time beyond three seconds as evidence of chronic airflow limitation.

Figure 4.21 *Respiratory System*

Sitting Up

1. GENERAL INSPECTION
    Sputum mug contents (blood, pus, etc.)
    Type of cough
    Rate and depth of respiration, and breathing pattern at rest
    Accessory muscles of respiration

2. HANDS
    Clubbing
    Cyanosis (peripheral)
    Nicotine staining
    Wasting, weakness—finger abduction and adduction (lung cancer involving the brachial plexus)
    Wrist tenderness (hypertrophic pulmonary osteoarthropathy)
    Pulse (tachycardia; pulsus paradoxus)
    Flapping tremor (CO_2 narcosis)

3. FACE
    Eyes—Horner's syndrome (apical lung cancer), anaemia
    Mouth—central cyanosis
    Voice—hoarseness (recurrent laryngeal nerve palsy)

4. TRACHEA

5. CHEST POSTERIORLY
    Inspect
       Shape of chest and spine
       Scars
       Prominent veins (determine direction of flow)
    Palpate
       Cervical lymph nodes
       Expansion
       Vocal fremitus

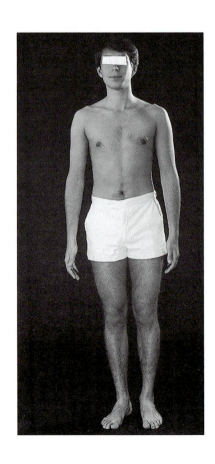

Percuss
 Supraclavicular region
 Back
 Axillae
 Tidal percussion (diaphragm
  paralysis)
Auscultate
 Breath sounds
 Adventitious sounds
 Vocal resonance

6. CHEST ANTERIORLY

 Inspect
  Radiotherapy marks, other signs as
   noted above
 Palpate
  Supraclavicular nodes
  Expansion
  Vocal fremitus
  Apex beat
 Percuss
 Auscultate
 Pemberton's sign (superior vena cava
  obstruction)

7. CARDIOVASCULAR SYSTEM

 (Lying at 45°)
  Jugular venous pressure
   (SVC obstruction, etc.)
  Cor pulmonale

8. FORCED EXPIRATORY TIME

9. OTHER
  Lower limbs—oedema, cyanosis
  Breasts
  Temperature chart (infection)
  Evidence of malignancy or pleural
   effusion: examine the breasts,
   abdomen, rectum, lymph nodes,
   etc.
  Respiratory rate after exercise

The next step is to examine the chest. You may wish to examine the front first, or go to the back to start. The advantage of the latter is that there are often more signs there, unless the trachea is obviously displaced.

Inspect the back. Look for kyphoscoliosis. Do not miss ankylosing spondylitis, which causes decreased chest expansion and upper lobe fibrosis. Look for thoracotomy scars and prominent veins. Also note any skin changes from radiotherapy.

Palpate first from behind for the cervical nodes. Then examine for expansion—first upper lobe expansion, which is best seen by looking over the patient's shoulders at clavicular movement during moderate respiration. The affected side will show a delay or decreased movement. Then examine lower lobe expansion by palpation. Note asymmetry and reduction of movement.

Now ask the patient to bring his or her elbows together in the front to move the scapulae out of the way. Examine for vocal fremitus, then percuss the back of the chest.

Auscultate the chest. Note breath sounds (whether normal or bronchial) and their intensity (normal or reduced). Listen for adventitious sounds (crackles and wheezes). Finally examine for vocal resonance. If a localised abnormality is found, try to determine the abnormal lobe and segment.

Return to the front of the chest. Inspect again for chest deformity, distended veins, radiotherapy changes and scars. Palpate the supraclavicular nodes carefully. Then proceed with percussion and auscultation as before. Listen high up in the axillae too. Before leaving the chest feel the axillary nodes and examine the breasts.

Lie the patient down at 45 degrees and measure the jugular venous pressure. Then examine the praecordium and lower limbs for signs of cor pulmonale. Finally examine the liver and take the temperature.

Suggested Reading

Original and Review Articles

Anonymous, Obtaining an exposure history. Agency for Toxic Substances and Disease Registry. United States Department of Health and Human Services, Public Health Service, Atlanta, Georgia. *Am Fam Phys* 1993; 48: 483–91.

Bassett AA. Technique of clinical screening for breast cancer. *N Engl J Med* 1982; 307: 826–827.

Forgacs P. The functional basis of pulmonary sounds. *Chest* 1978; 73: 399–405.

Hansen-Flaschen J, Nordberg J. Clubbing and hypertrophic osteoarthropathy. *Clin Chest Med* 1987; 8: 287–298.

Kramane SS. Lung sounds for the clinician. *Arch Intern Med* 1986; 146: 1411–1412.

Mannino DM, Etzel RA, Flanders WD, Do the medical history and physical examination predict low lung function? *Arch Intern Med* 1993; 153: 1892–7.

Schapira RM, Schapira MM, Funahashi A, McAuliffe TL, Varkey B. The value of the forced expiratory time in the physical diagnosis of obstructive airways disease. *JAMA* 1993; 270: 731–736.

Schmitt BP, Kushner MS, Wiener SL. The diagnostic usefulness of the history of the patient with dyspnea. *J Gen Intern Med* 1986; 1: 386–393.

Textbooks

Brewis RAL. Lecture notes on respiratory disease. 4th ed. Oxford: Blackwell, 1991.

Campbell IA, Schonell M. Respiratory medicine. 2nd ed. Edinburgh: Churchill Livingstone, 1984.

Fraser RS, Pare JAP, Pare PD, Genereux GP. Diagnosis of diseases of the chest. Philadelphia: WB Saunders, 1990.

James DG, Studdy PR. Color atlas of respiratory diseases. 2nd ed. Chicago: Mosby-Year Book, 1993.

Lillington GA. A diagnostic approach to chest diseases: differential diagnoses based on roentgenographic patterns. 3rd ed. Baltimore: Williams & Wilkins, 1987.

Seaton A, Seaton D, Leitch AG. Crofton and Douglas's respiratory diseases. 4th ed. Oxford: Blackwell, 1989.

Chapter 5

THE GASTROINTESTINAL SYSTEM

To study the phenomena of disease without books is to sail an uncharted sea, while to study books without patients is not to go to sea at all.

Sir William Osler (1849–1919)

Gastroenterologists and gastrointestinal surgeons concern themselves with the entire length of the gut, the liver, the exocrine pancreas and the peripheral effects of alimentary disease.

The Gastrointestinal History

Presenting Symptoms (Table 5.1)

Abdominal Pain

There are many causes of abdominal pain and careful history taking will often lead to the correct diagnosis. The following should be considered.

Frequency and Duration

Try to determine whether the pain is acute or chronic, when it began and how often it occurs.

Site and Radiation

The site of pain is important. Ask the patient to point to the area affected by pain and the point of maximum intensity. Parietal peritoneal inflammation which causes pain usually does so in a localised area. Ask about radiation of pain. Pain often radiates through to the back with pancreatic disease or a penetrating peptic ulcer. It may radiate to the shoulder with diaphragmatic irritation or to the neck with oesophageal reflux.

Character and Pattern

The pain may be colicky (which comes and goes in waves and is related to peristaltic movements) or steady. Colicky pain comes from obstruction of the bowel or the ureters. If the pain is chronic one should ask about the daily pattern of pain.

139

Table 5.1   *Gastrointestinal History*

Major Symptoms
Abdominal pain
Appetite and/or weight change
Nausea and/or vomiting
Heartburn and/or acid regurgitation
Waterbrash
Dysphagia
Disturbed defaecation (diarrhoea, constipation, faecal incontinence)
Bleeding (haematemesis, melaena, rectal bleeding)
Jaundice
Dark urine, pale stools
Abdominal swelling
Pruritus
Lethargy
Fever

Aggravating and Relieving Factors

Pain due to peptic ulceration may or may not be related to meals. Eating may precipitate ischaemic pain in the gut. Antacids or vomiting may relieve peptic ulcer pain or that of gastro-oesophageal reflux. Defaecation or passage of flatus may relieve the pain of colonic disease temporarily. Patients who get some relief by rolling around vigorously are more likely to have a colicky pain, while those who lie perfectly still are more likely to have peritonitis.

Patterns of Pain

Peptic Ulcer Disease

This is classically a dull or burning pain in the epigastrium that is relieved by food or antacids. It is typically episodic and may occur at night, waking the patient from sleep. This combination of symptoms is suggestive of the diagnosis. It is often unrelated to meals, despite classical teaching to the contrary. It is not possible to distinguish duodenal ulceration from gastric ulceration clinically.

Pancreatic Pain

This is a steady epigastric pain which may be partly relieved by sitting up and leaning forward. There is often radiation of the pain to the back, and vomiting is common.

Biliary Pain

Although usually called 'biliary colic' this is rarely colicky. With cystic duct obstruction there is often epigastric pain. It is usually a severe constant pain that can last for hours. There may be a history of episodes of similar pain in the past. If cholecystitis develops, the pain typically shifts to the right upper quadrant and becomes more severe.

Renal Colic

This is a colicky pain superimposed on a background of constant pain in the renal angle, often with radiation towards the groin. It can be very severe indeed.

Bowel Obstruction

This is colicky pain. Periumbilical pain suggests a small bowel origin but colonic pain can occur anywhere in the abdomen. Small bowel obstruction tends to cause more frequent colicky pain (with a cycle every 2 to 3 minutes) than large bowel obstruction (every 10 to 15 minutes). Obstruction is often associated with vomiting, constipation and abdominal distension.

Appetite or Weight Change

Loss of appetite (anorexia) and weight loss are important gastrointestinal symptoms. The presence of both anorexia and weight loss should make one suspicious of an underlying malignancy, but may also occur with depression and in other diseases (page 292). The combination of weight loss with an increased appetite suggests malabsorption of nutrients or a hypermetabolic state (e.g., thyrotoxicosis). It is important to document when the symptoms began and how much weight loss has occurred over this period. Liver disease can sometimes cause disturbance of taste. This may cause smokers with acute hepatitis and jaundice to give up smoking.

Nausea and Vomiting

Nausea is the sensation of wanting to vomit. Heaving and retching may occur but there is no expulsion of gastric contents. There are many possible causes for these complaints. Gastrointestinal tract infections (e.g., from food poisoning by *Staphylococcus aureus*) or small bowel obstruction can cause acute symptoms. In patients with chronic symptoms, pregnancy and drugs (e.g., digoxin, opiates, dopamine agonists, chemotherapy) should always be ruled out. In the gastrointestinal tract, peptic ulcer disease with gastric outlet obstruction, motor disorders (e.g., gastroparesis from diabetes mellitus, or after gastric surgery), acute hepatobiliary disease and alcoholism are important causes. Finally, psychogenic vomiting, eating disorders (e.g., bulimia) and, rarely, increased intracranial pressure should be considered in patients with chronic unexplained nausea and vomiting.

The timing of the vomiting can be helpful; vomiting delayed more than one hour after the meal is typical of gastric outlet obstruction or gastroparesis, while early morning vomiting before eating is characteristic of pregnancy, alcoholism and raised intracranial pressure. Also ask about the contents of the vomitus (e.g., bile indicates an open connection between the duodenum and stomach, old food suggests gastric outlet obstruction, while blood suggests ulceration).

Heartburn and Acid Regurgitation

Heartburn refers to the presence of a burning pain or discomfort in the retrosternal area. Typically, this sensation travels up towards the throat and occurs after meals or is aggravated by bending, stooping or lying supine. Antacids relieve the pain at least transiently. This symptom is due to regurgitation of stomach contents into the oesophagus. Usually these contents are acidic, although occasionally alkaline reflux can induce similar problems. Associated with gastro-oesophageal reflux may be *acid regurgitation* where the patient experiences a sour or bitter tasting fluid coming up into the mouth. This symptom strongly suggests that reflux is occurring. In patients with gastro-oesophageal reflux disease, the lower oesophageal sphincter muscle relaxes inappropriately. Reflux symptoms may be aggravated by alcohol, chocolate, caffeine, a fatty meal, theophylline, calcium channel blockers and anticholinergic drugs as these lower the oesophageal sphincter pressure.

Waterbrash refers to excessive secretion of saliva into the mouth and should not be confused with regurgitation; it may occur, uncommonly, in patients with peptic ulcer disease or oesophagitis.

Dysphagia

Dysphagia is difficulty swallowing. Such difficulty may occur with solids or liquids. The causes of dysphagia are listed in Table 5.2. If a patient complains of difficulty swallowing, it is important to differentiate painful swallowing from actual difficulty. Painful swallowing is termed 'odynophagia' and occurs with any severe inflammatory process involving the oesophagus. Causes include infectious oesophagitis (e.g., Candida, herpes simplex), peptic ulceration of the oesophagus, caustic damage to the oesophagus or oesophageal perforation.

If the patient complains of difficulty initiating swallowing or complains of fluid regurgitating into the nose or choking on trying to swallow, this suggests that the cause of the dysphagia is in the pharynx (pharyngeal dysphagia). Causes of pharyngeal dysphagia can include neurological disease (e.g., motor neurone disease, resulting in bulbar or pseudobulbar palsy) (page 366).

If the patient complains of food sticking in the oesophagus, it is important to consider a number of anatomical causes of oesophageal blockage. If there is a mechanical obstruction at the lower end of the oesophagus most often the patient will localise the dysphagia to the lower retrosternal area. However, obstruction higher in the oesophagus may be felt anywhere in the retrosternal area. If heartburn is also present, for example, this suggests that gastro-oesophageal reflux with

Table 5.2   *Causes of Dysphagia*

Mechanical Obstruction
Intrinsic (within oesophagus)
Reflux oesophagitis with stricture formation
Carcinoma of oesophagus or gastric cardia
Pharyngeal or oesophageal web
Pharyngeal pouch
Schatzki (lower oesophageal) ring
Foreign body
Extrinsic (outside oesophagus)
Goitre with retrosternal extension
Mediastinal tumours, bronchial carcinoma, vascular compression (rare)
Neuromuscular Motility Disorders
More common
Achalasia
Diffuse oesophageal spasm
Scleroderma
Less common
Neurological disorders: bulbar or pseudobulbar palsy, myasthenia gravis, polymyositis, myotonic dystrophy

stricture formation may be the cause of the dysphagia. The actual course of the dysphagia is also a very important part of the history to obtain. If the patient states that the dysphagia is intermittent or is present only with the first few swallows of food, this suggests either a lower oesophageal ring or oesophageal spasm. However, if the patient complains of progressive difficulty swallowing, this suggests a stricture, carcinoma or achalasia. If the patient states that both solids and liquids stick, then a motor disorder of the oesophagus is more likely, such as achalasia or diffuse oesophageal spasm.

Diarrhoea

The symptom diarrhoea can be defined in a number of different ways. Patients may complain of frequent stools (more than three per day being abnormal) or they may complain of a change in the consistency of the stools which have become loose or watery. There are a large number of possible causes of diarrhoea.

Some patients pass small amounts of formed stool more than three times a day because of an increased desire to defaecate. The stools are not loose and stool volume is not increased. This is not true diarrhoea. It can occur because of local rectal pathology, incomplete rectal emptying, or because of a psychological disturbance that leads to an increased interest in defaecation.

When a history of diarrhoea is obtained, it is also important to determine if this has occurred acutely or whether it is a chronic problem. Acute diarrhoea is more likely to be infectious in nature while chronic diarrhoea has a large number of causes.

Clinically, diarrhoea can be divided into a number of different groups based on the likely disturbance of physiology.

1. *Secretory diarrhoea* is likely if the diarrhoea is of high volume (commonly more than one litre per day) and persists when the patient fasts; there is no pus or blood, and the stools are not excessively fatty. Secretory diarrhoea occurs when net secretion in the colon or small bowel exceeds absorption; some of the causes include infections (e.g., *E. coli, Staphylococcus aureus, Vibrio cholerae*), hormonal (e.g., vasoactive intestinal polypeptide secreting tumour, Zollinger–Ellison* syndrome, carcinoid syndrome), and villous adenoma.

2. *Osmotic diarrhoea* is characterised by its disappearance with fasting and by large volume stools related to the ingestion of food. Osmotic diarrhoea occurs due to excessive solute drag; causes include lactose intolerance (disaccharidase deficiency), magnesium antacids or after gastric surgery.

3. *Abnormal intestinal motility* (e.g., thyrotoxicosis, the irritable bowel syndrome) can also cause diarrhoea.

4. *Exudative diarrhoea* occurs when there is inflammation in the colon. Typically the stools are of small volume but frequent, and there may be associated blood or mucus (e.g., inflammatory bowel disease, colon cancer).

5. *Malabsorption* of nutrients can result in steatorrhoea. Here the stools are fatty, pale coloured, extremely smelly, float in the toilet bowel and are difficult to flush away. Steatorrhoea is defined as the presence of more than 7 g of fat in a 24 hour stool collection. There are many causes of steatorrhoea (page 190).

---

*   Robert Milton Zollinger (b. 1903), American surgeon and Edwin H. Ellison (b. 1918), American physician. This syndrome is characterised by gastric acid hypersecretion, peptic ulceration and in 40% of cases diarrhoea due to a gastrinoma (gastrin secreting tumour).

Constipation

It is important to determine what patients mean if they say they are constipated. Constipation is a common symptom and can refer to the passage of infrequent stools (fewer than three times per week), hard stools or stools that are difficult to evacuate. This symptom may occur acutely or may be a chronic problem. In many patients chronic constipation arises because of habitual neglect of the impulse to defaecate leading to the accumulation of large, dry faecal masses. With constant rectal distension from faeces, the patient may grow less aware of rectal fullness leading to chronic constipation. Constipation may arise from ingestion of drugs (e.g., codeine, antidepressants and aluminium or calcium antacids), and with various metabolic or endocrine diseases (e.g., hypothyroidism, hypercalcaemia, diabetes mellitus, phaeochromocytoma, porphyria, hypokalaemia) and neurological disorders (e.g., aganglionosis, Hirschsprung's* disease, autonomic neuropathy, spinal cord injury, multiple sclerosis). Constipation can also arise after partial colonic obstruction from carcinoma; it is, therefore, very important to determine if there has been a recent change in bowel habit, as this may indicate development of a malignancy. Patients with very severe constipation in the absence of structural disease may be found to have slow colonic transit on a transit study; such slow-transit constipation is most common in young women.

Difficulty with evacuation of faeces may occur with disorders of the pelvic floor muscles or nerves, or anorectal disease (e.g., fissure, or stricture). Patients with this problem may complain of straining, a feeling of anal blockage or even the need to self-digitate.

A chronic but erratic disturbance in defaecation (typically alternating constipation and diarrhoea) associated with abdominal pain, in the absence of any structural or biochemical abnormality, is very common; such patients are classified as having the *irritable bowel syndrome*. Patients who report two or more of the following (abdominal pain relieved by defaecation, looser or more frequent stools with the onset of abdominal pain, passage of mucus per rectum, a feeling of incomplete emptying of the rectum following defaecation and visible abdominal distension) are more likely to have the irritable bowel syndrome than organic disease.

Mucus

The passage of mucus may occur because of a solitary rectal ulcer, fistula or villous adenoma, or in the irritable bowel syndrome.

Bleeding (Table 5.3)

Patients may present with the problem of haematemesis (vomiting blood), melaena (passage of jet black stools) or haematochezia (passage of bright red blood per rectum). Sometimes patients may present because routine testing for occult blood in the stools is positive (page 181). It is important to ensure that if vomiting of blood is reported this is not the result of bleeding from a tooth socket or the nose, or coughing up of blood. Haematemesis indicates that the site of the bleeding is proximal to or at the duodenum. Ask about symptoms of

---

* Harold Hirschsprung (1830–1916), physician, Queen Louise Hospital for Children, Copenhagen, described this disease in 1888.

Table 5.3   *Causes of Acute Gastrointestinal Bleeding*

Upper Gastrointestinal Tract

More Common

1. Chronic peptic ulcer: duodenal ulcer (40%), gastric ulcer (20%)
2. Acute peptic ulcer (erosions) (30%)

Less Common (10%)

3. Mallory-Weiss* syndrome (tear at the gastro-oesophageal junction)
4. Oesophageal and/or gastric varices
5. Erosive or ulcerative oesophagitis
6. Gastric carcinoma, polyp, other tumours
7. Dieulafoy's† ulcer (single defect that involves an ectatic submucosal artery)
8. Watermelon stomach (antral vascular ectasias)
9. Aortoenteric fistula (usually aorto-duodenal and after aortic surgery)
10. Vascular anomalies—angiodysplasia, arteriovenous malformations, blue rubber bleb naevus syndrome, hereditary haemorrhagic telangiectasia, CRST syndrome
11. Pseudoxanthoma elasticum, Ehlers-Danlos‡ syndrome
12. Amyloidosis
13. Vasculitis
14. Ménétrièr's§ disease
15. Bleeding diathesis
16. Pseudohaematemesis (nasopharyngeal origin)

Lower Gastrointestinal Tract

More Common

1. Angiodysplasia
2. Diverticular disease
3. Colonic carcinoma or polyp
4. Haemorrhoids or anal fissure

Less Common

5. Massive upper gastrointestinal bleeding
6. Inflammatory bowel disease
7. Ischaemic colitis
8. Meckel's diverticulum
9. Small bowel disease, e.g., tumour, diverticula, intussusception
10. Haemobilia (bleeding from the gallbladder)
11. Solitary colonic ulcer

---

* George Kenneth Mallory (b. 1926), Professor of Pathology and Medicine, and Soma Weiss (b. 1899), Professor of Medicine, Boston City Hospital.
† Georges Dieulafoy (b. 1839), Paris physician.
‡ Edvard Ehlers (1863–1937), German dermatologist, described the syndrome in 1901, and Henri Alexandre Danlos (1844–1912), French dermatologist, described the syndrome in 1908.
§ Pierre Ménétrièr (b. 1859), French physician.
′ Johann Friedrich Meckel (1781–1833), Professor of Surgery and anatomy at Halle.
CRST = Calcinosis, Raynaud's phenomenon, sclerodactyly and telangiectasia.

peptic ulceration; haematemesis is commonly due to bleeding chronic peptic ulceration, particularly duodenal ulcer. Acute peptic ulcers often bleed without abdominal pain. A Mallory-Weiss tear occurs with repeated vomiting; typically the patient reports first the vomiting of clear gastric contents and then the vomiting of blood. Less common causes of upper gastrointestinal bleeding are presented in Table 5.3.

Haemorrhoids and local anorectal diseases such as fissures will commonly present with passing small amounts of bright red blood per rectum. The blood is normally not mixed in the stools but is on the toilet paper, on top of the stools or in the toilet bowl. Melaena usually results from bleeding from the upper gastrointestinal tract, although right-sided colonic and small bowel lesions can occasionally be responsible. Massive rectal bleeding can occur from the distal colon or rectum, or from a major bleeding site higher in the gastrointestinal tract. With substantial lower gastrointestinal tract bleeding, it is important to consider the presence of angiodysplasia or diverticular disease (where bleeding more often occurs from the right rather than the left colon even though diverticula are more common in the left colon). Less common causes of lower gastrointestinal bleeding are presented in Table 5.3.

Spontaneous bleeding into the skin, or from the nose or mouth can be a problem for patients with coagulopathy resulting from liver disease.

Jaundice

Usually the relatives notice a yellow discoloration of the sclera or skin before the patient does. Jaundice is due to the presence of excess bilirubin being deposited in the sclera and skin. The causes of jaundice are described on page 185. If there is jaundice, ask about the colour of the urine and stools; pale stools and dark urine occur with obstructive or cholestatic jaundice because urobilinogen is unable to reach the intestine. Also ask about abdominal pain; gallstones, for example, can cause biliary pain and jaundice.

Pruritus

This symptom means itching of the skin and may be either generalised or localised. Cholestatic liver disease can cause pruritus which tends to be worse over the extremities. Other causes of pruritus are discussed on page 445.

Abdominal Swelling

Persistent swelling can be due to ascitic fluid accumulation; this is discussed on page 160. It may be associated with ankle oedema.

Lethargy

Tiredness and easy fatiguability are common symptoms for patients with acute or chronic liver disease, but the mechanism is not known. This can also occur because of anaemia due to gastrointestinal or chronic inflammatory disease.

Past History

Surgical procedures can result in jaundice from the anaesthesia (e.g., multiple uses of halothane), hypoxaemia of liver cells (hypotension during the operative or postoperative period), or direct damage to the bile duct during abdominal surgery. A history of relapsing and remitting epigastric pain in a patient who presents with severe abdominal pain may indicate that a peptic ulcer has perforated. A past history of inflammatory bowel disease (either ulcerative colitis or Crohn's disease) is important as these are chronic diseases that tend to flare up.

The treatment history is very important. Non-steroidal anti-inflammatory drugs including aspirin can induce bleeding from acute or chronic damage to the gastrointestinal tract. As described above, many drugs can result in disturbed defaecation. A large number of drugs are also known to affect the liver. For example, acute hepatitis can occur with halothane, phenytoin or chlorothiazide. Cholestasis may occur from a hypersensitivity reaction to chlorpromazine or other phenothiazines, sulphonamides, sulphonylureas, phenylbutazone, rifampicin or nitrofurantoin. Anabolic steroids and the contraceptive pill can cause dose-related cholestasis. Fatty liver can occur with alcohol use, tetracycline, valproic acid or amiodarone. Large blood-filled cavities in the liver called peliosis hepatis can occur with anabolic steroid use or the contraceptive pill. Acute liver cell necrosis can occur if an overdose of paracetamol (acetaminophen) is taken.

Social History

The patient's occupation may be relevant (e.g., health care workers may be exposed to hepatitis). Toxin exposure can also be important in chronic liver disease (e.g., carbon tetrachloride, vinyl chloride). Ask about recent travel to countries where hepatitis is endemic if a patient has symptoms suggestive of liver disease.

The alcohol history is very important, particularly as alcoholics often deny or understate the amount they consume (Table 1.3). Contact with any persons who have been jaundiced should always be noted. The sexual history should be obtained. A history of any injections (e.g., intravenous drugs, plasma transfusions, dental treatment or tattooing) in a patient who presents with symptoms of liver disease is important, particularly as hepatitis B or C may be transferred in this way.

Family History

A family history of bowel cancer or inflammatory bowel disease is important. A positive family history of jaundice, anaemia, splenectomy or cholecystectomy may occur in patients with haemolytic anaemia or congenital or familial hyperbilirubinaemia.

The Gastrointestinal Examination

Examination of the gastrointestinal system includes a complete examination of the abdomen. It is also important to search for the peripheral signs of gastrointestinal and liver disease.

Positioning the Patient

For the proper examination of the abdomen it is important that the patient be lying flat with the head resting on a single pillow (Figure 5.1). This relaxes the abdominal muscles and facilitates abdominal palpation. Helping the patient into this position affords the opportunity to make a general inspection.

General Appearance

Jaundice

The yellow discoloration of the sclerae and the skin that results from hyperbilirubinaemia is best observed in natural daylight (page 184). Whatever the underlying cause, the depth of jaundice can be quite variable.

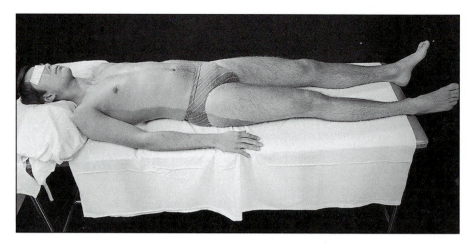

Figure 5.1 *Gastrointestinal examination: positioning the patient.*

Weight and Wasting

The patient's weight must be recorded. Failure of the gastrointestinal tract to absorb food normally may lead to loss of weight and cachexia. This may also be the result of gastrointestinal malignancy or alcoholic cirrhosis. Folds of loose skin may be visible hanging from the abdomen and limbs. These suggest recent weight loss. Obesity can cause fatty infiltration of the liver (non-alcoholic steatohepatitis) and result in abnormal liver function. Anabolic steroid use can induce increase in muscle bulk (sometimes considered desirable) and various liver tumours including adenomas or hepatocellular carcinomas (less desirable).

Skin

The gastrointestinal tract and the skin have a common origin from the embryoblast. A number of diseases can present with both skin and gut involvement (Table 5.4).

Pigmentation

Generalised skin pigmentation can result from chronic liver disease, especially in haemochromatosis (due to haemosiderin stimulating melanocytes to produce melanin). Malabsorption may result in Addisonian type pigmentation ('sunkissed' pigmentation) of the nipples, palmar creases, pressure areas and mouth (page 312).

Peutz-Jeghers* Syndrome

Freckle-like spots (discrete, brown-black lesions) around the mouth and on the buccal mucosa (Figure 5.2), and on the fingers and toes, are associated with hamartomas of the small bowel (50%) and colon (30%) which can present with

---

*   John Peutz (1886–1957), physician at St John's Hospital, The Hague, Holland, first described this condition in 1921. Harold Jeghers (b. 1904), Professor of Medicine, Boston City Hospital, USA.

Table 5.4 *The Skin and the Gut*

Disease	Skin	Gut	Other Associations
Gastrointestinal polyposis syndromes			
Peutz-Jeghers syndrome (autosomal dominant)	Pigmented macules on hands, feet, lips	Hamartomatous polyps (rarely adenocarcinoma) stomach, small bowel, large bowel	
Gardener's* syndrome (autosomal dominant)	Cysts, fibromas, lipomas (multiple)	Polyps, adenocarcinoma large bowel	Bone osteomas
Cronkhite-Canada syndrome	Alopecia, hyperpigmentation, glossitis, dystrophic nails	Hamartomatous polyps, diarrhoea, exocrine pancreatic insufficiency	
Hormone secreting tumours			
Carcinoid synodrome	Flushing, telangiectases	Watery diarrhoea, hepatomegaly	Wheeze, right heart murmurs
Systemic mastocytosis (due to mast cell proliferation and histamine release)	Telangiectases, flushing, pigmented papules, pruritus, dermographism, Darier's† sign (rub skin lesion with the blunt end of a pen: a palpable red wheal occurs minutes later)	Peptic ulcer, diarrhoea, malabsorption	Asthma, headache, tachycardia
Glucagonoma (glucagon secreting tumour)	Migratory necrolytic rash (on flexural and friction areas)	Glossitis, weight loss, diabetes mellitus	
Vascular disorders			
Hereditary haemorrhagic telangiectasia (autosomal dominant)	Telangiectases (especially nail beds, palms, feet)	Gastrointestinal bleeding	Nasopharyngeal bleeding, pulmonary arteriovenous fistulas, high output cardiac failure
Pseudoxanthoma elasticum (autosomal recessive)	Yellow plaques/papules in flexural areas	Bowel bleeding, ischaemia	Angioid streaks in fundus
Blue rubber bleb syndrome	Hemangiomas (e.g., tongue)	Bleeding into bowel or liver	

Table 5.4 *The Skin and the Gut (continued)*

Disease	Skin	Gut	Other Associations
Degos' disease (malignant atrophic papulosis)	Dome-shaped red papules (early), small procelain white atrophic scars (late)	Intestinal perforation, infarction (primarily in young men—very rare)	
Acanthosis nigricans	Brown to black skin papillomas (usually axillae)	Carcinoma	Acromegaly, diabetes mellitus
Dermatitis herpetiformis	Pruritic vesicles on knees, elbows, buttocks	Coeliac disease	
Zinc deficiency	Red, scaly, crusting lesions around mouth, eyes, genitalia; white patches on tongue	Diarrhoea (zinc deficiency occurs particularly in setting of Crohn's disease with fistulas, cirrhosis, parenteral nutrition, pancreatitis)	
Porphyria cutanea tarda	Vesicles on exposed skin (e.g., hands)	Alcoholic liver disease	
Systemic sclerosis	Skin that is thick and bound down, calcinosis, Raynaud's[‡] phenomenon, sclerodactyly, telangiectasias	Gastro-oesophageal reflux, oesophageal dysmotility, small bowel bacterial overgrowth with malabsorption	
Inflammatory bowel disease	Pyoderma gangrenosum Erythema nodosum Clubbing Mouth ulcers		
Haemochromatosis (autosomal recessive)	Skin pigmentation (bronze)	Hepatomegaly, signs of chronic liver disease	Diabetes mellitus, heart failure (cardiomyopathy, arthropathy, testicular atrophy)

[*] Eldon John Gardener (b. 1909), American geneticist.
[†] Ferdinand Jean Darier (b. 1856), Paris dermatologist.
[‡] Maurice Raynaud (b. 1834), Paris physician.

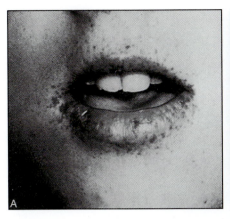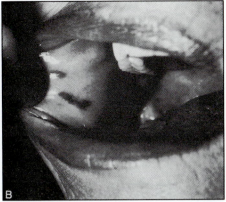

Figure 5.2   *Peutz-Jeghers syndrome, with discrete brown-black lesions.*

From Boland CR, et al. Colonic polyps and the gastrointestinal polyposis syndromes. In Sleisenger MH, Fordtran JS, editors. Gastrointestinal Disease. 4th ed. Philadelphia: WB Saunders, 1989. With permission.

bleeding or intussusception. In this autosomal dominant condition the incidence of gastrointestinal adenocarcinoma is increased.

Acanthosis Nigricans

These are brown to black velvety elevations of the epidermis due to confluent papillomas and are usually found in the axillae and nape of the neck. Acanthosis nigricans is associated rarely with gastrointestinal carcinoma (particularly stomach) and lymphoma, as well as with acromegaly, diabetes mellitus and other endocrinopathies.

Hereditary Haemorrhagic Telangiectasia (Rendu*-Osler-Weber[†] Syndrome)

Multiple small telangiectasiae occur in this disease. They are often present on the lips and tongue (Figure 5.3), but may be found anywhere on the skin. When they are present in the gastrointestinal tract they can cause chronic blood loss or even, occasionally, torrential bleeding. An associated arteriovenous malformation in the liver may be present. This is an autosomal dominant condition and is uncommon.

Porphyria Cutanea Tarda

Fragile vesicles appear on exposed areas of the skin and heal with scarring (Figure 5.4). The urine is dark in this chronic disorder of porphyrin metabolism associated with alcoholism, liver disease and hepatitis C.

Systemic Sclerosis

Tense tethering of the skin in systemic sclerosis is often associated with gastro-oesophageal reflux and gastrointestinal motility disorders (page 281).

---

*   Henri Rendu (1844–1902), French physician.
[†]   Frederick Weber (1863–1962), English physician.

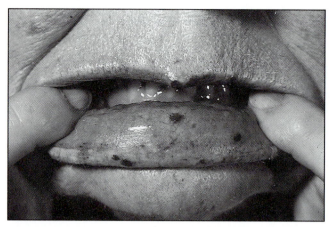

Figure 5.3
Hereditary haemorrhagic telangiectasia involving the lips.

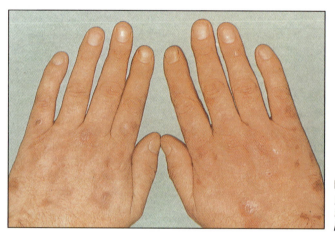

Figure 5.4
Porphyria cutanea tarda—scarring from photosensitivity.

Mental State

The syndrome of hepatic encephalopathy, due to decompensated advanced cirrhosis (chronic liver failure) or fulminant hepatitis (acute liver failure), is an organic neurological disturbance. The features depend on the aetiology and the precipitating factors (page 188). Patients eventually become stuporous and then comatose. The combination of hepatocellular damage and portosystemic shunting due to disturbed hepatic structure (both extrahepatic and intrahepatic) causes this syndrome. It is probably related to the liver's failure to remove toxic metabolites from the portal blood. These toxic metabolites may include ammonia, mercaptans, short chain fatty acids and amines.

The Hands

Even the experienced gastroenterologist must restrain his or her excitement and begin the examination of the gastrointestinal tract with the hands. The signs which may be elicited here give a clue to the presence of chronic liver disease. Whatever its aetiology, permanent diffuse liver damage results in similar peripheral signs. However, none of these signs alone is specific for chronic liver disease.

Nails

Leuconychia

When chronic liver or other disease results in hypoalbuminaemia, the nail beds opacify, often leaving only a rim of pink nail bed at the top of nail. The thumb and index nails bilaterally are most often involved. The exact mechanism is uncertain. It may be that compression of capillary flow by extracellular fluid is the explanation. Muehrcke's lines (transverse white lines) can also occur in hypoalbuminaemic states including cirrhosis. Blue lunulae may be seen in patients with Wilson's disease.

Clubbing

Of patients with cirrhosis up to one-third may have finger clubbing. This may be related in at least some cases to arteriovenous (AV) shunting in the lungs resulting in arterial oxygen desaturation. Cyanosis may be associated with severe long-standing chronic liver disease. The cause of this pulmonary AV shunting is unknown. Conditions such as inflammatory bowel disease and coeliac disease, which cause long-standing nutritional depletion, can also cause clubbing.

The Palms

Palmar Erythema ('Liver Palms')

This is reddening of the palms of the hands affecting the thenar and hypothenar eminences. Often the soles of the feet are also affected. This can be a feature of chronic liver disease. While the finding has been attributed to raised oestrogen levels, it has not been shown to be related to plasma oestradiol levels so the aetiology remains uncertain. Palmar erythema can also occur with pregnancy, thyrotoxicosis, rheumatoid arthritis, polycythaemia and rarely with chronic febrile diseases or chronic leukaemia. It may also be a normal finding.

Anaemia

Inspect the palmar creases for pallor suggesting anaemia (page 224), which may result from gastrointestinal blood loss, malabsorption (folate, vitamin B_{12}), haemolysis (e.g., hypersplenism) or chronic disease.

Dupuytren's Contracture*

This is a visible and palpable thickening and contraction of the palmar fascia causing permanent flexion, most often of the ring finger. It is often bilateral and occasionally may affect the feet. It is associated with alcoholism (not liver disease), but is also found in some manual workers; it may be familial. The palmar fascia of these patients contains abnormally large amounts of xanthine and this may be related to the pathogenesis.

Hepatic Flap (Asterixis)

Before leaving the hands one should ask the patient to stretch out the arms in front, separate the fingers and extend the wrists for 15 seconds. Jerky, irregular

---

* Baron Guillaume Dupuytren (1777–1835), French surgeon.

flexion-extension movement at the wrist and metacarpophalangeal joints, often accompanied by lateral movements of the fingers, constitute the flapping of hepatic encephalopathy (page 188). It is thought to be due to interference with the inflow of joint position sense information to the reticular formation in the brainstem. This results in rhythmical lapses of postural muscle tone. Occasionally the arms, neck, tongue, jaws and eyelids can also be involved. The flap is usually bilateral, tends to be absent at rest, and is brought on by sustained posture. The rhythmic movements are not synchronous on each side and the flap is absent when coma supervenes.

Although this flap is characteristic of liver failure, it is not diagnostic: it can also occur in cardiac, respiratory and renal failure, as well as in hypoglycaemia, hypokalaemia, hypomagnesaemia or barbiturate intoxication.

A tremor may occur in Wilson's disease and in alcoholism.

The Arms

Inspect the upper limbs for *bruising*. Large bruises (ecchymoses) may be due to clotting abnormalities. Hepatocellular damage can interfere with protein synthesis and therefore the production of all the clotting factors (except factor VIII which is made elsewhere in the reticuloendothelial system). Obstructive jaundice results in a shortage of bile acids in the intestine, and therefore may reduce absorption of vitamin K (a fat-soluble vitamin), which is essential for the production of clotting factors II (prothrombin), VII, IX and X.

Petechiae (pinhead sized bruises) may also be present (page 225). Chronic excessive alcohol consumption can sometimes result in bone marrow depression causing thrombocytopenia, which may be responsible for petechiae. In addition, splenomegaly secondary to portal hypertension can cause hypersplenism with resultant excessive destruction of platelets in the spleen; in severe liver disease (especially acute hepatic necrosis) diffuse intravascular coagulation can occur.

Look for muscle wasting which is often a late manifestation of malnutrition in alcoholic patients. Alcohol can also cause a proximal myopathy (page 402).

Scratch marks due to severe itch (pruritus) are often prominent in patients with obstructive or cholestatic jaundice. This is commonly the presenting feature of primary biliary cirrhosis* before other signs are apparent. The mechanism of pruritus is thought to be retention of an unknown substance normally excreted in the bile, rather than bile salt deposition in the skin as was earlier thought.

Spider naevi (Figure 5.5) consist of a central arteriole from which radiate numerous small vessels which look like spiders' legs. They range in size from just visible to half a centimetre in diameter. Their usual distribution is in the area drained by the superior vena cava, so they are found on the arms, neck and chest wall. They can occasionally bleed profusely. Pressure applied with a pointed object to the central arteriole causes blanching of the whole lesion. Rapid refilling occurs on release of the pressure.

The finding of more than two spider naevi anywhere on the body is likely to be abnormal. Spider naevi can be caused by cirrhosis, most frequently due to alcohol.

---

* Primary biliary cirrhosis (PBC) is an uncommon chronic non-suppurative destructive cholangitis of unknown aetiology; 90% of affected patients are female, and it is often associated with other autoimmune disease, e.g., CREST, Sjögren's syndrome, rheumatoid arthritis, thyroiditis.

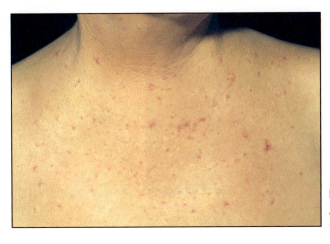

Figure 5.5

A large crop of spider naevi.

They may occur transiently with viral hepatitis. During the second to fifth months of pregnancy spider naevi frequently appear only to disappear again within eight weeks of delivery. It is not known why they occur only in the upper part of the body. Like palmar erythema they are traditionally attributed to oestrogen excess. Part of the normal hepatic function is the inactivation of oestrogens, which is impaired in chronic liver disease. Oestrogens are known to have a dilating effect on the spiral arterioles of the endometrium and this has been used to explain the presence of spider naevi, but changes in plasma oestradiol levels have not been found to correlate with the appearance and disappearance of spider naevi.

The differential diagnosis of spider naevi includes *Campbell de Morgan* spots,* venous stars and hereditary haemorrhagic telangiectasia. Campbell de Morgan spots are flat or slightly elevated red circular lesions which occur on the abdomen or the front of the chest. They do not blanch on pressure and are very common. *Venous stars* are 2 cm to 3 cm lesions which can occur on the dorsum of the feet, legs, back and the lower chest. They are due to elevated venous pressure and are found overlying the main tributary to a large vein. They are not obliterated by pressure. The blood flow is from the periphery to the centre of the lesion which is the opposite of the flow in the spider naevus. Lesions of *hereditary haemorrhagic telangiectasia* (page 226) occasionally resemble spider naevi.

Palpate the axillae for *lymphadenopathy* (page 227). Look in the axillae for acanthosis nigricans.

The Face

Eyes

Look first at the sclerae for signs of *jaundice* (Figure 5.6) (page 156) or *anaemia* (page 224). *Kayser-Fleischer[†] rings* are brownish green rings occurring at the

---

*   Campbell de Morgan (1811–1876), London surgeon.

[†]   Bernhard Kayser (1869–1954), German ophthalmologist, described these rings in 1902. Bruno Fleischer (1848–1904), German ophthalmologist.

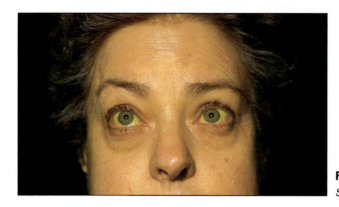

Figure 5.6
Scleral icterus.

periphery of the cornea, affecting the upper pole more than the lower. They are due to deposits of excess copper in Descemet's* membrane of the cornea. Slit-lamp examination is often necessary to show them. They are typically found in Wilson's[†] disease (page 413), a copper storage disease which causes cirrhosis and neurological disturbances. The Kayser-Fleischer rings are usually present by the time neurological signs have appeared. Patients with other cholestatic liver diseases, however, can also have these rings. *Iritis* may be seen in inflammatory bowel disease (page 191).

Xanthelasma are yellowish plaques in the subcutaneous tissues in the periorbital region and are due to deposits of lipids (Figure 3.8). They may indicate protracted elevation of the serum cholesterol. In patients with cholestasis an abnormal lipoprotein (lipoprotein X) is found in the plasma and is associated with elevation of the serum cholesterol. Xanthelasma are common in patients with primary biliary cirrhosis (see also Table 3.4).

Periorbital purpura following proctosigmoidoscopy ('black eye syndrome') is a characteristic sign of amyloidosis (perhaps related to factor X deficiency) but is exceedingly rare (Figure 5.7).

Parotids

Next inspect and palpate the cheeks over the parotid area for parotid enlargement (Table 5.5). Ask the patient to clench the teeth so that the masseter muscle is palpable; the parotid is best felt behind the masseter muscle and in front of the ear. It is normally impalpable. Parotidomegaly which is bilateral is associated with alcoholism rather than liver disease *per se*. It is due to fatty infiltration, perhaps secondary to alcohol toxicity with or without malnutrition. A tender swollen parotid suggests the diagnosis of parotititis following an acute illness or surgery.

The Mouth

The Teeth and Breath

The very beginning of the gastrointestinal tract is, like the very end of the tract, accessible to inspection without elaborate equipment. Look first briefly at the state

---

*   Jean Descemet (b. 1732), Paris surgeon and anatomist.

[†]   Samuel Alexander Wilson (b. 1877), London neurologist.

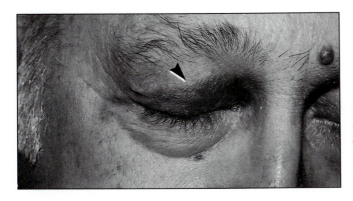

Figure 5.7
Amyloidosis: note the periorbital purpura that followed a proctoscopic examination, a characteristic (albeit rare) sign.

Table 5.5   *Causes of Parotid Enlargement*

Bilateral
1. Mumps (can be unilateral)
2. Sarcoidosis or lymphoma, which may cause painless bilateral enlargement
3. Mikulicz* syndrome: bilateral painless enlargement of all three salivary glands. This disease is probably an early stage of Sjögren's syndrome
5. Alcohol-associated parotitis
6. Malnutrition
7. Severe dehydration: as occurs in renal failure, terminal carcinomatosis and severe infections

Unilateral
1. Mixed parotid tumour (occasionally bilateral)
2. Tumour infiltration, which usually causes painless unilateral enlargement and may cause facial nerve palsy (page 358)
3. Duct blockage, e.g., salivary calculus

*   Johann von Mikulicz-Radecki (1850–1905), Professor of Surgery, Breslau.

of the teeth and note whether they are real or false. False teeth will have to be removed for complete examination of the mouth. Note if there is gum hypertrophy (Table 5.6) or pigmentation (Table 5.7). Loose-fitting false teeth may be responsible for ulcers and decayed teeth may be responsible for fetor.

Other causes of fetor are listed in Table 5.8. These must be distinguished from *fetor hepaticus* which is a rather sweet smell of the breath. It is an indication of severe hepatocellular disease and may be due to methylmercaptans. These substances are known to be exhaled in the breath and may be derived from methionine when this amino acid is not demethylated by a diseased liver. Severe fetor hepaticus which fills the patient's room is a bad sign and indicates a precomatose condition in many cases. The presence of fetor hepaticus in a patient with a coma of unknown cause may be a helpful clue to the diagnosis.

Unless the smell is obvious one should get a patient to exhale through the mouth while one sniffs a little of the exhaled air.

The Tongue

Thickened epithelium with bacterial debris and food particles commonly cause a *coating* over the tongue, especially in smokers. It is rarely a sign of disease and is more marked on the posterior part of the tongue where there is less mobility and

Table 5.6 *Causes of Gum Hypertrophy*

Phenytoin
Pregnancy
Scurvy (vitamin C deficiency: the gums become spongy, red, bleed easily and are swollen and irregular)
Gingivitis, e.g., from smoking, calculus, plaque, Vincent's* angina (fusobacterial membranous tonsillitis)
Leukaemia (usually monocytic)

*   Jean Hyacinthe Vincent (1862–1950), Professor of Forensic Medicine and French Army bacteriologist.

Table 5.7 *Causes of Pigmented Lesions in the Mouth*

1.	Heavy metals: lead or bismuth (blue-black line on the gingival margin), iron (haemochromatosis—blue-grey pigmentation of the hard palate)
2.	Drugs: antimalarials, the oral contraceptive pill (brown or black areas of pigmentation anywhere in the mouth)
3.	Addison's disease (blotches of dark brown pigment anywhere in the mouth)
4.	Peutz-Jeghers syndrome (lips, buccal mucosa or palate)
5.	Malignant melanoma (raised, painless black lesions anywhere in the mouth)

Table 5.8 *Causes of Fetor (bad breath)*

1.	Faulty oral hygiene
2.	Fetor hepaticus (a sweet smell)
3.	Ketosis (diabetic ketoacidosis results in excretion of ketones in exhaled air causing a sickly sweet smell)
4.	Uraemia (fish breath: an ammoniacal odour)
5.	Alcohol (distinctive)
6.	Paraldehyde
7.	Putrid (due to anaerobic chest infections with large amounts of sputum)
8.	Cigarettes

the papillae desquamate more slowly. It occurs frequently in respiratory tract infections, but is in no way related to constipation or any serious abdominal disorder.

Lingua nigra (black tongue) is due to elongation of papillae over the posterior part of the tongue which appears dark brown because of the accumulation of keratin. There is no known cause and apart from its aesthetic problems it is symptomless. Bismuth compounds may also cause a black tongue.

Geographical tongue is a term used to describe slowly changing red rings and lines which occur on the surface of the tongue. It is not painful, and the condition tends to come and go. It is not usually of any significance, but can be a sign of riboflavin (vitamin B₂) deficiency.

Leucoplakia is important to recognise. Here there is white coloured thickening of the mucosa of the tongue and mouth; the condition is premalignant. Most of the causes of leucoplakia begin with 'S': sore teeth (poor dental hygiene), smoking, spirits, sepsis or syphilis, but often no cause is apparent. Leucoplakia may also occur on the larynx, anus and vulva.

Table 5.9 *Causes of Mouth Ulcers*

Common	
Aphthous	
Drugs (e.g., gold, steroids)	
Trauma	
Uncommon	
Gastrointestinal disease:	Crohn's disease, ulcerative colitis
	Coeliac disease
Rheumatological disease:	Behçet's* syndrome
	Reiter's† syndrome
Erythema multiforme	
Infection: Viral—herpes zoster, herpes simplex	
Bacterial—syphilis (primary chancre, secondary snail track ulcers, mucous patches), tuberculosis	
Self-inflicted	

* Hulusi Behçet (b. 1889), Turkish dermatologist.
† Hans Reiter (b. 1881), Berlin bacteriologist.

The term *'glossitis'* is generally used to describe a smooth appearance of the tongue which may also be erythematous. The appearance is due to atrophy of the papillae, and in later stages there may be shallow ulceration. These changes occur in the tongue often as a result of nutritional deficiencies to which the tongue is sensitive because of the rapid turnover of mucosal cells. Deficiencies of iron, folate and the vitamin B group, especially vitamin B_{12}, are common causes. Glossitis is common in alcoholics and can also occur in the rare carcinoid syndrome. However, many cases, especially those in elderly people, are impossible to explain.

Enlargement of the tongue *(macroglossia)* may occur in congenital conditions such as Down's syndrome (page 317) or in endocrine disease including acromegaly (page 308). Tumour infiltration (e.g., haemangioma or lymphangioma) or infiltration of the tongue with amyloid material in amyloidosis can also be responsible for macroglossia.

Mouth Ulcers

This is an important topic because a number of systemic diseases can present with ulcers in the mouth (Table 5.9). *Aphthous ulceration* is the commonest type seen. This begins as a small painful vesicle on the tongue or mucosal surface of the mouth which may break down to form a painful shallow ulcer. These ulcers heal without scarring. The cause is completely unknown. They usually do not indicate any serious underlying systemic disease, but may occur in Crohn's* disease or coeliac disease. The acquired immunodeficiency syndrome (AIDS) may be associated with a number of mouth lesions (page 463). *Angular stomatitis* refers to cracks at the corners of the mouth; causes include vitamin B_6, B_{12}, folate and iron deficiency.

---

*   Burrill Bernard Crohn (b. 1884), American gastroenterologist at Mount Sinai Hospital, New York, described this disease in 1932.

Candidiasis

Fungal infection with *Candida albicans* (thrush) causes creamy white curd-like patches in the mouth which are removed only with difficulty and leave a bleeding surface. The infection may spread to involve the oesophagus causing dysphagia or odynophagia. Moniliasis is associated with immunosuppression (steroids, tumour chemotherapy, alcoholism or an underlying immunological abnormality such as AIDS, or haematological malignancy), where it is due to decreased host resistance. Broad-spectrum antibiotics, which inhibit the normal oral flora, are also a common cause because fungal overgrowth is permitted. Faulty oral hygiene, iron deficiency and diabetes mellitus can also be responsible. Rarely, chronic mucocutaneous candidiasis, a distinct syndrome comprising recurrent or persistent oral thrush, finger or toe nail bed infection and skin involvement, occurs; in some of these patients, endocrine diseases such as hypoparathyroidism, hypothyroidism, or Addison's disease are associated (page 313).

The Neck and Chest

Palpate the cervical lymph nodes (page 229). It is particularly important to feel for the supraclavicular nodes especially on the left side. These may be involved with advanced gastric or other gastrointestinal malignancy, or with lung cancer. The presence of a large left supraclavicular node in combination with carcinoma of the stomach is called Troisier's* sign. Look for spider naevi.

In males, *gynaecomastia* may be a sign of chronic liver disease (page 319). Gynaecomastia may be unilateral or bilateral and the breasts may be tender. This may be a sign of cirrhosis, particularly alcoholic cirrhosis, or of chronic active hepatitis. In chronic liver disease, changes in the oestradiol to testosterone ratio may be responsible. In cirrhotic patients, spironolactone, used to treat ascites, is also a common cause. Gynaecomastia may also occur in alcoholics without liver disease because of damage to the Leydig[†] cells of the testis from alcohol. A number of drugs may rarely cause gynaecomastia (e.g., digoxin, cimetidine).

The Abdomen

Self-restraint is no longer required and it is now time to examine the abdomen itself.

Inspection

The patient should lie flat, with one pillow under the head and the abdomen exposed from the nipples to the pubic symphysis (Figure 5.1). Don't be too eager to begin palpation, as inspection is very often helpful. Inspection begins with a careful look for abdominal *scars* which may indicate previous surgery or trauma (Figure 5.8). Look in the area around the umbilicus for laparoscopic surgical scars. Older scars are white and recent scars are pink because the tissue remains vascular. Note the presence of stomas (end-colostomy, loop colostomy, ileostomy or ileal conduit) or fistulae.

Generalised abdominal *distension* (Figure 5.9) may be present. All the causes of this sound as if they begin with the letter 'F': fat (gross obesity), fluid (ascites),

---

[*]   Charles Émile Troisier (1844–1919), Professor of Pathology in Paris described this sign in 1886.

[†]   Franz von Leydig (b. 1821), Bonn anatomist and zoologist.

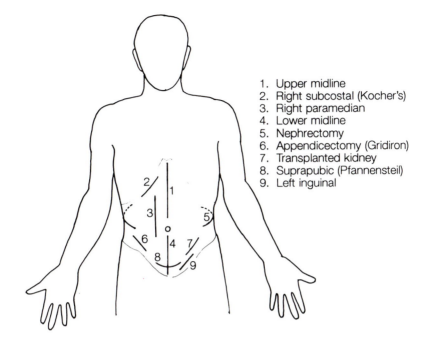

1. Upper midline
2. Right subcostal (Kocher's)
3. Right paramedian
4. Lower midline
5. Nephrectomy
6. Appendicectomy (Gridiron)
7. Transplanted kidney
8. Suprapubic (Pfannensteil)
9. Left inguinal

Figure 5.8   *Abdominal scars.*

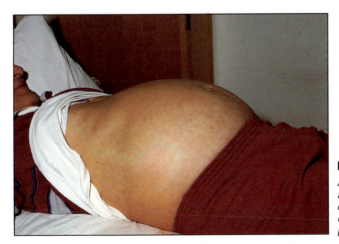

Figure 5.9

Abdomen distended with ascites: umbilicus points downwards, unlike cases of distension due to a pelvic mass.

fetus, flatus (gaseous distension due to bowel obstruction), faeces, 'filthy' big tumour (eg. ovarian tumour or hydatid cyst) or 'phantom' pregnancy. Look at the shape of the umbilicus which may give a clue to the underlying cause. An umbilicus buried in fat suggests that the patient eats too much. However, when the peritoneal cavity is filled with large volumes of fluid (ascites) from whatever cause, the abdominal flanks and wall appear tense and the umbilicus is shallow or everted and points downward. In pregnancy the umbilicus is pushed upwards by the uterus enlarging from the pelvis. This appearance may also result from a huge ovarian cyst.

Local swellings may indicate enlargement of one of the abdominal or pelvic organs. A hernia is a protrusion of an intra-abdominal structure through an abnormal opening; this may occur because of previous surgery weakening the abdominal wall (incisional hernia), a congenital abdominal wall defect or from chronically increased intra-abdominal pressure.

Prominent *veins* may be obvious on the abdominal wall. If these are present the direction of venous flow should be elicited at this stage. A finger is used to occlude the vein and blood is then emptied from the vein below the occluding finger with a second finger. The second finger is removed and, if the vein refills, flow is occurring towards the occluding finger (Figure 5.10). Flow should be tested separately in veins above and below the umbilicus. In patients with severe portal hypertension, portal to systemic flow occurs through the umbilical veins which may, rather rarely, become engorged and distended. The direction of flow then is away from the umbilicus. Because of their engorged appearance they have been likened to the mythical Medusa's hair after Minerva had turned it into snakes; this sign is called a *caput Medusae* (head of Medusa) but is very rare (Figure 5.11). More often only one or two veins (often epigastric) are visible. Engorgement can also occur because of inferior vena caval obstruction, usually due to a tumour or thrombosis but sometimes because of tense ascites. In this case the abdominal veins enlarge to provide collateral blood flow from the legs, avoiding the blocked inferior vena cava. The direction of flow is then upwards towards the heart. Therefore, to distinguish caput Medusae from inferior vena caval obstruction, determine the direction of flow *below* the umbilicus; it will be towards the legs in

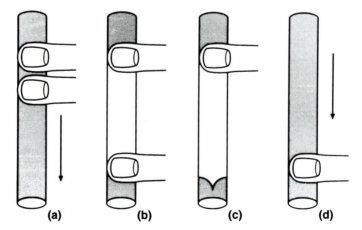

(a)   (b)   (c)   (d)

Figure 5.10   *Detecting the direction of flow of a vein: (a) place two fingers firmly on the vein; (b) the second finger is moved along the vein to empty it of blood and keep it occluded; (c) the second finger is removed but the vein does not refill; (d) at repeat testing and removing the first finger, filling occurs indicating the direction of flow.*

Adapted from Swash M, editor. Hutchison's Clinical Methods. 19th ed. Philadelphia: Balliére Tindall, 1989, with permission.

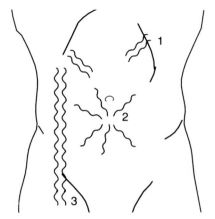

Figure 5.11   *Prominent veins on the abdominal wall: 1 = thin veins over the costal margin—not of clinical relevance; 2 = caput Medusae (rare); 3 = inferior vena caval obstruction.*

From Swash M, editor. Hutchison's Clinical Methods. 19th ed. Philadelphia: Balliére Tindall, 1989, with permission.

the former and towards the head in the latter. Prominent superficial veins can occasionally be congenital.

Pulsations may be visible. An expanding central pulsation in the epigastrium suggests an abdominal aortic aneurysm. However, the abdominal aorta can often be seen to pulsate in normal thin people.

Visible peristalsis may occur in very thin normal people occasionally; however, it usually suggests intestinal obstruction. Pyloric obstruction due to peptic ulceration or tumour may cause visible peristalsis seen as a slow wave of movement passing across the upper abdomen from left to right. Obstruction of the distal small bowel can cause similar movements in a ladder pattern in the centre of the abdomen.

Skin lesions should also be noted on the abdominal wall. These include the vesicles of herpes zoster, which occur in a radicular pattern (they are localised to only one side of the abdomen in the distribution of a single nerve root). Herpes zoster may be responsible for severe abdominal pain which is of mysterious origin until the rash appears. The Sister Joseph* nodule is a metastatic tumour deposit in the umbilicus, the anatomical region where the peritoneum is closest to the skin. Discoloration of the umbilicus where a faintly bluish hue is present is very rarely found in cases of extensive haemoperitoneum and acute pancreatitis (Cullen's[†] sign—the umbilical 'black eye'). Skin discoloration may also rarely occur in the flanks in severe cases of acute pancreatitis (Grey-Turner's[‡] sign).

---

*   Sister Joseph of St Mary's Hospital, Rochester, described this sign to Dr William Mayo (1861–1939) of the Mayo Clinic.

†   Thomas S Cullen (1869–1953), Professor of Gynaecology who originally described this sign as an indication of a ruptured ectopic pregnancy.

‡   George Grey-Turner (b. 1877), English surgeon.

Stretching of the abdominal wall severe enough to cause rupture of the elastic fibres in the skin produces pink linear marks with a wrinkled appearance which are called *striae*. When these are wide and purple-coloured, Cushing's syndrome may be the cause (page 310). Ascites, pregnancy or recent loss of weight are much more common causes of striae.

Next, squat down beside the bed so that the patient's abdomen is at eye level. Ask him or her to take slow deep breaths through the mouth and watch for evidence of asymmetrical movement, indicating the presence of a mass. In particular a large liver may be seen to move below the right costal margin or a large spleen below the left costal margin.

Palpation

This part of the examination often reveals the most information. Successful palpation requires relaxed abdominal muscles. To this end, reassure the patient that the examination will not be painful and use warm hands. Ask the patient if any particular area is tender and examine this area last. Encourage the patient to breathe gently through the mouth. If necessary, ask the patient to bend the knees to relax the abdominal wall muscles.

For descriptive purposes the abdomen has been divided into nine areas or regions (Figure 5.12). Palpation in each region is performed with the palmar surface of the fingers acting together. For the palpation of the edges of organs or masses the lateral surface of the forefinger is the most sensitive part of the hand.

Palpation should begin with light pressure in each region. All the movements of the hand should occur at the metacarpophalangeal joints and the hand should be moulded to the shape of the abdominal wall. Note the presence of any tenderness or lumps in each region. As the hand moves over each region the mind should be considering the anatomical structures that underlie it. Deep palpation of the abdomen is performed next, though care should be taken to avoid the tender areas until the end of the examination. Deep palpation is used to detect deeper masses

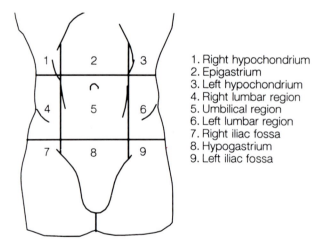

1. Right hypochondrium
2. Epigastrium
3. Left hypochondrium
4. Right lumbar region
5. Umbilical region
6. Left lumbar region
7. Right iliac fossa
8. Hypogastrium
9. Left iliac fossa

Figure 5.12   *Regions of the abdomen.*

Table 5.10 *Descriptive Features of Intra-abdominal Masses*

For any abdominal mass all the following should be determined.
1. Site: the region involved
2. Tenderness
3. Size (which must be measured) and shape
4. Surface, which may be regular or irregular
5. Edge, which may be regular or irregular
6. Consistency, which may be hard or soft
7. Mobility and movement with inspiration
8. Whether it is pulsatile or not
9. Whether one can get above the mass

and to define those already discovered. Any mass must be carefully characterised and described (Table 5.10).

Guarding of the abdomen, when resistance to palpation occurs due to contraction of the abdominal muscles, may result from tenderness or anxiety, and may be voluntary or involuntary. The latter suggests peritonitis. *Rigidity* is a constant involuntary contraction of the abdominal muscles always associated with tenderness and indicates peritoneal irritation. *Rebound tenderness* is said to be present when the abdominal wall, having been compressed slowly, is released rapidly and a sudden stab of pain results. This may make the patient wince so the face should be watched while this manoeuvre is performed. It strongly suggests the presence of peritonitis and should be performed if there is doubt about the presence of localised or generalised peritonitis.*

The Liver

Feel for hepatomegaly (Figure 5.13). With the examining hand aligned parallel to the right costal margin, and beginning in the right iliac fossa, ask the patient to breathe in and out slowly through the mouth. With each expiration the hand is advanced by 1 or 2 cm closer to the right costal margin. During inspiration the hand is kept still and the lateral margin of the forefinger waits expectantly for the liver edge to strike it.

If the liver edge has been identified, an attempt should be made to feel the surface of the liver. The edge of the liver and the surface itself may be hard or soft, tender or non-tender, regular or irregular, and pulsatile or non-pulsatile. The normal liver edge may be just palpable below the right costal margin on deep inspiration, especially in thin people. The edge is then felt to be soft and regular with a fairly sharply defined border and the surface of the liver itself is smooth. Sometimes only the left lobe of the liver may be palpable (to the left of the midline) in patients with cirrhosis.

If the liver edge is palpable the total *liver span* should be measured Remember that the liver span varies with height and that inter-observer error is quite large for this measurement. The normal upper border of the liver is level with the sixth rib in about the midclavicular line. At this point the percussion note over the chest

---

* Be careful not to surprise your patient by a sudden jabbing and release movement: rebound tenderness should be elicited slowly. If you suspect the patient may be feigning a tender abdomen, test for rebound with your stethoscope after telling the patient to lie still and quiet so that you can hear.

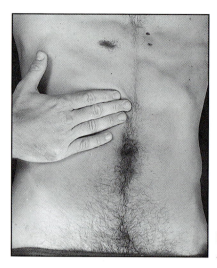

Figure 5.13
Abdominal examination: the liver.

changes from resonant to dull. To estimate the liver span percuss down along the right midclavicular line until the liver dullness is encountered and measure from here to the palpable liver edge. The normal span is less than 12.5 cm. Other causes of a normal but palpable liver include ptosis due to emphysema, asthma or a subdiaphragmatic collection, or a Riedel's* lobe. The Riedel's lobe is a tongue-like projection of the liver from the right lobe's inferior surface; it can be quite large and rarely extends as far as the right iliac fossa. It can be confused with an enlarged gallbladder or right kidney.

Many diseases cause hepatic enlargement and these are listed in Table 5.11. Remember the diseased liver is not always enlarged; a small liver is common in advanced cirrhosis, and the liver shrinks rapidly with acute hepatic necrosis (due to liver cell death and collapse of the reticulin framework).

The Gallbladder

The gallbladder is occasionally palpable below the right costal margin where this crosses the lateral border of the rectus muscles. If biliary obstruction or acute cholecystitis is suspected, the examining hand should be oriented perpendicular to the costal margin, feeling from medial to lateral. Unlike the liver edge, the gallbladder if palpable will be a bulbous, focal rounded mass which moves downwards on inspiration. The causes of an enlarged gallbladder are listed in Table 5.12.

Murphy's[†] *sign* should be sought if cholecystitis is suspected. On taking a deep breath, the patient catches his or her breath when an inflamed gallbladder presses on the examiner's hand which is lying at the costal margin.

The clinician examining for an enlarged gallbladder must always be mindful of *Courvoisier's*[‡] *law* which states that, if the gallbladder is enlarged and the patient

---

*   Bernhard Riedel (1846–1916), German surgeon, described this in 1888.

†   John Murphy (1857–1916), American surgeon.

‡   Ludwig Courvoisier (1843–1918), Professor of Surgery, Switzerland.

Table 5.11   *Differential Diagnosis in Liver Palpation*

Hepatomegaly

1. Massive
Metastases
Alcoholic liver disease with fatty infiltration
Myeloproliferative disease
Right heart failure
Hepatocellular cancer

2. Moderate
The above causes
Haemochromatosis
Haematological disease—e.g., chronic leukaemia, lymphoma
Fatty liver—secondary to, e.g., diabetes mellitus
Infiltration—e.g., amyloid

3. Mild
The above causes
Hepatitis
Biliary obstruction
Hydatid disease
Human immunodeficiency virus (HIV) infection

Firm and Irregular Liver

Hepatocellular carcinoma
Metastatic disease
Cirrhosis
Hydatid disease, granuloma (e.g., sarcoid), amyloid, cysts, lipoidoses

Tender Liver

Hepatitis
Rapid liver enlargement—e.g., right heart failure, Budd-Chiari* syndrome (hepatic vein
    thrombosis)
Hepatocellular cancer
Hepatic abscess
Biliary obstruction/cholangitis

Pulsatile Liver

Tricuspid regurgitation
Hepatocellular cancer
Vascular abnormalities

*   George Budd (1808–1882), Professor of Medicine, King's College Hospital, London. Hans Chiari (1851–1916), Professor of Pathology, Prague.

is jaundiced, the cause is unlikely to be gallstones. Rather, carcinoma of the pancreas or lower biliary tree resulting in obstructive jaundice is likely to be present. This is because the gallbladder with stones is usually chronically fibrosed and therefore incapable of enlargement. Note that if the gallbladder is not palpable, and the patient is jaundiced, some cause other than gallstones is still possible, since at least 50% of dilated gallbladders are impalpable.

The Spleen

The spleen enlarges inferiorly and medially (Figure 5.14). Its edge should be sought below the umbilicus in the midline initially. A two-handed technique is

Table 5.12 *Gallbladder Enlargement*

With Jaundice

1. Carcinoma of the head of the pancreas
2. Carcinoma of the ampulla of Vater*
3. In-situ gallstone formation in the common bile duct
4. Mucocele of the gallbladder due to a stone in Hartmann's[†] pouch and a stone in the common bile duct (very rare)

Without Jaundice

1. Mucocele or empyema of the gallbladder
2. Carcinoma of the gallbladder (stone hard, irregular swelling)
3. Acute cholecystitis

* Abraham Vater (b. 1864), Wittenberg anatomist and botanist.
† Henri Hartmann (b. 1860), Paris surgeon.

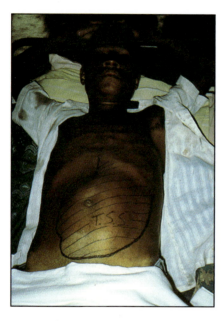

Figure 5.14
Massive splenomegaly: note the splenic notch.

recommended (Figure 5.14). The left hand is placed posterolaterally over the left lower ribs and the right hand is placed on the abdomen parallel to the left costal margin. Don't start palpation too near the costal margin or a large spleen will be missed. As the right hand is advanced closer to the left costal margin, the left hand compresses firmly over the rib cage so as to produce a loose fold of skin; this removes tension from the abdominal wall and enables a slightly enlarged soft spleen to be felt as it moves down towards the right iliac fossa at the end of inspiration.

If the spleen is not palpable, the patient must be rolled on to the right side towards the examiner and palpation repeated. Here one begins close to the left costal margin (Figure 5.15). As a general rule, splenomegaly becomes just detect-

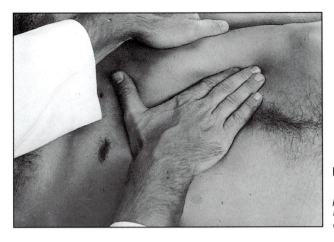

Figure 5.15

The spleen: bimanual palpation with the patient rolled towards the examiner.

Table 5.13   *Causes of Hepatosplenomegaly*

Chronic liver disease with portal hypertension
Haematological disease, e.g., myeloproliferative disease, lymphoma, leukaemia,
    pernicious anaemia, sickle cell anaemia
Infection, e.g., acute viral hepatitis, infectious mononucleosis, cytomegalovirus
Infiltration, e.g., amyloid, sarcoid
Connective tissue disease, e.g., systemic lupus erythematosus
Acromegaly
Thyrotoxicosis

able if the spleen is one-and-a-half to two times enlarged. The causes of splenomegaly are listed in Table 7.6 (page 232). The causes of hepatosplenomegaly are listed in Table 5.13.

The Kidneys

The first important differential diagnosis to consider, if a right or left subcostal mass is palpable, must be a kidney. An attempt to palpate the kidney should be a routine part of the examination. The bimanual method is the best. The patient lies flat on his or her back. To palpate the right kidney, the examiner's left hand slides underneath the back to rest with the heel of the hand under the right loin. The fingers remain free to flex at the metacarpophalangeal joints in the area of the renal angle. The flexing fingers can push the contents of the abdomen anteriorly. The examiner's right hand is placed over the right upper quadrant.

First an attempt should be made to capture the kidney between the two hands. It is more often possible to feel a kidney by ballotting. In this case the renal angle is pressed sharply by the flexing fingers of the posterior hand. The kidney can be felt to float upwards and strike the anterior hand. The opposite hands are used to palpate the left kidney.

When palpable, the kidney feels like a swelling with a rounded lower pole and a medial dent (the hilum). However, it is unusual for a normal kidney to be felt as clearly as this. The lower pole of the right kidney may be palpable in thin, normal persons. Both kidneys move downwards with inspiration. The causes of kidney enlargement are listed in Table 6.4.

It is particularly common to confuse a large left kidney with splenomegaly. The major distinguishing features are: (i) the spleen has no palpable upper border—one cannot feel the space between the spleen and the costal margin, which is present in renal enlargement; (ii) the spleen, unlike the kidney, has a notch which may be palpable; (iii) the spleen moves inferomedially on inspiration while the kidney moves inferiorly; (iv) the spleen is not usually ballottable unless gross ascites is present, but the kidney is, again because of its retroperitoneal position; (v) the percussion note is dull over the spleen but is usually resonant over the kidney as the latter lies posterior to loops of gas-filled bowel; (vi) a friction rub may occasionally be heard over the spleen, but never over the kidney because it is too posterior.

Other Abdominal Masses

The causes of a mass in the abdomen, excluding the liver, spleen and kidneys, are summarised in Table 5.14.

Stomach and duodenum: although many clinicians palpate the epigastrium to elicit tenderness in patients with suspected peptic ulcer, the presence or absence of tenderness is not helpful in making this diagnosis. With gastric outlet obstruction due to a peptic ulcer or gastric carcinoma (page 196), the 'succussion splash' (the sign of Hippocrates) may occasionally be present. In a case of suspected gastric outlet obstruction, after warning the patient what is to come, grasp one iliac crest with each hand, place your stethoscope close to the epigastrium and shake the patient vigorously from side to side. The listening ears eagerly await a splashing noise due to excessive retained fluid in an obstructed stomach. The test is not useful if the patient has just drunk a pint of milk or other fluid for his or her ulcer. The clinician must then return three hours later, having forbidden the patient to drink anything further.

Pancreas: a pancreatic pseudocyst following acute pancreatitis may, if large, be palpable as a rounded swelling above the umbilicus. It is characteristically tense, does not descend with inspiration and feels fixed. Occasionally a pancreatic carcinoma may be palpable in thin patients.

Aorta: arterial pulsation from the abdominal aorta may be present, usually in the epigastrium, in thin normal people. The problem is to determine whether such a pulsation represents an aortic aneurysm (usually due to atherosclerosis) or not. Measure the width of the pulsation gently with two fingers by aligning these parallel to the aorta and placing them at the outermost palpable margins. With an aortic aneurysm the pulsation is expansile (i.e., it enlarges appreciably with systole) (Figure 5.16). If an abdominal aortic aneurysm is larger than 5cm in diameter it usually merits surgical repair.

Bowel: particularly in severely constipated patients with soft abdominal walls and hard faeces, the sigmoid colon is often palpable. Unlike other masses, faeces can usually be indented by the examiner's finger. Rarely, carcinoma of the bowel may be palpable, particularly in the caecum where masses can grow to a large size before they cause obstruction. Such a mass does not move on respiration. In the examination of children or adults with chronic constipation and a megarectum, the enlarged rectum containing impacted stool may be felt above the symphysis pubis, filling a variable part of the pelvis in the middle line.

Table 5.14   *Causes of Abdominal Masses*

Right Iliac Fossa

Appendiceal abscess or mucocele of the appendix
Carcinoma of the caecum or caecal distension due to distal obstruction
Crohn's disease (usually when complicated by an abscess)
Ovarian tumour or cyst
Carcinoid tumour
Amoebiasis
Psoas abscess
Ileocaecal tuberculosis
Hernia
Transplanted kidney

Left Iliac Fossa

Faeces (NB: can often be indented)
Carcinoma of sigmoid or descending colon
Diverticular abscess
Ovarian tumour or cyst
Psoas abscess
Hernia
Transplanted kidney

Upper Abdomen

Retroperitoneal lymphadenopathy (e.g., lymphoma, teratoma)
Left lobe of the liver
Abdominal aortic aneurysm (expansile)
Carcinoma of the stomach
Pancreatic pseudocyst or tumour
Gastric dilatation (e.g., pyloric stenosis, acute dilatation in diabetic ketoacidosis or after
    surgery)
Carcinoma of the transverse colon
Omental mass (e.g., metastatic tumour)
Small bowel obstruction

Pelvis

Bladder
Ovarian tumour or cyst
Uterus (e.g., pregnancy, tumour, fibroids)
Small bowel obstruction

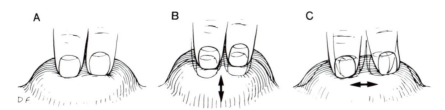

Figure 5.16   *Detecting an expansile impulse: A = no impulse; B = transmitted pulsation from a neighbouring artery; C = expansile impulse, the sign of an aneurysm.*

Adapted from Clain A, editor. Hamilton Bailey's physical signs in clinical surgery. 17th ed. John Wright and Sons, 1986, with permission.

Table 5.15   *Some Causes of Anterior Abdominal Wall Masses*

Lipoma
Sebaceous cyst
Dermal fibroma
Malignant deposits—e.g., melanoma, carcinoma
Epigastric hernia
Umbilical or para-umbilical hernia
Incisional hernia
Rectus sheath haematoma

Bladder: an empty bladder is impalpable. If there is urinary retention, the full bladder may be palpable above the pubic symphysis. It forms part of the differential diagnosis of any swelling arising out of the pelvis. It is characteristically impossible to feel the bladder's lower border. The swelling is typically regular, smooth, firm and oval-shaped. The bladder may sometimes reach as high as the umbilicus. It is unwise to make a definite diagnosis concerning a swelling coming out of the pelvis until one is sure the bladder is empty. This may require the insertion of a urinary catheter.

Inguinal lymph nodes: these are described on page 231.

Testes: palpation of the testes is part of the routine abdominal examination (page 217). Testicular atrophy occurs in chronic liver disease (e.g. alcoholic liver disease, haemochromatosis); its mechanism is believed to be similar to that responsible for gynaecomastia (page 319).

Anterior abdominal wall: the skin and muscles of the anterior abdominal wall are prone to the same sorts of lumps that occur anywhere on the surface of the body (Table 5.15). So to avoid embarrassment it is important not to confuse these with intra-abdominal lumps. To determine whether a mass is in the abdominal wall ask the patient to fold the arms across the upper chest and sit halfway up. An intra-abdominal mass disappears or decreases in size, but one within the layers of the abdominal wall will remain unchanged.

Pain can arise from the abdominal wall; this can cause confusion with intra-abdominal causes of pain. To test for *abdominal wall pain*, feel for an area of localised tenderness that reproduces the pain while the patient is supine. If this is found, ask the patient to fold the arms across the upper chest and sit halfway up, then palpate again (Carnett's* test). If the tenderness disappears, this suggests that the pain is in the abdominal cavity (as the tensed abdominal muscles are protecting the viscera), but if the tenderness persists or is greater, this suggests that the pain is arising from the abdominal wall (e.g., muscle strain, nerve entrapment, myositis). However, the Carnett test may occasionally be positive when there is visceral disease with involvement of the parietal peritoneum producing inflammation of the overlying muscle (e.g., appendicitis).

Percussion

Percussion is used to define the size and nature of organs and masses, to detect fluid in the peritoneal cavity, and to elicit tenderness in patients with peritonitis.

---

*   B Carnett described this in 1926.

Liver

The liver borders should be percussed routinely to determine the liver span. If the liver edge is not palpable and there is no ascites, the right side of the abdomen should be percussed in the midclavicular line up to the right costal margin until dullness is encountered. This defines the liver's lower border even when it is not palpable. The upper border of the liver must always be defined by percussing down the midclavicular line (page 111). Loss of normal liver dullness may occur in massive hepatic necrosis, or with free gas in the peritoneal cavity (e.g., perforated bowel).

Spleen

If the spleen seems impalpable, occasionally percussion over the left costal margin will detect enlargement. If the percussion note is dull over the lower left ribs in the midaxillary line, this suggests splenomegaly, but is unreliable. In these cases palpation should be repeated.

Kidneys

Percussion over a right or left subcostal mass can help distinguish hepatic or splenic from renal masses: in the latter case there will usually be a resonant area because of overlying bowel (be warned, however, that sometimes a very large renal mass may displace overlying bowel).

Bladder

An area of suprapubic dullness may indicate the upper border of an enlarged bladder or pelvic mass.

Ascites

The percussion note over most of the abdomen is resonant due to air in the intestines. The resonance is detectable out to the flanks. When peritoneal fluid (ascites) collects, the influence of gravity causes this to accumulate first in the flanks in a supine patient. Thus, a relatively early sign of ascites (when at least two litres of fluid have accumulated) is a dull percussion note in the flanks. With gross ascites abdominal distension and umbilical eversion occur (Figure 5.8) and dullness is detectable closer to the midline. However, an area of central resonance will always persist. Routine abdominal examination should include percussion starting in the midline with the finger pointing towards the feet; the percussion note is tested out towards the flanks on each side.

If dullness in the flanks is detected the sign of **shifting dullness** should be sought. To detect this sign, while standing on the right side of the bed, percuss out to the left flank until dullness is reached. This point should be marked and the patient rolled towards the examiner. Ideally 30 seconds to one minute should then pass so that fluid can move inside the abdominal cavity and then percussion is repeated over the marked point.

Shifting dullness is present if the area of dullness has changed to become resonant. This is because peritoneal fluid moves under the influence of gravity to the right side of the abdomen when this is the lowermost point. Very occasionally, fluid and air in dilated small bowel in small intestinal obstruction, or a massive ovarian cyst filling the whole abdomen, can cause confusion.

To detect a **fluid thrill** (or wave) the clinician asks an assistant to place the edge of the palm firmly on the centre of the abdomen with the fingers pointing towards the groin. The examiner flicks the side of the abdominal wall, and a pulsation (thrill) is felt by the hand placed on the other abdominal wall. A fluid thrill is only of value in massive ascites, and is not performed routinely. Interestingly it may also occur when there is a massive ovarian cyst or a pregnancy with hydramnios.

The causes of ascites are listed in Table 5.16.

When significant ascites is present, abdominal masses may be difficult to feel by direct palpation. Here is the opportunity to practise **dipping**. Using the hand placed flat on the abdomen, the fingers are flexed at the metacarpophalangeal joints rapidly so as to displace the underlying fluid. This enables the fingers to reach a mass covered in ascitic fluid. In particular, this should be attempted to palpate an enlarged liver or spleen. The liver and spleen may become ballottable when gross ascites is present.

Auscultation

While some cardiologists believe that the sounds produced in the abdominal cavity are not as varied or as interesting as those one hears in the chest, they are important.

Bowel Sounds

Place the diaphragm of the stethoscope just below the umbilicus. Bowel sounds can be heard over all parts of the abdomen in normal healthy people. They have a soft gurgling character and occur only intermittently. Bowel sounds should be described as either present or absent; the terms 'decreased' or 'increased' are meaningless because the sounds vary depending upon when a meal was last eaten.

Complete absence of bowel sounds over a three-minute period indicates paralytic ileus (this is complete absence of peristalsis in a paralysed bowel). As only liquid is present, the heart sounds may be audible over the abdomen, transmitted by the dilated bowel.

Table 5.16 *Classification of Ascites by the Serum Albumin to Ascites Albumin Concentration Gradient*

High gradient (≥11 gm/L)
1.   Cirrhosis*
2.   Alcoholic hepatitis,
3.   Fulminant hepatic failure
4.   Congestive heart failure, constrictive pericarditis (cardiac ascites)
5.   Budd-Chiari syndrome (hepatic vein thrombosis) or veno-occlusive disease
6.   Myxoedema
7.   Massive liver metastases

Low gradient (<11 gm/L)
1.   Peritoneal carcinomatosis
2.   Tuberculosis
3.   Pancreatic ascites
4.   Nephrotic syndrome

*   NB. Patients with a high serum to ascites albumin concentration gradient most often have portal hypertension.

The bowel that is obstructed produces a louder and more high pitched sound with a tinkling quality due to the presence of air and liquid ('obstructed bowel sounds'). Intestinal hurry or rush, which occurs in diarrhoeal states, causes loud gurgling sounds often audible without the stethoscope. These bowel sounds are called borborygmi.

Friction Rubs

These indicate an abnormality of the parietal and visceral peritoneum due to inflammation, but are very rare. They may be audible over the liver or spleen. A rough creaking or grating noise is heard as the patient breathes. Hepatic causes include a tumour within the liver (hepatocellular cancer or metastases), a liver abscess, a recent liver biopsy, a liver infarct, or gonococcal or chlamydial perihepatitis due to inflammation of the liver capsule (Fitz-Hugh-Curtis* syndrome). A splenic rub indicates a splenic infarct.

Venous Hums

A venous hum is typically heard between the xiphisternum and the umbilicus in cases of portal hypertension, but is rare. It may radiate to the chest or over to the liver. Large volumes of blood flowing in the umbilical or para-umbilical veins in the falciform ligament are responsible. These channel blood from the left portal vein to the epigastric or internal mammary veins in the abdominal wall. A venous hum may occasionally be heard over the large vessels such as the inferior mesenteric vein or after portacaval shunting. Sometimes a thrill is detectable over the site of maximum intensity of the hum. The Cruveilhier-Baumgarten† syndrome is the association of a venous hum at the umbilicus and dilated abdominal wall veins. It is almost always due to cirrhosis of the liver. It occurs when patients have a patent umbilical vein which allows portal-to-systemic shunting at this site. The presence of a venous hum or a caput Medusae suggests that the site of portal obstruction is intrahepatic rather than in the portal vein itself.

Bruits

Uncommonly, an arterial systolic bruit can be heard over the liver. This is usually due to a hepatocellular cancer but may occur in acute alcoholic hepatitis, with an arteriovenous malformation or transiently after a liver biopsy. Auscultation for renal bruits on either side of the midline above the umbilicus is indicated if renal artery stenosis is suspected (page 210). A bruit in the epigastrium may be heard in patients with chronic intestinal ischaemia from mesenteric arterial stenosis, but may also occur in the absence of pathology. A bruit may occasionally be audible over the spleen when there is a tumour of the body of the pancreas or a splenic arteriovenous fistula.

Hernias

Chiefly of surgical importance, inguinal and femoral hernias should not be missed during an abdominal examination. Look for an obvious swelling. Asking the

---

*   A H Curtis described hepatic adhesions associated with pelvic inflammatory disease in 1930, while T Fitz-Hugh described right upper abdominal acute gonococcal peritonitis in 1934. However, this syndrome was actually first described by C Stajano in 1920.

†   Jean Cruveilhier (1791–1874), Professor of Pathological Anatomy, Paris, and Paul von Baumgarten (1848–1928), German pathologist.

Table 5.17 *Differential Diagnosis of a Solitary Groin Lump*

Above the inguinal ligament
Inguinal hernia
Undescended testis
Cyst of the canal of Nuck
Encysted hydrocele or lipoma of the cord
Iliac node
Large femoral hernia (rare)

Below the inguinal ligament
Femoral hernia
Lymph node
Saphena varix (sensation of a 'jet of water' on palpation, disappears when supine)
Femoral aneurysm (pulsatile)
Psoas abscess (associated with fever, flank pain and flexion deformity)

patient to cough may make the hernia appear. In the patient with an acute abdomen, a strangulated hernia must be excluded as a cause in all cases. Complete examination requires that the patient be examined while standing.

Inguinal Hernias

First decide if the swelling in the groin is above or below the inguinal ligament, which lies between the anterior superior iliac spine and the pubic tubercle (Table 5.17). The pubic tubercle is found just above the attachment of the adductor longus tendon to the pubic bone, which can be felt on the upper medial aspect of the thigh. If the swelling lies medial to and above the pubic tubercle it is likely to be an inguinal hernia. The characteristic inguinal hernia is a soft lump which can be pushed back into the abdominal cavity (i.e., is reducible) and an impulse is palpable if the patient coughs. The cough impulse must always be sought. *An indirect inguinal hernia* passes through the internal inguinal ring, which lies 1cm above the femoral pulse at the mid-inguinal point* (Figure 5.17) and descends through the inguinal canal. In males a small indirect inguinal hernia may be palpated by gently invaginating the scrotum and feeling an impulse when the patient coughs (Figure 5.18). Remember that, when examining a male, one should count the number of testes in the scrotum (normally two) as a maldescended testis may be confused with an inguinal hernia. Indirect hernias are more likely to strangulate than *direct inguinal hernias*, which protrude forward through the inguinal (Hesselbach's[†]) triangle. A direct inguinal hernia appears immediately on standing and disappears on lying down (Figure 5.17). Although examiners will expect students to try to differentiate direct and indirect inguinal hernias, ultimately differentiation can only be made at operation.

Femoral Hernias

These occur lateral to and below the pubic tubercle, 2cm medial to the femoral pulse, and do not involve the inguinal canal. There may not be a cough impulse

---

[*] The mid-inguinal point is halfway between the anterior superior iliac spine and the symphysis pubis.

[†] Franz Hesselbach (1759–1816), Professor of Surgery, Germany, described this triangle bounded by the inguinal ligament, the inferior epigastric artery and the rectus abdominis.

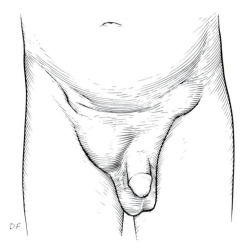

Figure 5.17   *Note the elliptical swelling of an indirect inguinal hernia descending into the scrotum on the right side. Also note the globular swelling of a direct inguinal hernia on the left side.*

Adapted from Dunphy JE, Botsford TW. Physical examination of the surgical patient. An introduction to clinical surgery. 4th ed. Philadelphia: WB Saunders, 1975, with permission.

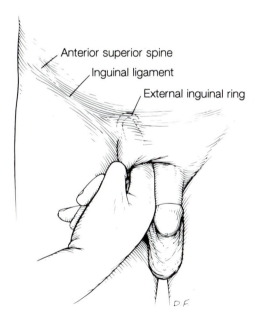

Figure 5.18   *To examine the inguinal canal in a male, the scrotum can be invaginated as shown.*

Adapted from Dunphy JE, Botsford TW. Physical examination of the surgical patient. An introduction to clinical surgery. 4th ed. Philadelphia: WB Saunders, 1975, with permission.

because of the presence of an omental plug or strangulation. Do not confuse an impulse conducted by the femoral vein during coughing with a femoral hernia. A femoral hernia is usually small and firm and can be mistaken for a lymph node.

If a hernia strangulates the overlying skin may become red and tense, and the lump is usually tender. The cough impulse is lost. Remember that hernias are often bilateral, that two different types may occur on the same side, and that there may be an associated hydrocele (one can get above a hydrocele in the inguinal canal but not a hernia). The differential diagnosis of a lump in the groin is given in Table 5.17.

Rectal Examination

The examining physician often hesitates to make the necessary examination because it involves soiling the finger.

William Mayo (1861–1939)

The abdominal examination is not complete without the performance of a rectal examination. It should be performed in all patients admitted to hospital, unless the examiner has no fingers or acute illness such as myocardial infarction presents a temporary contraindication. Following an explanation as to what is to happen, the patient lies on his or her left side with the knees drawn up and back to the examiner. This is called the left lateral position.

The examiner dons a pair of gloves and begins the inspection of the anus and perianal area by separating the buttocks. The following must be looked for.

1. Thrombosed external haemorrhoids (piles): small (less than 1cm), tense bluish swellings may be seen on one side of the anal margin. They are painful and are due to rupture of a vein in the external haemorrhoidal plexus. They are also called perianal haematomas.
2. Skin tags: these look like tags elsewhere on the body and can be an incidental finding or occur with haemorrhoids or Crohn's disease.
3. Rectal prolapse: circumferential folds of red mucosa are visible protruding from the anus. These may only become apparent when the patient is asked to strain as if to pass stool. A gaping anus suggests loss of internal and external sphincter tone. This may co-exist with prolapse.
4. Anal fissure (fissure-in-ano): this is a crack in the anal wall which may be painful enough to prevent rectal examination with the finger. Fissures-in-ano usually occur directly posteriorly and in the midline. A tag of skin may be present at the base: this is called a sentinel pile. It indicates that the fissure is chronic. It may be necessary to get the patient to bear down for a fissure to become visible. Multiple or broad-based fissures may be present in patients with inflammatory bowel disease, malignancy or venereal disease.
5. Fistula-in-ano: the entrance of this tract may be visible, usually within 4cm of the anus. The mouth has a red pouting appearance caused by granulation tissue. This may occur with Crohn's disease or peri-anal abscess (page 183).
6. Condylomata accuminata (anal warts) may be confused with skin tags, but are in fact pedunculated papillomas with a white surface and red base. They may surround the anus.

Table 5.18   *Causes of a Palpable Mass in the Rectum*

Rectal carcinoma
Rectal polyp
Hypertrophied anal papilla
Diverticular phlegmon (recent or old)
Sigmoid colon carcinoma (prolapsing into the pouch of Douglas*)
Metastatic deposits in the pelvis (Blumer's shelf)
Uterine or ovarian malignancy
Prostatic or cervical malignancy (direct extension)
Endometriosis
Pelvic abscess or sarcoma
Amoebic granuloma
Foreign body

NB: Faeces, while palpable, also indent.
*   James Douglas (b. 1675), Scottish anatomist and surgeon in London.

7. Carcinoma of the anus: may be visible as a fungating mass at the anal verge.

8. Pruritus ani: the appearance of this irritating anal condition varies from weeping red dermatitis to a thickened white skin.

9. Excoriation from diarrhoea.

Next ask the patient to strain: incontinence and leakage of faeces or mucus, abnormal descent of the perineum, the presence of a patulous anus or pain are noted. Internal haemorrhoids prolapse in the right anterior, right posterior and left lateral positions

Now the time for action has come. The tip of the gloved right index finger is lubricated and placed over the anus. Ask the patient to breathe in and out quietly through the mouth, as a distraction and to aid relaxation. Slowly increasing pressure is applied with the pulp of the finger until the sphincter is felt to relax slightly. At this stage the finger is advanced into the rectum slowly. During entry, external sphincter tone should be assessed as normal or reduced.

Palpation of the anterior wall of the rectum for the *prostate gland* in the male and for the *cervix* in the female is performed first. The normal prostate is a firm rubbery bi-lobed mass with a central furrow. It becomes firmer with age. With prostatic enlargement, the sulcus becomes obliterated and the gland is often asymmetrical. A very hard nodule is apparent when a carcinoma of the prostate is present. The prostate is boggy and tender in prostatitis. A mass above the prostate or cervix may indicate a metastatic deposit on Blumer's* shelf. The finger is then rotated clockwise so that the left lateral wall, posterior wall and right lateral wall of the rectum can be palpated in turn. Then the finger is advanced as high as possible into the rectum and slowly withdrawn along the rectal wall. A soft lesion, such as a small rectal carcinoma or polyp, is more likely to be felt this way (Table 5.18).† Ask the patient to squeeze your finger with the anal muscles as a further test of anal tone.

---

*   George Blumer (1858–1940) described in 1909 cancer in the pouch of Douglas forming a shelf-like structure.

†   It can be useful to perform the rectal examination with the patient supine and the head of the bed elevated; this allows the intra-abdominal contents to descend and a bimanual examination (using the opposite hand to compress the lower abdomen) is possible.

After the finger has been withdrawn the glove is inspected for bright blood or melaena, mucus or pus, and the colour of the faeces is noted. Haemorrhoids are not palpable unless thrombosed. The occurrence of significant pain during the examination suggests an anal fissure, an ischiorectal abscess, a recently thrombosed external pile, proctitis or anal ulcers.

Proctosigmoidoscopy

The examination of the rectum with a sigmoidoscope is an essential part of the physical examination of any patient with symptoms referable to the anorectal region or large bowel. The principal indications include rectal bleeding, chronic diarrhoea, constipation or change in bowel habit. It should also be performed in some patients with abdominal pain, before treatment is begun for any anorectal condition, and before a barium enema is ordered for any reason.

The examination can be performed without anaesthesia, except in patients who have a very painful anal condition.

Procedure

Begin by inspecting the anal area as outlined earlier. Then a digital examination of the rectum is performed.

Explain to the patient what is about to happen. Warn him or her that there will be a feeling of fullness and the desire to defaecate, and possibly cramps in the rectal region. The patient is then placed in the left lateral position and asked to relax and breathe quietly through the mouth.

If a rigid sigmoidoscope is to be used, it is warmed slightly and, with the obturator in place, is inserted into the rectum in the direction of the umbilicus until the rectal ampulla is reached (4 to 5 cm). This is the only part of the examination that is performed blind. The obturator is then removed. The tip of the sigmoidoscope is gently swung posteriorly under direct vision to follow the curve of the sacrum. The important landmarks to note during sigmoidoscopy are the anal verge, the dentate line, the anorectal junction, the lowest and middle rectal valves, and finally the rectosigmoid junction. Small amounts of air may be insufflated to assist with this. At about 12 to 15cm, smooth rectal mucosa gives way to the concentric rugae of the distal sigmoid. It is possible to advance the rigid instrument into the distal sigmoid in the majority of men and in many women. The flexible sigmoidoscope often can examine the entire left colon in skilled hands. The instrument must *never* be advanced unless the lumen is clearly visible and the patient is not experiencing pain.

Once the sigmoidoscope has been advanced as far as possible it should be withdrawn gradually while the circumference of the mucosa is inspected carefully. Look behind for the valves of Houston.* It is possible to sample faeces from areas away from the anal margin, which can be tested for occult blood and subjected to microbiological examination. Mucosal lesions can also be biopsied.

Common Abnormalities Seen on Sigmoidoscopy

1.   Blood, seen to be arising from above the highest level examined, indicates that a total examination of the colon by colonoscopy is essential.

---

*   The middle one of three transverse folds of mucous membrane in the rectum, described by John Houston (1802–1845), Irish surgeon.

2. Erythematous and ulcerated areas indicating inflammation, which may be local or diffuse.
3. Mucosal oedema, where there is loss of the normal vascular pattern of the colon, may be seen in mild inflammatory bowel disease.
4. Polyps, which may be sessile or pedunculated, solitary or multiple.
5. Carcinoma.
6. Strictures, which may be due to carcinoma, Crohn's disease, trauma, ischaemia, radiation, or (very rarely) tuberculosis.
7. The orifices of diverticula.
8. Fissures.

If an abnormality of the anal canal is suspected this is best seen using *ano-oscopy*, which can be carried out after sigmoidoscopy. Lesions to look for in the anal canal include swellings, masses, fissures, the internal openings of fistulae, squamous metaplasia and haemorrhoids. Haemorrhoids appear as swellings at the site of the normal anal cushions at 3, 7 and 11 o'clock and they descend on straining. Remember that haemorrhoids are common and may coexist with more sinister bowel disease.

Testing of the Stools for Blood

Testing of the stools for blood can sometimes be helpful particularly in the assessment of anaemia, iron deficiency, gastrointestinal bleeding or symptoms suggesting colonic cancer. In the guaiac test, stool is placed on a guaiac-impregnated paper; blood results in phenolytic oxidation, causing a blue colour. Newer tests can quantitate the amount of blood in the stool.

Unfortunately, both false-positive and false-negative results occur with the occult blood tests. Peroxidase and catalase, present in various foods (e.g., fresh fruit, uncooked vegetables), and haem in red meat can cause false-positive results as can aspirin, anticoagulants or oral iron. Vitamin C can reduce the sensitivity of guaiac results, and should not be taken prior to testing.

False-negative results are not uncommon with colorectal neoplasms because they bleed intermittently. Hence the value of testing for occult blood in screening any population for cancer remains controversial.

Other

Complete the examination of the gastrointestinal tract by weighing the patient. Examine the legs for bruising or oedema, which may be the result of liver disease. Neurological signs of alcoholism (e.g., a coarse tremor) or evidence of thiamine deficiency (peripheral neuropathy or memory loss) may also be present.

Examination of the cardiovascular system may be helpful in patients with hepatomegaly. Cardiac failure is a common cause of liver enlargement and can even cause cirrhosis. Measurement of the patient's temperature is important, especially in an acute abdominal case or if there is any suggestion of infection.

Examine with particular care all lymph node groups, the breasts and chest if there is any evidence of malignant disease such as firm, irregular hepatomegaly (Table 7.7, page 232).

Examination of the Gastrointestinal Contents

Faeces

Never miss an opportunity to inspect a patient's faeces because considerable information about the gastrointestinal tract can be obtained in this way.

Melaena

Melaena stools are poorly formed, black and have a tarry appearance. They have a very characteristic and offensive smell. The cause is the presence of blood digested by gastric acid and colonic bacteria. Melaena usually indicates bleeding from the oesophagus, stomach or duodenum. The most common cause is acute or chronic peptic ulceration. Less often, right-sided colonic bleeding and (rarely) small bowel bleeding can cause melaena. The differential diagnosis of dark stools includes ingestion of iron tablets, bismuth, liquorice or charcoal. However, these tend to result in small well-formed non-tarry stools and the offensive smell is absent.

Bright Red Blood (Haematochezia)

This appearance usually results from haemorrhage from the rectum or left colon. Blood loss may result from a carcinoma or polyp, an arteriovenous malformation, inflammatory bowel disease or diverticular disease. Beetroot ingestion can sometimes cause confusion. It can occasionally occur with massive upper gastrointestinal bleeding. The blood is mixed in with the bowel motion if it comes from above the anorectum, but if blood appears on the surface of the motion or only on the lavatory paper, this suggests, but does not guarantee, that bleeding is from a local rectal cause such as internal haemorrhoids or a fissure. Dark red jelly-like stools may be seen with ischaemic bowel.

Steatorrhoea

The stools are usually very pale, offensive, smelly and bulky. They float and are difficult to flush away. However, the commonest cause of floating stools is gas and water rather than fat.

Steatorrhoea results from malabsorption of fat. In severe pancreatic disease oil (triglycerides) may be passed per rectum and this is virtually pathognomonic of pancreatic steatorrhoea.

'Toothpaste' Stools

Here the faeces are expressed like toothpaste from a tube: the condition is usually due to severe constipation with overflow diarrhoea. It may, however, also occur in the irritable bowel syndrome, with a stricture or in Hirschsprung's disease.

Rice-water Stools

Cholera causes massive excretion of fluid and electrolytes from the bowel, which results in a severe secretory diarrhoea. The pale watery stools are of enormous volume and contain mucous debris.

Vomitus

The clinician who is fortunate enough to have vomitus available for inspection (ill-informed staff may throw out this valuable substance) should not lose the opportunity of a detailed examination. There are a number of interesting types of vomitus.

'Coffee-ground'

Old blood clot in vomitus has the appearance of the dregs of a good cup of coffee. Unfortunately, all darker vomitus is often described as having this appearance. This emphasises the need for personal inspection. Iron tablets and red wine can also have the same effect on the vomitus, not to mention coffee ingestion.

Bright Red Blood (Haematemesis)

Look for the presence of fresh clot. It indicates fresh bleeding from the upper gastrointestinal tract.

Yellow-green Vomitus

This results from the vomiting of bile and upper small bowel contents, often when there is obstruction.

Faeculent Vomiting

Here brown offensive material from the small bowel is vomited. It is a late sign of small intestinal obstruction. Recently ingested tea can have the same appearance but lacks the smell.

Brownish-black fluid in large volumes may be vomited in cases of acute dilatation of the stomach. A succussion splash will usually be present. Acute dilatation may occur in association with diabetic ketoacidosis or following abdominal surgery. It represents a medical emergency because of the risk of aspiration; there is a need for urgent placement of a nasogastric tube (page 196).

Projectile Vomiting

This term describes the act of vomiting itself and may indicate pyloric stenosis. It may also occur with raised intracranial pressure.

Urinalysis

Note that testing of the urine can be very helpful in diagnosing liver disease.

Strip colour tests can detect bilirubin and urobilinogen in the urine. False-positive or negative results can occur with vitamin C or even exposure to sunlight.

An understanding of the reasons for the presence of bilirubin or urobilinogen in the urine necessitates an explanation of the metabolism of these substances (Figure 5.19).

Red blood cells are broken down by the reticuloendothelial system causing the release of haem, which is converted to biliverdin and then *unconjugated bilirubin*, a water-insoluble compound. For this reason unconjugated bilirubin

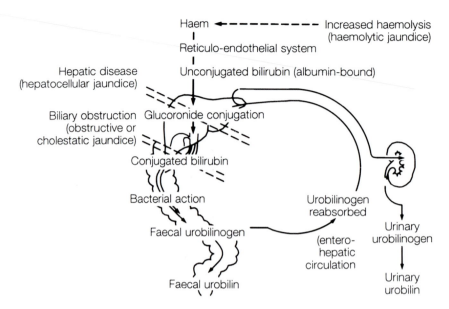

Figure 5.19 *Bile pigment pathway and the enterohepatic circulation.*

From Bouchier IAD, Morris JS, editors. Clinical skills. A system of clinical examination. 2nd ed. London: WB Saunders, 1982, with permission.

released with haemolytic anaemia will not appear in the urine (termed *acholuric jaundice*).

Unconjugated bilirubin is transported in the blood bound largely to albumin, but also to other plasma proteins. Unconjugated bilirubin is then taken up by the liver cells and transported to the endoplasmic reticulum, where glucuronyl transferases conjugate bilirubin with glucuronide. This results in the formation of *conjugated bilirubin* which is water-soluble. Conjugated bilirubin is then concentrated and excreted by the liver cell into the canaliculus.

Conjugated bilirubin is virtually all excreted into the small bowel; it is converted in the terminal ileum and colon to *urobilinogen*, and then to *stercobilin*. Stercobilin is responsible for the normal colour of the stools with other non-bilirubinoid dietary pigments. Up to 20% of urobilinogen is reabsorbed by the bowel, and small amounts are excreted in the urine as urinary urobilinogen. This can often be normally detected by reagent strips.

Total biliary obstruction from whatever cause results in absence of urinary urobilinogen, as no conjugated bilirubin reaches the bowel resulting in pale stools (absence of stercobilin). The conjugated bilirubin, unable to be excreted (the rate-limiting step), leaks from the hepatocytes into the blood and from there is excreted into the urine (normally there is no bilirubin detected in urine). This results in dark urine (excess conjugated bilirubin). Acute liver damage, as in viral hepatitis, may sometimes initially result in excessive urinary urobilinogen because the liver is unable to re-excrete the urobilinogen reabsorbed from the bowel. These changes are summarised in Table 5.19.

Table 5.19 *Changes in Urine and Faeces with Jaundice*

Substance and Site	Cause of Jaundice		
	Haemolysis	Obstruction or Cholestasis	Hepatocellular Liver Disease
Urine			
Bilirubin (conjugated)	Normal*	Raised	Normal or raised
Urobilinogen	Raised	Absent or decreased	Normal or raised
Faeces			
Stercobilinogen	Raised	Absent or decreased	Normal
Causes	Haemolytic anaemia	Extrahepatic biliary obstruction (e.g., gall-stones, carcinoma of pancreas or bile duct, strictures of the bile duct), intrahepatic cholestasis (e.g., drugs, recurrent jaundice of pregnancy)	Hepatitis, cirrhosis, drugs, venous obstruction

* Unconjugated bilirubin levels are elevated in the serum.

Examination of the Acute Abdomen

It is very important to try to determine whether a patient who presents with acute abdominal pain requires an urgent operation or whether careful observation with reassessment is the best course of action. An operation is most often indicated in those patients who clinically have peritonitis or major blood loss.

Assess the patient's *vital signs* (pulse rate, blood pressure, respiratory rate and temperature) immediately and recheck these at frequent intervals. Signs of a reduced circulating blood volume progressing to shock (page 19) include tachycardia, orthostatic hypotension, tachypnoea, peripheral vasoconstriction and sweating; with sepsis there is also usually a fever. Shock may occur with major gastrointestinal bleeding, severe acute pancreatitis, a ruptured aortic aneurysm or sepsis. Severe sepsis most frequently follows a perforated viscus and subsequent generalised peritonitis.

Inspect the abdomen. Look particularly for lack of movement with respiration, distension, visible peristalsis of bowel loops (in bowel obstruction) and for hernias or masses.

Palpate very gently to assess if there is tenderness or rigidity and whether these signs are localised or generalised (Table 5.20). Do not miss a pulsatile mass in the epigastrium (abdominal aortic aneurysm). In the patient with a very tender abdomen, testing for rebound tenderness by palpation is unnecessary (and cruel); in such a case, *percuss* lightly over any areas of tenderness to determine if this produces pain (a sign of peritonitis).

Examine for hernias. If a hernia is found, determine if this is tender or reducible. A tender, reducible hernia can occur in peritonitis (because the hernial sac con-

Table 5.20 *Differential Diagnosis of the Acute Abdomen*

Severe abdominal pain with rigidity of the entire abdominal wall and prostration

Perforated peptic ulcer
Perforation of other intra-abdominal organs
Dissecting aneurysm
Severe pancreatitis

Tenderness and rigidity in the right hypochondrium

Acute cholecystitis
Appendicitis in a high appendix
Perforated or penetrating duodenal ulcer
Pleurisy, pneumonitis
Subphrenic abscess
Acute pyelonephritis
Cholangitis
Bleed into an hepatic tumour

Tenderness and rigidity in the left hypochondrium

Pancreatitis
Subphrenic abscess
Diverticulitis
Ruptured spleen
Acute pyelonephritis
Leaking aneurysm of the splenic artery
Acute gastric distension

Tenderness and rigidity in the right iliac fossa

Appendicitis
Perforated or penetrating duodenal ulcer
Crohn's disease or inflamed ileocaecal glands
Inflamed Meckel's diverticulum
Cholecystitis with a low gallbladder

Tenderness and rigidity in the left iliac fossa

Diverticulitis
Colitis
Colonic cancer
Pelvic peritonitis, ruptured ovarian cyst

Periumbilical pain without abdominal signs

Acute small bowel ischaemia
Acute appendicitis
Acute small bowel obstruction
Acute pancreatitis

Obstetric and gynaecological causes

Ectopic pregnancy
Torsion of, or haemorrhage into, an ovarian cyst
Acute salpingitis
Ruptured uterus

tains peritoneum). A tender non-reducible hernia suggests bowel obstruction; however, a femoral hernia causing small bowel obstruction may not be tender.

Auscultate for bowel sounds which may be louder, more high pitched and tinkling in bowel obstruction or absent in ileus.

Rectal and vaginal examinations are essential; note any tenderness (and its location), masses or blood loss. A purulent vaginal discharge suggests salpingitis.

Urinalysis may show glycosuria and ketonuria in diabetic ketoacidosis (which can cause acute abdominal pain), haematuria in renal colic, bilirubinuria in cholangitis or proteinuria in pyelonephritis (page 212).

Examine the *respiratory system* for signs of consolidation, a pleural rub or pleural effusion, and examine the *cardiovascular system* for atrial fibrillation (a major cause of embolism to a mesenteric artery) or signs of myocardial infarction. Examine the *back* for evidence of spinal disease that may radiate to the abdomen.

Note: Herpes zoster may cause abdominal pain before the typical vesicles erupt.

Correlation of Physical Signs and Gastrointestinal Disease

Liver Disease

Signs of chronic liver disease include:
Hands: leuconychia, clubbing, palmar erythema, bruising, asterixis.
Face: jaundice, scratch marks, spider naevi, fetor hepaticus.
Chest: gynaecomastia, loss of body hair, spider naevi, bruising, pectoral muscle wasting.
Abdomen: hepatosplenomegaly, ascites, signs of portal hypertension, testicular atrophy.
Legs: oedema, muscle wasting, bruising.
Fever: may occur in up to one-third of patients with advanced cirrhosis (particularly when this is secondary to alcohol) or if there is infected ascites.

The presence of three or more of the following signs strongly suggests cirrhosis: (i) spider naevi; (ii) palmar erythema; (iii) hepatomegaly (firm, non-tender, irregular edge); (iv) splenomegaly or ascites; (v) abnormal collateral veins on the abdomen.

Portal Hypertension

Signs

Splenomegaly: correlates poorly with the degree of portal hypertension.
Collateral veins: haematemesis (from oesophageal or gastric varices).
Ascites.

Causes of Portal Hypertension

1. Cirrhosis of the liver
2. Other causes:
    (a) **Presinusoidal**: (i) portal vein compression (e.g., lymphoma, carcinoma); (ii) intravascular clotting (e.g., in polycythaemia); (iii) umbilical vein phlebitis.
    (b) **Intrahepatic**: (i) sarcoid, lymphoma or leukaemic infiltrates; (ii) congenital hepatic fibrosis.
    (c) **Postsinusoidal**: (i) hepatic vein outflow obstruction (Budd-Chiari syndrome) may be idiopathic, or caused by myeloproliferative disease, can-

cer (kidney, pancreas, liver), the contraceptive pill or pregnancy, paroxysmal nocturnal haemoglobinuria (PNH), fibrous membrane, trauma, schistosomiasis; (ii) veno-occlusive disease; (iii) constrictive pericarditis; (iv) chronic cardiac failure.

Hepatic Encephalopathy

Grading

Grade 0: normal mental state.
Grade 1: mental changes (lack of awareness, anxiety, euphoria, reduced attention span, impaired ability to add and subtract).
Grade 2: lethargy, disorientation (for time), personality changes, inappropriate behaviour.
Grade 3: stupor, but responsive to stimuli; gross disorientation, confusion.
Grade 4: coma.

Causes of Hepatic Encephalopathy

These include: (i) acute liver failure (e.g., post-viral hepatitis, alcoholic hepatitis); (ii) cirrhosis; and (iii) chronic portosystemic encephalopathy, e.g., from a portocaval shunt.

Encephalopathy may be precipitated by: (i) diarrhoea, diuretics or vomiting (resulting in hypokalaemia which may increase renal ammonia and other toxin production, or alkalosis which may increase the amount of ammonia and other toxins that cross the blood-brain barrier); (ii) gastrointestinal bleeding or a relatively high protein diet (causing an acute increase in nitrogenous contents in the bowel); (iii) infection (e.g., urinary tract, chest or spontaneous bacterial peritonitis); (iv) acute liver cell decompensation (e.g., from an alcoholic binge or a hepatoma); (v) sedatives; (vi) metabolic disturbances such as hypoglycaemia.

Dysphagia

Dysphagia (difficulty in swallowing) and odynophagia (pain on swallowing) are important symptoms of underlying organic disease. It is important to examine such patients carefully for likely causes (see Table 5.2).

Signs

General inspection: note weight loss, due to decreased food intake or oesophageal cancer *per se*.

The hands: inspect the nails for koilonychia (page 224), and the palmar creases for pallor indicative of anaemia. Iron deficiency anaemia can be associated with an upper oesophageal web, which is a thin structure consisting of mucosa and submucosa but not muscle. Iron deficiency anaemia and dysphagia due to an upper oesophageal web is called the Plummer-Vinson*(/)Paterson-Brown-Kelly[†] syndrome. Also examine the hands for signs of scleroderma (page 281).

---

* Henry Plummer (1874–1936), Physician at the Mayo Clinic, Porter Vinson (1890–1959), Physician, Medical College Virginia, described the syndrome in 1921.

[†] Donald Paterson (1863–1939), Cardiff otolaryngologist, and Adam Brown-Kelly (1865–1941), Glasgow otolaryngologist, described this syndrome in 1919.

The mouth: inspect the mucosa for ulceration or infection (e.g., candidiasis) which can cause odynophagia. Examine the lower cranial nerves for evidence of bulbar or pseudobulbar palsy (page 366).

The neck: palpate the supraclavicular nodes, which may occasionally be involved with oesophageal cancer (page 229). Examine for evidence of retrosternal thyroid enlargement (page 296). A mass on the left side of the neck which is accompanied by gurgling sounds may rarely be caused by a Zenker's* diverticulum, an outpouching of the posterior hypopharyngeal wall.

The lungs: examine for evidence of aspiration into the lungs (due to overflow of retained material, gastro-oesophageal reflux or, rarely, the development of a tracheo-oesophageal reflux from oesophageal cancer).

The abdomen: feel for hepatomegaly due to secondary deposits from oesophageal cancer and for an epigastric mass from a gastric cancer. Perform a rectal examination to exclude melaena (albeit uncommon with oesophageal disease).

Assessment of Gastrointestinal Bleeding

Haematemesis, melaena or massive rectal bleeding are dramatic signs of gastrointestinal haemorrhage. It is important in such a case to assess the amount of blood loss and attempt to determine the likely site of bleeding. Haematemesis indicates bleeding from a site proximal to, or in, the duodenum.

Assessing Degree of Blood Loss

First take the pulse rate and the blood pressure lying and sitting. As a general rule loss of one-and-a-half litres or more of blood volume over a few hours results in a fall in cardiac output causing hypotension and tachycardia. A pulse rate of more than 100 a minute or a systolic blood pressure of less than 100 mmHg , or a 15 mmHg postural fall in systolic blood pressure, suggests significant recent blood loss. These are indications for blood transfusion. The signs depend to some extent on the state of the patient's cardiovascular system. Those with pre-existing cardiovascular disease will become shocked much earlier than young fit patients with a normal cardiovascular system.

Once signs of shock are present massive blood loss has occurred. These signs include peripheral cyanosis with cold extremities, clammy skin, dyspnoea and air hunger; the patients are anxious. The blood pressure is low, with a compensating tachycardia, and the urine output is reduced or absent. These are ominous signs in patients with gastrointestinal haemorrhage. Urgent resuscitative measures must be instituted.

Determining the Possible Bleeding Site

The causes of acute gastrointestinal haemorrhage are listed in Table 5.3.

Examine the patient with **acute upper gastrointestinal bleeding** for signs of chronic liver disease and portal hypertension. Part of the assessment should include inspection of the vomitus and stools (page 182) and a rectal examination. Remember that, of patients with chronic liver disease and upper gastrointestinal bleeding, only about half are bleeding from varices. The others are usually bleeding from peptic ulceration (either acute or chronic). Look for evidence of a bleeding diathesis.

---

* Friedrich Albert Zenker (b. 1825), Erlangen pathologist.

Finally, examine the patient for any evidence of skin lesions that can be associated with vascular anomalies in the gastrointestinal tract, though these are rare (Tables 5.3, 5.4). For example, pseudoxanthoma elasticum is an autosomal recessive disorder of elastic fibres which results in xanthoma-like yellowish nodules, particularly in the axillae or neck. These patients may also have angioid streaks of the optic fundus (page 309) and angiomatous malformations of blood vessels which can bleed into the gastrointestinal tract. Ehlers-Danlos syndrome is a group of connective tissue disorders resulting in fragile and hyperextensible skin. In a number of types blood vessels are involved. Type IV is characterised by gastrointestinal tract bleeding, spontaneous bowel perforation, minimal skin hyperelasticity and minimal joint hyperextension.

Examine the patient with **acute lower gastrointestinal bleeding** as described above paying close attention to the abdominal examination and the rectal examination. Inspect the stools and test them for blood. Sigmoidoscopy is essential in all these patients.

Malabsorption

Numerous diseases can cause maldigestion or malabsorption of food. Fat, protein and/or carbohydrate absorption may be affected.

Signs of Malabsorption

General: wasting (protein and fat malabsorption), folds of loose skin (recent weight loss), pallor (anaemia) or pigmentation (e.g., Whipple's disease).

   Stools: steatorrhoea (pale, bulky and offensive stools).

   Mouth: glossitis and angular stomatitis (vitamin B_2, B_6, B_{12}, folate or niacin deficiency), intra-oral purpura (vitamin K deficiency) or hyperkeratotic white patches (vitamin A deficiency).

   Limbs: bruising (vitamin K deficiency), oedema (protein deficiency), peripheral neuropathy (vitamin B_{12} or thiamine deficiency), rash, bone pain (vitamin D deficiency).

   Signs suggesting the underlying cause: in the abdomen these include scars from previous surgery, such as a gastrectomy, operations for Crohn's disease or massive small bowel resection; on the skin dermatitis herpetiformis (itchy red lumps on the extensor surfaces) may be found—this condition is strongly associated with coeliac disease and the histocompatibility antigen HLA-B8; there may be *signs of chronic liver disease*; or *signs of inflammatory bowel disease*.

Causes of Malabsorption

Common causes include coeliac disease, chronic pancreatitis, and a previous gastrectomy.

Classification of Malabsorption

Lipolytic phase defects (pancreatic enzyme deficiency): (i) chronic pancreatitis; (ii) cystic fibrosis.

   Micellar phase defects (bile salt deficiency): (i) extrahepatic biliary obstruction; (ii) chronic liver disease; (iii) bacterial overgrowth; (iv) terminal ileal disease such as Crohn's disease or resection.

Mucosal defects (diseased epithelial lining): (i) coeliac disease; (ii) tropical sprue; (iii) lymphoma; (iv) Whipple's disease*; (v) bowel ischaemia or resection; (vi) amyloidosis; (vii) hypogammaglobulinaemia; (viii) AIDS.

Delivery phase defects (inability to transport fat out of cells to lymphatics): (i) intestinal lymphangiectasia; (ii) abetalipoproteinaemia; (iii) carcinomatous infiltration of lymphatics.

Inflammatory Bowel Disease

Inflammatory bowel disease refers to two chronic idiopathic diseases of the gastrointestinal tract, ulcerative colitis and Crohn's disease.

Ulcerative Colitis

In the gastrointestinal tract only the large bowel is affected. Occasionally the terminal ileum can be secondarily involved (backwash ileitis). The disease almost always involves the rectum and may extend, without skip areas, to involve a variable part of the colon.

Abdominal signs: if there is proctitis only, there are usually no abnormal external findings (except at sigmoidoscopy and biopsy). Occasionally, anal fissures may be present.

With colitis, in the uncomplicated case the abdominal examination may be normal or there may be tenderness and guarding over the affected colon.

Signs of complications: local signs include the following: (i) *toxic dilatation (megacolon)*—one of the most feared complications in which there are signs of distension, generalised guarding and rigidity (peritonism), pyrexia and tachycardia; (ii) *massive bleeding or perforation*; (iii) *carcinoma*—there is an increased incidence of colonic cancer in extensive, long-standing ulcerative colitis.

Systemic signs include: (i) *chronic liver disease*—primary sclerosing cholangitis or cirrhosis; (ii) *anaemia*—due to chronic disease *per se*, or blood loss, or autoimmune haemolysis; (iii) *arthritis*—there may be a peripheral non-deforming arthropathy affecting particularly the knees, ankles and wrists (10%), and there may be signs of ankylosing spondylitis in 3%; (iv) *skin manifestations*—• erythema nodosum (2%) consists of tender red nodules usually on the shins (Figure 5.20), • pyoderma gangrenosum (rare) starts as a tender red raised area which becomes bullous and ulcerates (Figure 5.21); it may occur anywhere but is often on the anterior aspects of the legs; • mouth ulcers are common and are due to aphthous ulceration (5%); • finger clubbing may be present; (v) *ocular changes* include conjunctivitis, iritis and episcleritis, which are strongly associated with arthritis and skin rash. Conjunctivitis is an inflammation of the conjunctiva which then appears red and swollen. The eye itself is not tender. Iritis is an inflammation of the iris with central scleral injection, which radiates out from the pupil and the eye is tender. Episcleritis is a nodule of inflammation on the scleral surface.

Crohn's Disease

The whole of the gastrointestinal tract may be affected from the mouth to the anus. However, most commonly the terminal ileum, with or without the colon, is involved.

---

* George Hoyt Whipple (b. 1878), Baltimore pathologist, described this rare disease characterised by diarrhoea, arthralgia, central nervous system signs and pigmentation.

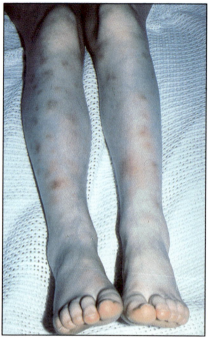

Figure 5.20   *Erythema nodosum.*   **Figure 5.21**   *Pyoderma gangrenosum.*

Abdominal signs: if the condition affects only the terminal ileum there are often no abnormal findings, although tenderness, fullness or a mass (either soft or firm) in the right iliac fossa may be present. Occasionally there may be signs of an abdominal abscess: these patients may have a high swinging fever, localised tenderness, a palpable mass, and evidence of bowel obstruction (pain, vomiting and constipation with dehydration, abdominal distension and tenderness, and an empty rectum).

Anal disease occurs in up to 75% of patients with small bowel disease and in up to 95% with large bowel disease. The commonly associated conditions are fissures, fistulae and abscesses.

Colonic involvement produces the same signs as ulcerative colitis.

Signs of complications: these are similar to those of ulcerative colitis with the following exceptions. (i) *Liver disease*—primary sclerosing cholangitis is less common. (ii) *Osteomalacia*, which may occur in patients with extensive terminal ileal involvement, results in bone tenderness and fracture. (iii) *Signs of malabsorption*. (iv) *Finger clubbing* is more common. (v) *Signs of gastrointestinal malignancy* (small bowel or colonic carcinoma) are uncommon but the incidence is increased. (vi) The incidence of *gallstones and renal stones* is increased. (vii) *Renal disease* due to pyelonephritis, hydronephrosis or very rarely secondary amyloidosis may occur.

The Abdominal X-ray: A Systematic Approach

Interpretation of the plain radiograph requires knowledge of basic anatomy and pathological processes.

The soft tissue density of the abdominal organs is similar to that of water. Therefore they are usually not visible unless outlined by fat or adjacent gas. For example, fluid-filled bowel is not visible, but the bowel walls are outlined by the contained gas.

Because of this intrinsic lack of contrast in the abdomen, radio-opaque contrast media are introduced to show up various organs. Barium meals, barium enemas, oral cholecystograms, intravenous urograms and arteriograms are contrast studies.

Radiography

As with the chest X-ray the name and date should be checked. The left and right sides should be easily distinguished by the stomach gas on the left and the triangular bulky soft tissue of the liver seen in the right hypochondrium.

Review of an Abdominal X-ray

Boundaries: diaphragm, psoas muscles, the extraperitoneal fat ('flank lines').
Bones: lower ribs and costal cartilages, lumbar spine, pelvis.
Hollow viscera gas: check gas outlining the stomach, small bowel and large bowel.
Solid organs: size of liver, spleen and kidneys.
Pelvic organs: bladder size.
Vascular: aortic calcification.
Abnormalities: renal or biliary calculi, dilated bowel, free peritoneal gas (Figure 5.22).

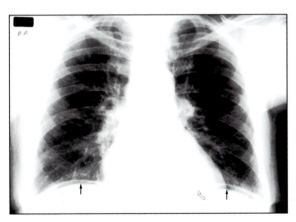

Figure 5.22 *Free peritoneal gas. The erect chest X-ray is superior to an erect abdominal film for the demonstration of free gas.*

On the erect chest X-ray, free peritoneal gas is seen below the hemidiaphragm (black arrows). The free gas on the left must be distinguished from gas in the gastric fundus (open arrow). This free gas (black arrow) on the left is crescentic in shape because it outlines the spleen and lies at the apex of the hemidiaphragm. It indicates a perforation of a hollow abdominal viscus unless there has been recent surgery or penetrating trauma.

Bowel Gas Pattern

Supine films are taken in most conditions to show the distribution of the bowel gas. In patients with an acute abdomen, a horizontal beam film, usually an erect view, is also taken to show air-fluid levels.

With obstruction, there is an accumulation of fluid and gas proximally.

In inflammatory or ischaemic colitis the swollen bowel mucosa will be outlined by gas ('thumb-printing').

Bowel Dilatation

When an ileus (Figure 5.23) or obstruction (Figures 5.24, 5.25) is present, it is possible to distinguish small from large bowel dilatation. The *large bowel loops* are peripheral, few in number, have diameters greater than 5cm, contain faeces, and have haustral margins which do not extend across the bowel lumen. In contrast, the *small bowel loops* are central, multiple, between 3 and 5cm in diameter, and do not contain faeces. Valvulae conniventes which extend completely across the bowel lumen are seen in the jejunal loops.

With gastric dilatation the stomach may be massively enlarged and distended with air (Figure 5.26).

Calcification

Calcification shows up well against the grey soft tissue densities.

About 90% of renal stones are calcified (Figure 6.1, page 208), whereas only 10% of gallstones are calcified. To show radiolucent gallstones, an ultrasound examination is the test of choice.

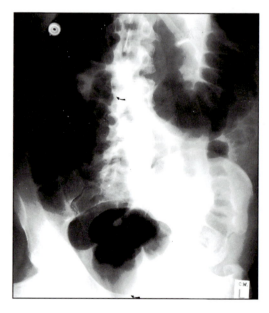

Figure 5.23   *Generalised ileus. The large bowel is filled with gas and is dilated except in the descending colon. Dilated small bowel is also seen in the right hypochondrium (arrow).*
    Since gas is seen around to the rectum (arrow), mechanical obstruction is excluded.

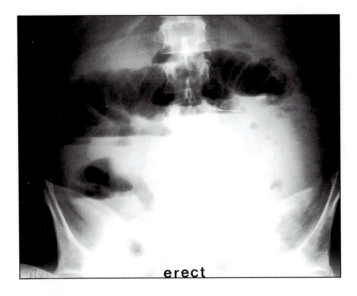

erect

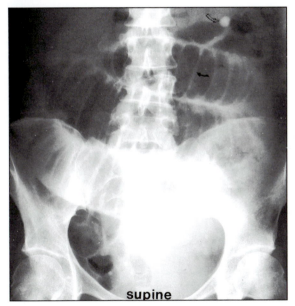

supine

Figure 5.24 *Small bowel obstruction. There is gross dilatation of the small bowel. It is recognised as small bowel from its central position and its transverse mucosal bands—the valvulae conniventes (black arrow).*

Air-fluid levels are seen on the erect view. The supine view gives a better view of the distribution of the dilated loops. From the number and position of the displayed dilated loops, the obstruction would be at the level of the mid-small bowel.

The round radio-opaque shadow in the left hypochondrium is a tablet (open arrow).

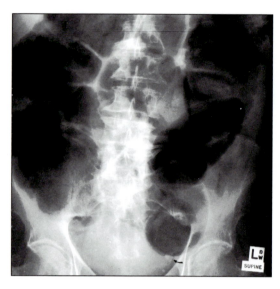

Figure 5.25

Large bowel obstruction. The large bowel is markedly distended around to the sigmoid colon where it abruptly stops (arrow). The common causes of obstruction are carcinoma or diverticular stricture.

The increased peristalsis occurring at the onset of obstruction can remove the gas and faeces distal to the obstruction. Therefore no gas is seen in this patient.

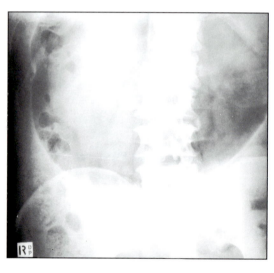

Figure 5.26

Gastric dilatation. The stomach is massively enlarged and distended with air. When this occurs acutely, prompt nasogastric aspiration is necessary.

Mechanical obstruction due to a pyloric ulcer or carcinoma needs exclusion. Atonic dilatation is usually a postoperative complication, but may occur with diabetic coma, trauma, pancreatitis or hypokalaemia.

Calcification may be seen in the pancreas in chronic pancreatitis (Figure 5.27).

Costal cartilage calcification is commonly seen in elderly patients, projected over the hypochondrial regions.

Calcification in the walls of an abdominal aortic aneurysm may be seen on a lateral abdominal film. Splenic and renal artery aneurysms are also often calcified.

Vascular calcification is often seen in the elderly.

Ascites

With accumulation of peritoneal fluid within the peritoneal cavity, the film looks generally grey and lacks detail. On the supine film the bowel loops float towards the middle of the abdomen.

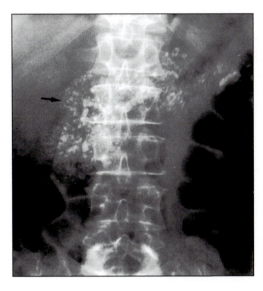

Figure 5.27

Pancreatic calcification. Stippled calcification is seen in the region of the pancreas (arrow), indicating chronic calcific pancreatitis. The most likely cause is alcohol excess.

Summary

The Gastrointestinal Examination: A Suggested Method
(Figure 5.28)

Position the patient correctly with one pillow for the head and complete exposure of the abdomen. Look briefly at the general appearance and inspect particularly for signs of chronic liver disease.

Examine the hands. Ask the patient to extend his or her arms and hands and look for hepatic flap. Look also at the nails for clubbing and for white nails and note any palmar erythema or Dupuytren's contractures. The arthropathy of haemochromatosis may also be present. Look now at the arms for bruising, scratch marks and spider naevi.

Then go to the face. Note any scleral abnormality (jaundice, anaemia or iritis). Look at the corneas for Kayser-Fleischer rings. Feel for parotid enlargement, then inspect the mouth with a torch and spatula for angular stomatitis, ulceration, telangiectasias and atrophic glossitis. Smell the breath for fetor hepaticus. Now look at the chest for spider naevi and in men for gynaecomastia and loss of body hair.

Inspect the abdomen from the side, squatting to the patient's level. Large masses may be visible. Ask the patient to take slow deep breaths and look especially for the hepatic, splenic and gallbladder outlines. Now stand up and look for scars, distension, prominent veins, striae, hernia, bruising and pigmentation.

Palpate lightly in each region for masses, having asked first if any area is particularly tender. This will avoid causing the patient pain and may also provide a clue to a site of possible pathology. Next palpate more deeply each region, then feel specifically for hepatomegaly and splenomegaly. If there is hepatomegaly confirm this with percussion and estimate the span. This procedure is repeated for splenomegaly. Always roll the patient on to the right side and palpate again if the

Figure 5.28 *Gastrointestinal system*

Lying flat (1 pillow)

GENERAL INSPECTION
  Jaundice (liver disease)
  Pigmentation
      (haemóchromatosis,
      Whipple's disease)
  Xanthomata
      (chronic cholestasis)
  Mental state
      (encephalopathy)

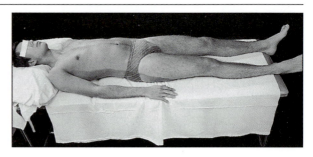

HANDS
  Nails—Clubbing
      —Leuconychia
  Palmar erythema
  Dupuytren's contractures (alcohol)
  Arthropathy
  Hepatic flap

ARMS
  Spider naevi
  Bruising
  Wasting
  Scratch marks (chronic cholestasis)

FACE
  Eyes—Sclera: jaundice, anaemia, iritis
      —Cornea: Kayser-Fleischer rings
      (Wilson's disease)
  Parotids (alcohol)
  Mouth—Breath: fetor hepaticus
      —Lips: stomatitis, leucoplakia,
      ulceration, localised pigmentation
      (Peutz-Jeghers syndrome),
      telangiectasia (hereditary
      haemorrhagic telangiectasia)
      —Gums: gingivitis, bleeding,
      hypertrophy, pigmentation, monilia
      —Tongue: atrophic glossitis,
      leucoplakia, ulceration

CERVICAL/AXILLARY LYMPH NODES

CHEST
  Gynaecomastia
  Spider naevi
  Body hair

ABDOMEN
  Inspect
    Scars
    Distension

  Prominent veins—determine direction of
      flow (caput Medusae; IVC obstruction)
    Striae
    Bruising
    Pigmentation
    Localised masses
    Visible peristalsis
  Papate
    Superficial palpation—tenderness,
      rigidity, outline of any mass
    Deep palpation—organomegaly (liver,
      spleen, kidney), abnormal masses
  Roll on to right side (spleen)
  Percuss
    Viscera outline
    Ascites—shifting dullness
  Auscultate
    Bowel sounds
    Bruits, hums
    Rubs

GROIN
  Genitalia
  Lymph nodes
  Hernial orifices (standing up)

LEGS
  Bruising
  Oedema
  Neurological signs (alcohol)

OTHER
  Rectal examination (PR)—inspect (fistulae,
      tags, blood, mucus), palpate (masses)
  Urine analysis (bile)
  Blood pressure (renal disease)
  Cardiovascular system (cardiomyopathy,
      cardiac failure
  Temperature chart (infection)

spleen is not felt initially. Attempt now to feel the kidneys bimanually. Remember the important distinguishing features of a spleen as opposed to a kidney.

Percuss routinely for ascites. If the abdomen is resonant right out to the flanks do not roll the patient over. Otherwise test for shifting dullness. This is performed by percussing away from your side of the bed until you reach a dull note. Then roll the patient towards you and, after waiting a minute or so, begin percussing again for resonance.

By auscultation note the presence of bowel sounds, listening for bruits, hums and rubs. Always also auscultate briefly over the liver, spleen and renal areas.

Examine the groins next. Palpate for inguinal lymphadenopathy. Examine for hernias by asking the patient to stand and then cough. The testes must always be palpated. Now look at the legs for oedema and bruising. Neurological examination of the legs may be indicated if there are signs of chronic liver disease.

If the liver is enlarged or cirrhosis is suspected the patient should be sat up to 45 degrees and the jugular venous pressure estimated. This will avoid missing constrictive pericarditis or chronic cardiac failure as a cause of liver disease, or haemochromatosis which can cause a dilated cardiomyopathy. While the patient is sitting up palpate in the supraclavicular fossae for lymph nodes and feel at the back for sacral oedema. If ascites is present it is necessary to examine the chest for a pleural effusion. If malignant disease is suspected, examine all lymph node groups, the breasts and the lungs.

A rectal examination should always be performed and specimens of the patient's vomitus or faeces should be inspected if available. Perform a urinalysis (for bilirubin and urobilinogen, and glucose) and check the temperature.

Suggested Reading

Original and Review Articles

Chervu A, Clagett GP, Valentine RJ, Myers SI. Rossi PJ, Role of physical examination in detection of abdominal aortic aneurysms. *Surgery* 1995; 117: 454–7.

Drossman DA, Talley NJ, Leserman J, Olden KW, Barreiro MA, Sexual and physical abuse and gastrointestinal illness. Review and recommendations. *Ann Intern Med* 1995; 123: 782–94.

Editorial. Abdominal wall tenderness test: could Carnett cut costs? *Lancet* 1991; 337: 1134.

Espinoza P, Ducot B, Pelletier G, et al. Interobserver agreement in the physical diagnosis of alcoholic liver disease. *Dig Dis Sci* 1987; 32: 244–247.

Hendrix TR, Art and science of history taking in the patient with difficulty swallowing. *Dysphagia* 1993; 8: 69–73.

Muris JW, Starmans R, Wolfs GG, Pop P, Knottnerus JA, The diagnostic value of rectal examination. *Family Practice* 1993; 10: 34–7.

Murtagh J, Acute abdominal pain: a diagnostic approach. *Aust Fam Phys* 1994; 23: 358–61, 364–74.

Naylor CD, Physical examination of the liver. *JAMA* 1994; 271: 1859–65.

Rosen L. Physical examination of the anorectum: a systematic technique. *Dis Colon Rectum* 1990; 33: 439–440.

Sharpstone D, Colin-Jones DG, Chronic, non-visceral abdominal pain. *Gut* 1994; 35: 833–6.

Sherman HI, Hardison JE. The importance of a coexistent hepatic rub and bruit: a clue to the diagnosis of cancer in the liver. *JAMA* 1979; 241: 1495.

Theodossi A, Knill-Jones RP, Skene A. Interobserver variation of symptoms and signs in jaundice. *Liver* 1981; 1: 21–32.

Walton S, Bennett JR. Skin and gullet. *Gut* 1991; 32: 694–697.

Williams JW Jr, Simel DL. Does this patient have ascites? How to divine fluid in the abdomen. *JAMA* 1992; 267: 2645–2648.

Zoli M, Magalotti D, Grimaldi M, Gueli C, Marchesini G, Pisi E, Physical examination of the liver: is it still worth it? *Am J Gastroenterol* 1995; 90: 1428–32.

Textbooks

Ellis H, Calne RY. Lecture notes on general surgery. 8th ed. Oxford: Blackwell, 1993.

Sherlock S. Diseases of the liver and biliary system. 9th ed. Oxford: Blackwell, 1994.

Silen W. Cope's early diagnosis of the acute abdomen. 18th ed. New York: Oxford University Press, 1991.

Sleisenger MH, Fordtran JS, editors. Gastrointestinal disease. 6th ed. Philadelphia: Saunders, 1997.

Talley NJ, Martin CJ, editors. Clinical gastroenterology. A practical problem-based approach. MacLennan & Petty, 1996.

Yamada T, editor. Textbook of gastroenterology. 2nd ed. Philadelphia: JB Lippincott, 1995.

Chapter 6

THE GENITOURINARY SYSTEM

You know my method. It is founded upon the observation of trifles.

Sherlock Holmes, created by Sir Arthur Conan Doyle (1859–1930)

The Genitourinary History

Presenting Symptoms (Table 6.1)

These may include a change in the appearance of the urine, abnormalities of micturition, suprapubic or flank pain or the systemic symptoms of renal failure. Some patients have no symptoms but are found to be hypertensive or to have abnormalities on routine urinalysis or serum biochemistry. Others may feel unwell without localising symptoms.

Change in Appearance of the Urine

Some patients present with discoloured urine. A red discoloration suggests haematuria (blood in the urine). Urethral inflammation or trauma, or prostatic disease, can cause haematuria at the beginning of micturition which then clears, or haematuria only at the end of micturition. Patients with porphyria can have urine which changes colour on standing. Consumption of certain drugs (e.g., rifampicin) or of large amounts of beetroot, and rarely, haemoglobinuria (due to destruction of red blood cells and release of free haemoglobin) can cause red discoloration of the urine (page 212). Patients with severe muscle trauma may have myoglobinuria as a result of muscle breakdown. This can also cause red discoloration. It is worth noting that the colour of the urine is not a reliable guide to its concentration.

Urinary Obstruction

Urinary obstruction is a common symptom in elderly men and is most often due to prostatism. The patient may have noticed hesitancy (difficulty starting micturition) followed by a decrease in the size of the stream of urine and terminal dribbling of urine. With complete obstruction, overflow incontinence of urine can occur. This is associated with an increased risk of urinary infection.

Renal calculi can cause ureteric obstruction. The presenting symptom here, however, is usually severe loin pain with radiation of the pain down towards the symphysis pubis or perineum or testis (renal colic). Other causes of urinary obstruction are presented in Table 6.2.

201

Table 6.1 *Genitourinary History*

Major Symptoms

Change in appearance of urine, e.g., haematuria, stones, gravel
Change in urine volume or stream
  Polyuria
  Nocturia
  Anuria
  Decrease in stream size
  Hesitancy
  Dribbling
  Urine retention
  Incontinence of urine
  Double voiding (incomplete bladder emptying)
  Renal colic
  Dysuria (painful micturition), frequency, urgency
  Fever, loin pain
  Urethral discharge
Symptoms suggestive of chronic renal failure (uraemia)
  Oliguria, nocturia, polyuria
  Anorexia, a metallic taste, vomiting, fatigue, hiccup, insomnia
  Itch, bruising, oedema
Menses
  Date of onset
  Regularity
  Last period (date)
  Dysmenorrhoea, menorrhagia
Impotence
Loss of libido
Infertility
Pregnancies: number and any complications
Urethral or vaginal discharge
Genital rash

Urinary Incontinence

This is the inability to hold urine in the bladder voluntarily. The problem can occur transiently with urinary tract infections, delirium, excess urine output (e.g. from the use of diuretics), immobility (because patients are unable to reach the toilet), atrophic urethritis or vaginitis, or stool impaction. Common causes of established urinary incontinence include: (i) *stress incontinence* (instantaneous leakage after the stress of coughing or after a sudden rise in intra-abdominal pressure of any cause)—this problem is more common in women; (ii) *overactivity of the detrusor muscle* (characterised by an intense urge to urinate and then leakage of urine in the absence of cough or other stressors)—this occurs in men and women; (iii) *detrusor underactivity*—this is rare and is characterised by urinary frequency, nocturia and the frequent leaking of small amounts of urine; and (iv) *urethral obstruction*—this occurs typically in men with disease of the prostate, and is characterised by dribbling incontinence after incomplete urination.

Table 6.2 *Causes of Acute Renal Failure*

This is defined as a rapid deterioration in renal function severe enough to cause accumulation of waste products, especially nitrogenous wastes, in the body. Usually the urine flow rate is less than 20mL/hour or 400mL/day, but occasionally it is normal or increased (high output renal failure).

Prerenal

Fluid loss: blood (haemorrhage), plasma or water and electrolytes (diarrhoea and
    vomiting, dehydration)
Hypotension: myocardial infarction, septicaemic shock, drugs
Renovascular disease: embolus, dissection or atheroma
Increased renal vascular resistance: hepatorenal syndrome

Renal

Acute-on-chronic renal failure (precipitated by infection, dehydration, obstruction or
    nephrotoxic drugs)—see Table 6.3
Acute renal disease:
  e.g., primary or secondary glomerulonephritis, connective tissue diseases
Acute tubular necrosis secondary to:
  ischaemia (hypovolaemia)
  toxins and drugs (e.g., aminoglycoside antibiotics, contrast material, heavy metals)
  rhabdomyolysis, haemoglobinuria
Tubulointerstitial disease:
  e.g., drugs (e.g., sulphonamides, cyclosporin A)
  urate or calcium deposits
Vascular disease:
  e.g., vasculitis, scleroderma
Myeloma
Acute pyelonephritis (rare)

Postrenal (complete urinary tract obstruction)

Urethral obstruction:
  calculus or blood clot, sloughed papillae, trauma, phimosis or paraphimosis
At the bladder neck:
  e.g., calculus or blood clot, prostatic hypertrophy or cancer
Bilateral ureteric obstruction:
  intraureteric, e.g., clot, pyogenic, debris, calculi
  extraureteric, e.g., retroperitoneal fibrosis (e.g., due to radiation, methysergide or
    idiopathic), pelvic tumour or surgery, uterine prolapse

NB: Anuria may be due to urinary obstruction, bilateral renal artery occlusion, rapidly progressive (crescentic) glomerulonephritis, renal cortical necrosis or a renal stone in a single kidney.

Chronic Renal Failure

The clinical features of chronic renal failure are due to the accumulation of 'uraemic toxins'. The symptoms of renal failure can be deduced in part by considering the normal functions of the kidneys.

1. Urinary concentrating ability is lost early, leading to the risk of dehydration; nocturia is thus an early symptom.
2. Failure to excrete sodium may lead to hypertension.
3. Damage to the renal tubules may lead to sodium loss and hypotension.

4. Excretion of potassium depends largely on urine volume. Hyperkalaemia usually becomes a problem when a patient is oliguric (passes less than 400mL of urine a day).

5. Failure of acid excretion leads to metabolic acidosis.

6. Failure to hydroxylate vitamin D_3 causes vitamin D deficiency, compensating (secondary) hyperparathyroidism and therefore a fall in serum calcium and rise in phosphate. This is responsible for renal bone disease.

7. Failure to excrete erythropoietin leads to normochromic normocytic anaemia.

Adequacy of renal function is defined by the glomerular filtration rate (GFR). This is the volume of blood filtered by the kidneys per unit of time. The normal range is 90-120mL/min. The GFR is estimated by calculating the clearance of creatinine (a normal breakdown product of muscle) from the blood. The serum creatinine and urea levels also provide a measure of accumulation of uraemic toxins and therefore of renal function.

A uraemic patient may present with anuria (defined as failure to pass more than 50mL urine daily), oliguria (<400mL urine daily), nocturia (the need to get up during the night to pass urine) or polyuria (the passing of abnormally large volumes of urine) (page 294). Nocturia may be an indication of failure of the kidneys to concentrate urine normally, and polyuria may indicate complete inability to concentrate the urine.

The more general symptoms of renal failure include anorexia, vomiting, fatigue, hiccup and insomnia. Pruritus (a general itchiness of the skin), bruising and oedema due to fluid retention may also be present. Other symptoms indicating complications include bone pain, fractures because of renal bone disease and the symptoms of hypercalcaemia (including anorexia, nausea, vomiting, constipation, increased urination, mental confusion) because of tertiary (or primary) hyperparathyroidism (page 313). Patients may also present with the features of pericarditis (page 67), hypertension (page 69), cardiac failure (page 65), ischaemic heart disease (page 66), neuropathy (page 394) or peptic ulceration (page 140).

N.B. In secondary hyperparathyroidism serum calcium is low and phosphate is high. In tertiary hyperparathyroidism where parathyroid function has become autonomous, serum calcium and phosphate levels are both high.

Find out if the patient is undergoing dialysis and whether this is haemodialysis or peritoneal dialysis. There are a number of important question that must be asked of dialysis patients.

1. What fluid restriction has been recommended?

2. Have phosphate binding drugs been prescribed?

3. How much weight does the patient gain between each haemodialysis?

4. Does the patient still pass any urine?

5. Is the patient on a renal transplant list?

6. Is the patient compliant with his or her recommended dietary restrictions?

The patient should be well informed about the techniques involved and of any complications that have occurred including recurrent peritonitis with peritoneal dialysis or problems with vascular access for haemodialysis.

A common form of treatment for renal failure is renal transplantation. A patient may know how well the graft is functioning, and what the most recent renal function tests have shown. Find out whether the patient knows of rejection episodes, how these were treated, and if there has been more than one renal transplant. It is necessary to ascertain if there have been any problems with recurrent infection, urine leaks or side effects of treatment. Long-term problems with immunosuppression may have occurred including the development of cancers, chronic nephrotoxicity (e.g., from cyclosporin), obesity and hypertension from steroids, or recurrent infections. The patient should be aware of the need to avoid skin exposure to the sun and women should know that they need regular Papanicolaou (Pap) smears.

Menstrual History

A menstrual history should always be obtained. The menarche or date of the first period is important (page 294). The regularity of the periods over the preceding months or years and the date of the last period are both relevant. The patient may complain of dysmenorrhoea (painful menstruation) or menorrhagia (an abnormally heavy period or series of periods). Vaginal discharge can occur in patients with infections of the genital tract. Sometimes the type of discharge is an indication of the type of infection present (page 219). The history of the number of pregnancies and births is relevant; gravidity refers to the number of times a woman has conceived while parity refers to the number of babies delivered (live births or stillbirths). One should also ask about any complications that occurred during pregnancy (e.g., hypertension).

Ask about contraceptive methods.

Past History

Find out if there have been previous or recurrent urinary tract infections or renal calculi. There may have been operations to remove urinary tract stones, or pelvic surgery may have been performed because of urinary incontinence in women or prostatism in men. The patient may know about the previous detection of proteinuria or microscopic haematuria at a routine examination. Glomerulonephritis will usually have been diagnosed by renal biopsy, a procedure which is often a memorable event. Histories of diabetes mellitus or gout are relevant since these diseases may lead to renal complications. It is most important to find out about hypertension since this may not only cause renal impairment but is also a common complication of renal disease. A history of childhood enuresis (bedwetting) beyond the age of three years may be relevant as this can be associated with vesicoureteric reflux and subsequent renal scarring. Renovascular disease is more likely if there is a history of vascular disease elsewhere, such as myocardial ischaemia or cerebrovascular disease.

Social History

Patients with chronic renal failure may have many social problems. There may be a need for access to equipment at home for dialysis. One must ask detailed questions to find out how the patient is coping with the chronic illness and its complications. Determine if there is a history of analgesic abuse which may be the cause of the renal failure (page 7). Find out how well informed the patient is about the transplant, if this has been the treatment. Also find out what sort of support the patient has obtained from relatives and friends.

The sexual history is also relevant; ask women about infections of the urinary tract (page 4) and men about impotence.

Treatment

A detailed drug history must be taken. Note all the drugs, including steroids and immunosuppressants and their dosages. In patients with decreased renal function, the dosages of many drugs that are cleared by the kidneys must be adjusted. The patient with chronic renal failure should be well informed about the need for protein, fluid or salt restriction. Patients with urinary tract infections may have had a number of courses of antibiotics, and may know of sensitivities to these drugs. Treatment of hypertension should be documented. Patients should know which drugs to avoid. For example, tetracycline antibiotics and non-steroidal anti-inflammatory drugs can worsen renal function where this is already abnormal.

Family History

Some forms of renal disease are inherited. Polycystic kidney disease, for example, is an autosomal dominant condition. Ask about diabetes and hypertension in the family. A family history of deafness and renal impairment suggests Alport's syndrome, an hereditary form of nephritis.

The Genitourinary Examination

A set examination of the genitourinary system is not routinely performed. However, if renal disease is suspected or known to be present then certain signs must be sought. These are mostly the signs of chronic renal failure (uraemia), acute renal failure (Tables 6.2 and 6.3) or infection. On the other hand, examination of the male genitalia or female pelvis is part of the routine general examination.

Table 6.3 *Causes of Chronic Renal Failure*

This is defined as a severe reduction in nephron mass over a variable period of time resulting in uraemia
1. Glomerulonephritis
2. Diabetes mellitus
3. Systemic vascular disease
4. Analgesic nephropathy
5. Reflux nephropathy
6. Hypertensive nephrosclerosis
7. Polycystic kidneys
8. Obstruction
9. Amyloid

Clinical Features Suggesting that Renal Failure is Chronic Rather than Acute

Small kidney size (except with polycystic kidneys, diabetes, amyloid and myeloma)
Renal bone disease
Anaemia (with normal red blood cell indices)
Peripheral neuropathy

General Appearance

The general inspection remains crucial. Look for hyperventilation, which may indicate an underlying metabolic acidosis. Hiccupping may be present and can be an ominous sign of terminal uraemia. There may be a uraemic fetor present. This musty smell is not easy to describe but once detected is easily remembered. Patients with chronic renal failure commonly have a sallow complexion (a dirty brown appearance). This may be due to impaired excretion of urinary pigments (urochromes) combined with anaemia. The skin colour may be anything from slate grey to bronze, due to iron deposition in dialysis patients who have received multiple blood transfusions, but these signs are becoming less frequent with the use of exogenous erythropoietin. In terminal renal failure patients become drowsy and finally sink into a coma due to nitrogen or toxin retention. Twitching due to myoclonic jerks, and tetany and epileptic seizures due to a low serum calcium level and to nitrogen retention, occur late in renal failure. Over-vigorous correction of acidosis (e.g., with bicarbonate infusions) may also precipitate seizures and coma (page 414). There may be subcutaneous nodules due to calcium phosphate deposition.

It is essential to assess the state of hydration in all patients with renal disease (page 20). Severe dehydration can be a cause of acute renal failure and can cause precipitous decompensation in patients with chronic renal failure. Conversely, overhydration can result from intravenous infusions of fluid used in an attempt to correct acute renal failure, resulting in pulmonary oedema (page 65).

The Hands

The *nails* should be inspected look for leuconychia (page 153); white transverse opaque bands occur in hypoalbuminaemia (e.g., nephrotic syndrome). Muehrcke's* nails refer to paired white transverse lines near the end of the nails; these occur in hypoalbuminaemia. Half and half nails occur in up to one-third of patients with chronic renal failure—a distal brown arc at least 1mm wide is present (Terry's[†] nails). A single transverse white band (Mee's[‡] lines) may occur in arsenic poisoning, as well as in renal failure. Non-pigmented indented transverse bands can occur with any cause of a catabolic state (Beau's[§] lines).

Anaemia is common and causes palmar crease pallor. There are a number of causes of anaemia in patients with chronic renal failure, including poor nutrition (especially folate deficiency), blood loss, erythropoietin deficiency, haemolysis, bone marrow depression and the chronic disease state.

Asterixis (page 153) may be present in terminal chronic renal failure.

At the wrist and forearms inspect for scars and palpate for surgically created arteriovenous fistulae or shunts, used for haemodialysis access. There is a longitudinal swelling and a palpable continuous thrill present over the fistula. There may be scars from previous thrombosed shunts or carpal tunnel syndrome surgery present on either side. Look for signs of the carpal tunnel syndrome (page 261, 333).

---

*   R C Muehrcke reported this in the *British Medical Journal* in 1956.
†   R Terry described this sign in the *Lancet* in 1954.
‡   R A Mees reported this in 1919.
§   Joseph Honoré Simon Beau (b. 1806). Paris physician.

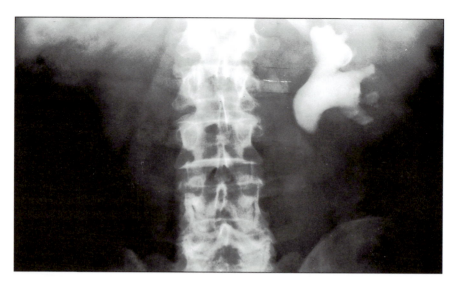

Figure 6.1 *Phleboliths (calcifications related to blood vessels) are rounded opacities seen in the pelvis below the level of the ischial spines, whereas ureteric calculi lie above this level, in the line of the ureters.*

The large Staghorn calculus shown here is occupying the calyces of the left renal pelvis. This type of calculus is almost always radio-opaque.

An intravenous urogram or abdominal ultrasound examination is necessary to check that there is no obstruction at the ureteropelvic junction.

In general, 90% of renal calculi are radio-opaque and visible on plain films. One-quarter of patients presenting with renal colic due to calcific calculi have hyperparathyroidism.

The Arms

Bruising occurs because of nitrogen retention causing impaired prothrombin consumption, a defect in platelet factor III, and abnormal platelet aggregation in chronic renal failure. *Skin pigmentation* is common reflecting a failure to excrete urinary pigments. *Scratch marks*, due to pruritus from calcium deposition (which results from secondary hyperparathyroidism), may be present. *Uraemic frost* is a fine white powder present on the skin where very high concentrations of urea have precipitated out of the sweat in terminal chronic renal failure; it is very rare. Evidence of *vasculitis*, which can cause renal disease, should also be looked for (page 285).

Look for signs of *peripheral neuropathy* in the limbs. Sensory impairment is more marked than motor impairment initially (page 394). Myopathy (page 402) and bone tenderness can also occur due to osteomalacia, which results from low 1,25-dihydroxyvitamin D and calcium levels.

The Face

The eyes are important; look for signs of *anaemia* and, rarely, *jaundice* (retention of nitrogenous wastes can cause haemolysis). *Band keratopathy* is a calcium deposition beneath the corneal epithelium in line with the interpalpebral fissure—it is due to secondary or tertiary hyperparathyroidism (page 313), or excessive replacement of calcium in patients with chronic renal failure.

The mouth should always be examined. A uraemic *fetor* may be present. This is an ammoniacal odour due to breakdown of urea to ammonia in the saliva. Mucosal *ulcers* can occur as there is a decrease in saliva flow, and patients with chronic renal failure are prone to infection, (e.g., thrush), due to decreased acute inflammatory responses as a result of nitrogen retention.

The presence of a *rash* or skin tethering may indicate an underlying connective tissue disease such as systemic lupus erythematosus or systemic sclerosis (page 277).

The Neck

Carefully assess the jugular venous pressure (page 45). Auscultate for carotid artery bruits; these provide a clue that there may be generalised atherosclerotic disease (which can cause renal artery stenosis).

The Chest

Examine the heart and lungs. In chronic renal failure there may be *congestive cardiac failure* due to fluid retention, and *hypertension* as a result of sodium and water retention and excess renin production. Signs of *pulmonary oedema* may also be present due to uraemic lung disease (a type of non-cardiogenic pulmonary oedema), volume overload or uraemic cardiomyopathy.

Pericarditis, which can be fibrinous or haemorrhagic in chronic renal failure, is secondary to retained metabolic toxins and can cause a pericardial rub or signs of cardiac tamponade (page 67). Lung infection is also common due to the immunosuppression present from the chronic renal failure itself or as a result of treatment.

The Abdominal Examination

Abdominal examination is performed as described on page 160. However, particular attention must be paid to the following.

Inspection

It is important to look for nephrectomy *scars* (Figure 5.7). These are often more posterior than one might expect. It may be necessary to roll the patient over and look in the region of the loins. Renal transplant scars are usually found in the right or left iliac fossae. A *transplanted kidney* may be visible as a bulge under the scar, as it is placed in a relatively superficial plane. Peritoneal dialysis results in small scars from catheter placement in the peritoneal cavity; these are situated on the lower abdomen, at or near the midline.

The abdomen may be distended because of large polycystic kidneys or *ascites* (as a result of the nephrotic syndrome, or dialysis fluid).

Inspect the scrotum for masses (see page 217) and genital oedema.

Palpation

Particular care is required here so that renal masses (Table 6.4) are not missed (page 169). Remember an enlarged kidney usually bulges forwards, while perinephric abscesses or collections tend to bulge backwards. Transplanted kid-

Table 6.4   *Renal Masses*

Unilateral Palpable Kidney

Renal cell carcinoma
Hydronephrosis or pyonephrosis
Polycystic kidneys (with asymmetrical enlargement)
Normal right kidney or solitary kidney
Acute renal vein thrombosis (unilateral)
Acute pyelonephritis
Renal abscess

Bilateral Palpable Kidneys

Polycystic kidneys
Hydronephrosis or pyonephrosis bilaterally
Renal cell carcinoma bilaterally
Diabetic nephropathy (early)
Nephrotic syndrome (Table 6.8)
Infiltrative disease, e.g., amyloid, lymphoma
Acromegaly

Table 6.5   *Adult Polycystic Kidney Disease*

If you find polycystic kidneys remember these very important points.
1. Take the blood pressure (75% have hypertension).
2. Examine the urine for haematuria (due to haemorrhage into a cyst) and proteinuria (usually less than 2g/day).
3. Look for evidence of anaemia (due to chronic renal failure) or polycythaemia (due to high erythropoietin levels). Note that the haemoglobin level is higher than expected for the degree of renal failure.
4. Note the presence of hepatomegaly or splenomegaly (due to cysts). These may cause confusion when one is examining the abdomen.
5. Tenderness on palpation may indicate an infected cyst.

NB: Subarachnoid haemorrhage occurs in 3% of patients due to rupture of an intracranial aneurysm. As this is an autosomal dominant condition, all family members should also be assessed.

neys in the right or left iliac fossa may be palpable as well. In polycystic kidney disease, hepatomegaly from hepatic cysts may be found (Table 6.5). Feel for the presence of an enlarged bladder (page 172). Also palpate for an abdominal aortic aneurysm.

Percussion

This is necessary to confirm the presence of ascites by examining for shifting dullness. Also percuss for an enlarged bladder.

Auscultation

The important sign here is the presence of a renal bruit. Renal bruits are best heard above the umbilicus, about 2cm to the left or right of the midline. Listen with the diaphragm of the stethoscope over both these areas. Next ask the patient to sit up and listen in both flanks. The presence of a systolic and diastolic bruit is important. A diastolic component makes the bruit more likely to be haemodynamically significant. Its presence suggests renal artery stenosis due to fibromuscular dysplasia or atherosclerosis. Approximately 50% of patients with renal artery stenosis will have a bruit. On the other hand, if a bruit is audible at least half these patients do not have any significant renal artery stenosis. In such cases the aorta or splenic artery may be the source of the sound. The absence of hypertension makes the diagnosis of renal artery stenosis less likely.

Rectal and Pelvic Examination

Here the presence of prostatomegaly in males and a frozen pelvis from cervical cancer in females is important, as this may be a cause of urinary tract obstruction and secondary renal failure. Feel for uterine prolapse.

The Back

Strike the vertebral column gently with the base of the fist to elicit bony tenderness. This may be due to renal osteodystrophy from osteomalacia or secondary hyperparathyroidism.

Gentle use of the clenched fist to strike the patient in the renal angle is known as Murphy's kidney punch and is designed to elicit renal tenderness in patients with renal infection. One should also look for sacral oedema in a patient confined to bed, particularly if the nephrotic syndrome or congestive cardiac failure is suspected.

The Legs

The important signs here are oedema, purpura (page 225), pigmentation, scratch marks and signs of peripheral vascular disease. Examination for peripheral neuropathy and myopathy is indicated, as in the arms. Gouty tophi or the presence of gouty arthropathy (page 276) may very occasionally provide an explanation for the patient's renal failure (although secondary uric acid retention is common with chronic renal failure, it rarely causes clinical gout).

The Blood Pressure

It is of the utmost importance to take the blood pressure in every patient with renal disease. This is because hypertension can be the cause of renal disease or one of its complications. Test for postural hypotension, as hypovolaemia may precipitate acute renal failure.

The Fundi

Examination of the fundi is important. Look especially for hypertensive changes (page 69) and diabetic changes (page 324). Diabetes can be a cause of chronic renal failure.

The Urine

*The ghosts of dead patients that haunt us do not ask
why we did not employ the latest fad of clinical investigation;
they ask why did you not test my urine?*

Sir Robert Hutchison (1871–1960)

This valuable fluid must not be discarded in any patient in whom a renal, diabetic, gastrointestinal or other major system disease is suspected.

Colour

Look at the colour of the urine and see Table 6.6.

Transparency

Phosphate or urate deposits can occur normally and produce white (phosphate) or pink (urate) cloudiness.

Fainter cloudiness may be due to bacteria. Pus, chyle or blood can cause a more turbid appearance.

Smell

A mild ammoniacal smell is normal. A urinary tract infection causes a fishy smell, and antibiotics can sometimes be smelt in the urine, as can asparagus.

Table 6.6 *Some Causes of Urine Colour Changes*

Colour	Underlying Causes
Very pale or colourless	Dilute urine (e.g., overhydration, recent excessive beer consumption, diabetes insipidus, post-obstructive diuresis)
Yellow-orange	Concentrated urine (e.g., dehydration) bilirubin tetracycline, anthracene, sulfasalazine, riboflavine
Brown	Bilirubin nitrofurantoin, phenothiazines
Pink	Beetroot consumption phenindione, phenolphthalein (laxatives)
Red	Haematuria, haemoglobinuria, myoglobinuria porphyrins, rifampicin, pyridium
Green	Methylene blue
Black	Severe haemoglobinuria methyldopa melanoma, ochronosis

Specific Gravity

A urinometer, which is a weighted float with a scale, is used to measure specific gravity. The depth to which the float sinks in the urine indicates the specific gravity which is read off the scale on the side. Water has a specific gravity of one and the presence of solutes (especially heavy solutes such as glucose or an iodine-contrast medium) in urine increases the specific gravity. The normal range is 1.002 to 1.025. A consistently low specific gravity suggests chronic renal failure (as there is failure of the kidneys to concentrate the urine) or diabetes insipidus (where there is a deficiency of antidiuretic hormone resulting in passage of a large volume of dilute urine). A high specific gravity suggests dehydration, or diabetes mellitus with the presence of large amounts of glucose in the urine.

There is a rough correlation between the specific gravity of the urine and its osmolality. For example, a specific gravity of 1.002 corresponds to an osmolality of 100 mOsm/kg, while a specific gravity of 1.030 corresponds to 1200 mOsm/kg.

The specific gravity can also be estimated by dipstick methods.

Chemical Analysis

A chemical reagent colour strip allows simultaneous multiple analyses of pH, protein, glucose, ketones, blood, nitrite, specific gravity, presence of leucocytes, bile and urobilinogen. The strip is dipped in the urine and colour changes are measured after a set period. The colours are compared with a chart provided.

pH

Normal urine is acid, except after meals when for a short time it becomes alkaline (the alkaline tide). Measuring the pH of urine is helpful in a number of critical circumstances. Sometimes the urine has to be made alkaline for therapeutic purposes, such as treating myoglobinuria or recurrent urinary calculi (due to uric acid or cystine). Distal renal tubular acidosis should be suspected if the early morning urine is consistently alkaline and cannot be acidified. Urinary tract infections with urea-splitting organisms, such as *Proteus mirabilis*, can also cause an alkaline urine which, in turn, favours renal calcium stone formation.

Protein

The colours are compared with a chart provided. The strip tests give only a semiquantitative measure of urinary protein (+ to ++++) and if positive must be confirmed by other tests. One-third of measured urinary protein is albumin and two-thirds is globulin. A reading of + of proteinuria may be normal, as up to 150 mg of protein a day is lost in the urine. Causes of abnormal amounts of protein in the urine are listed in Tables 6.7 and 6.8. Chemical dipsticks do not detect the presence of Bence-Jones* proteinuria (immunoglobulin light chains).

If proteinuria is detected on dipstick testing, this should be quantified with a 24-hour urinary collection, and careful urine (phase-contrast) microscopy should be carried out to look for evidence of active renal disease.

---

* Henry Bence-Jones (b. 1813), London physician.

Table 6.7   *Causes of Proteinuria*

Persistent Proteinuria

1. Renal disease

Almost any renal disease may cause a trace of proteinuria. Moderate or large amounts tend to occur with glomerular disease (Table 6.8).

2. No renal disease (functional)

Exercise
Fever
Hypertension (severe)
Congestive cardiac failure
Burns
Blood transfusion
Postoperative
Acute alcohol abuse

Orthostatic Proteinuria

Proteinuria which occurs when a patient is standing but not when recumbent is called orthostatic proteinuria. In the absence of abnormalities of the urine sediment, diabetes mellitus, hypertension or reduced renal function, this entity probably has a benign prognosis.

Table 6.8   *The Nephrotic Syndrome*

Definition

1. Proteinuria (>3.5g per 24 hours)
2. Hypoalbuminaemia (serum albumin <30g/L, due to proteinuria)
3. Oedema (due to hypoalbuminaemia)
4. Hyperlipidaemia (due to increased LDL and cholesterol, possibly from loss of plasma factors regulating lipoprotein synthesis)

Causes

Primary Renal Pathology

1. Membranous glomerulonephritis
2. Minimal change glomerulonephritis
3. Focal and segmental hyalinosis and sclerosis
4. Mesangiocapillary (membranoproliferative) glomerulonephritis
5. Crescentic glomerulonephritis

Secondary Renal Pathology

1. Drugs: e.g., penicillamine, probenecid, gold, captopril, heroin, non-steroidal anti-inflammatory drugs
2. Systemic disease: e.g., SLE, diabetes mellitus, hypertension, amyloid
3. Malignancy: e.g., carcinoma, lymphoma, multiple myeloma
4. Infections: e.g., hepatitis B, infective endocarditis, malaria, AIDS
5. Allergy: e.g., vaccines, bee sting

LDL = low density lipoprotein
SLE = systemic lupus erythematosus
AIDS = acquired immunodeficiency syndrome

Glucose and Ketones

A semi-quantitative measurement of glucose and ketones is available. Glycosuria usually indicates diabetes mellitus, but can occur with other diseases (Table 6.9). False-positive or negative results can occur with vitamin C (large doses), tetracyclines or levodopa ingestion.

Ketones in the urine of patients with diabetes mellitus are an important indication of the presence of diabetic ketoacidosis (Table 6.9). The three ketone bodies are acetone, beta-hydroxybutyric acid and acetoacetic acid. Lack of glucose (starvation), or lack of glucose availability for the cells (diabetes mellitus) causes activation of carnitine acetyl transferase, which accelerates fatty acid oxidation in the liver. However, the pathway for the conversion of fatty acids becomes saturated leading to ketone body formation. The strip colour tests only react to acetoacetic acid.

Blood

Blood in the urine (haematuria) is abnormal and can be seen with the naked eye if 0.5mL is present per litre of urine (Table 6.10). A positive dipstick test is abnormal and suggests haematuria, haemoglobinuria (uncommon) or myoglobinuria (also uncommon). The presence of more than a trace of protein in the urine in addition suggests that the blood is of renal origin. False-positive or negative results can occur if vitamin C is being taken.

Nitrite

If positive, this usually indicates infection with bacteria which produce nitrite. False-positive or negative results occur with vitamin C ingestion. More specific dipstick tests for white cells are now available.

The Urine Sediment

Every patient with suspected renal disease should have the urine sediment from the first morning urine sample (to avoid dilute urine) examined. Centrifuge 10 mL of the urine at 2000 rpm for four minutes. Remove the supernatant, leaving 0.5 mL—shake well to resuspend, then place one drop on a slide with a coverslip. Look at the slide using a low-power microscope, and at specific formed elements

Table 6.9 *Causes of Glycosuria and Ketonuria*

Glycosuria

Diabetes mellitus

Other reducing substances (false positives): metabolites of salicylates, ascorbic acid, galactose, fructose

Impaired renal tubular ability to absorb glucose (renal glycosuria)
  e.g., Fanconi* syndrome (proximal renal tubular disease)

Ketonuria

Diabetic ketoacidosis

Starvation

* Guido Fanconi (b. 1892), Zürich paediatrician.

Table 6.10 *Causes of Positive Dipstick Test for Blood in the Urine*

Haematuria

Renal

Glomerulonephritis
Polycystic renal disease
Pyelonephritis
Renal cell carcinoma
Analgesic nephropathy
Malignant hypertension
Renal infarction, e.g., infective endocarditis, vasculitis
Bleeding disorders

Renal Tract

Cystitis
Calculi
Bladder or ureteric tumour
Prostatic disease, e.g., cancer, benign prostatic hypertrophy
Urethritis

Haemoglobinuria

Intravascular haemolysis, e.g., microangiopathic haemolytic anaemia, march
haemoglobulinuria, prosthetic heart valve, paroxysmal nocturnal haemoglobinuria, chronic
cold agglutinin disease

Myoglobinuria

This is due to rhabdomyolysis (muscle destruction):
  Muscle infarction, e.g., trauma
  Excessive muscle contraction, e.g., convulsions, hyperthermia, marathon running
  Viral myositis, e.g., influenza, Legionnaires' disease
  Drugs or toxins, e.g., alcohol, snake venom
  Idiopathic

under the high-power field (hpf) for identification. There is a significant false-negative rate when there are low numbers of formed elements in the urine.

Look for the following.

Red Blood Cells (RBCs)

These appear as small circular objects without a nucleus. Usually none are seen, although up to 5 RBCs/low power field (lpf) may be normal in very concentrated urine. If their numbers are increased, try to determine if the RBCs originate from the glomeruli (more than 80% of the RBCs are dysmorphic—irregular in size and shape) or the renal tract (the RBCs are typically uniform).

White Blood Cells (WBCs)

These cells have lobulated nuclei. Usually fewer than 6 WBCs/hpf are present, although up to 10 may be normal in very concentrated urine. Tubular epithelial cells have a compact nucleus and are larger. Pyuria indicates urinary tract inflammation. Bacteria may also be seen if there is infection, but bacterial contamination is more likely if squamous epithelial cells (which are larger and have single nuclei) are prominent. Urine culture is essential, as pyuria is an insensitive guide to infection. Sterile pyuria is characteristic of tuberculosis.

Casts

Casts are cylindrical moulds formed in the lumen of the renal tubules or collecting ducts. They are signs of a damaged glomerular basement membrane or damaged tubules. The size of a cast is determined by the dimension of the lumen of the nephron in which it forms.

Hyaline casts are long cylindrical structures. One or two RBCs or WBCs may be present in the cast. Normally there are fewer than one per low power field. They consist largely of Tamm-Horsfall mucoprotein secreted by the renal tubules.

Granular casts: these cylindrical granular structures are abnormal and arise from the tubules, usually in patients with proteinuria. They consist of hyaline material containing fragments of serum proteins.

Red cell casts are always abnormal and indicate primary glomerular disease (haematuria of glomerular origin). They contain 10 to 50 red cells which are well defined.

White cell casts: here many WBCs are adherent to or inside the cast. These are abnormal, indicating bacterial pyelonephritis or, less commonly, glomerulonephritis, kidney infarction or vasculitis.

Fatty casts: the presence of fat in casts is indicative of the nephrotic syndrome.

Male Genitalia

Inspect the genitals for evidence of mucosal ulceration. This can occur in a number of systemic diseases, including Reiter's syndrome (page 275) and the rare Behçet's syndrome (page 286). If necessary, retract the foreskin to expose the glans penis. For aesthetic and protective reasons it is essential to wear gloves for this examination. This mucosal surface is prone to inflammation or ulceration in both infective and connective tissue diseases (Table 6.11). Look also for urethral discharge. If there is a history of discharge, attempt to express fluid by compressing or 'milking' the shaft. Any fluid obtained must be sent for microscopic examination and culture.

Examine the scrotum with the patient standing. Usually the left testis hangs lower than the right. This is the only part of the body which consistently does not appear bilaterally symmetrical on inspection. Inspect for oedema of the skin, sebaceous cysts or scabies.

Table 6.11   *Causes of Genital Lesions*

Ulcerative
Herpes simplex (vesicles followed by ulcers: tender)
Syphilis (non-tender)
Malignancy (squamous cell carcinoma: non-tender)
Chancroid (*Haemophilus ducreyi* infection: tender)
Behçet's syndrome
Non-ulcerative
Balanitis, due to Reiter's syndrome or poor hygiene
Venereal warts
Primary skin disease, e.g., psoriasis
NB: Always consider AIDS

Palpate each testis gently using the fingers and thumb of the right hand. The testes are normally equal in size, smooth and relatively firm. Absence of one or both testes may be due to previous excision, failure of the testis to descend, or a retractile testis. An undescended testis may be palpable in the inguinal canal, usually at or above the external inguinal ring. The presence of small firm testes suggests an endocrine disease (hypogonadism) or testicular atrophy due to alcohol or drug ingestion. A left varicocele is sometimes found when there is underlying left renal vein thrombosis.

Differential Diagnosis of a Scrotal Mass (Figure 6.2)

If a mass is palpable in the scrotum decide first whether it is possible to get above it. Have the patient stand up. If no upper border is palpable, it must be descending down the inguinal canal from the abdomen and is therefore an inguinoscrotal hernia (page 175).

If it is possible to get above the mass, it is necessary to decide whether it is separate from or part of the testis, and to test for translucency. This is performed using a transilluminoscope (a torch). With the patient in a darkened room a small torch is applied to the posterior part of the swelling by invaginating the scrotal wall. A cystic mass will light up while a solid mass remains dark.

A mass which is part of the testis and which is solid (non-translucent) is likely to be a tumour, or rarely a syphilitic gumma. A mass which is cystic (translucent) with the testis within it is a hydrocele (a collection of fluid in the tunica vaginalis of the testis). A mass which appears separate from the testis and transilluminates is probably a cyst of the epididymis, while a similar mass which fails to

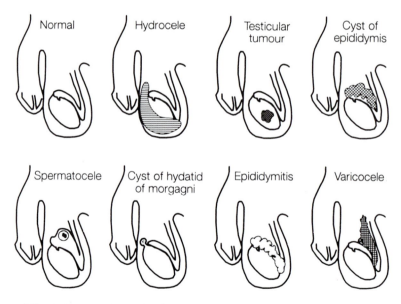

Figure 6.2 *Differential diagnosis of a scrotal mass.*

From Dunphy JE, Botsford TW. Physical examination of the surgical patient. An introduction to clinical surgery. 4th ed. Philadelphia: WB Saunders, 1975, with permission.

transilluminate is probably the result of chronic epididymitis. By feeling along the testicular-epididymal groove one can usually separate an epididymal mass from the testis itself.

Pelvic Examination

Never insult the vagina by examining the rectum first.

Old Axiom

Actually it is immaterial which of the examinations is done first; the important point is to change the glove.

Hamilton Bailey (1894–1961)

The pelvic examination should be performed as the final part of any complete physical examination. The patient should have first emptied her bladder. She should be on her back with her legs apart and her knees bent (the lithotomy position). The left lateral position (page 178) is used when the woman cannot assume the lithotomy position or when a view of the anterior vaginal wall is required; for example, when a urinary fistula is suspected. The perineum should be brightly illuminated by a lamp. Place a glove on each hand. Inspect first the external genitalia. Note any rash (e.g., sclerotic white areas of leukoplakia, or redness, swelling and excoriation from thrush or trichomoniasis), ulceration, warts, scars, sinus openings or other lesions. Separate the labia with the thumb and forefinger of the right hand. Note the size and shape of the clitoris, and the presence or absence of a discharge from the urethral orifice and vaginal outlet. A bloody vaginal discharge suggests menstruation, a miscarriage, cancer or a cervical polyp or erosion. A purulent discharge suggests vaginitis, cervicitis or endometritis (e.g., gonorrhoea) or a retained tampon. *Trichomonas vaginalis* causes a frothy, watery, pale, yellow-white discharge, while thrush (*Candida albicans*) causes a thick cheesy discharge associated with excoriations and pruritus. Ask the patient to bear down; a cystocele (descent of the bladder through the anterior vaginal wall) or rectocele (descent of the rectum through the posterior vaginal wall) or uterine prolapse may become apparent. Then ask the patient to cough; this may demonstrate stress incontinence. Note the presence of vaginal atrophy in older women.

A Bartholin* cyst or abscess is palpated between the thumb and index finger in the posterior part of the labia major; the normal gland is impalpable. Next insert the lubricated index and middle finger into the vagina. Locate the cervix first: it

---

* Caspar Bartholin Jr (b. 1655), Copenhagen anatomist.

normally points toward the posterior vaginal wall. Note the position, size, shape, consistency, tenderness and mobility. Next palpate the anterior, posterior and lateral fornices. Usually the ovaries are not palpable. If a mass is palpable its characteristics and location should be noted. Bimanual palpation of the uterus is now performed; the fingers in the vagina are kept high up while the left hand presses downwards and backwards above the pubic symphysis. Note whether the uterus is anterior (anteverted) or posterior (retroverted). Also note its size, shape and consistency and feel for tenderness and mobility. A large nodular mobile uterus suggests fibroids, while smooth enlargement of the uterus suggests pregnancy, adenomyosis or submucous fibroids.

A speculum examination of the vagina and cervix is made by introducing a well-lubricated warm bivalve speculum in a upwards direction and with the blades closed , while the other hand separates the labia. The blades are opened once the speculum is fully introduced, and the vagina and cervix are inspected. A smear for cervical cytology (Papanicolaou* or 'Pap' smear) can be taken to detect cervical dysplasia or cancer. This is done using a spatula that is placed firmly against the cervical os and rotated through 360°. The test is more accurate if some endocervical cells are also obtained. This can be done with a separate brush designed to fit into the os. A smear of vaginal wall cells for hormonal assessment can be taken with the other end of the spatula. The samples are smeared thinly on microscopic slides and placed immediately in fixative. Wet slides can also be prepared for *Trichomonas* or thrush, and cultures obtained for gonorrhoea if indicated.

Summary

Examination of a Patient with Chronic Renal Failure: A Suggested Method (Figure 6.3)

Lie the patient flat in bed while performing the usual general inspection. Note particularly the patient's mental state and the presence of a sallow complexion, whether the patient appears properly hydrated and whether there is any hyperventilation or hiccupping.

The detailed examination begins with the hands and the examination of the nails which may reveal leuconychia, white transverse lines or a distal brown arc. Examine the wrists and arms for vascular access. Get the patient to hold out the hands and look for asterixis. Then inspect the arms for bruising, subcutaneous nodules (calcium phosphate deposits), pigmentation, scratch marks and gouty tophi.

Go on now to the face and begin by examining the eyes for anaemia, jaundice or band keratopathy. Examine the mouth for dryness, ulcers or fetor, and note the presence of any vasculitic rash on the face.

The patient should be lying flat while the abdomen is examined for scars indicating peritoneal dialysis or operations, including renal transplants. Palpate for the kidneys, including transplanted kidneys, then examine the liver and spleen. Feel for an abdominal aortic aneurysm. Percuss over the bladder, determine if there is ascites, and listen for renal bruits. Rectal examination is indicated to detect prostatomegaly, frozen pelvis or bleeding.

---

* George N Papanicolaou (b. 1883), Greek physician in America.

Figure 6.3 *Chronic Renal Failure*

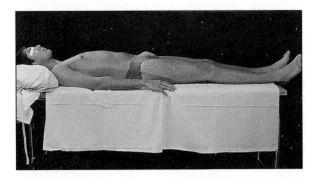

1. GENERAL INSPECTION
   Mental state
   Hyperventilation (acidosis), hiccups
   Sallow complexion
   Hydration
   Subcutaneous nodules (calcium
     phosphate deposits)

2. HANDS
   Nails—leuconychia; brown lines; distal
     brown arc
   Vascular shunts
   Asterixis
   Neuropathy

3. ARMS
   Bruising
   Pigmentation
   Scratch marks
   Myopathy

4. FACE
   Eyes—anaemia, jaundice, band
     keratopathy
   Mouth—dryness, ulcers, fetor
   Rash (vasculitis, etc.)

5. ABDOMEN
   Scars—dialysis, operations
   Kidneys—transplant kidney
   Bladder
   Liver
   Lymph nodes

   Ascites
   Bruits
   Rectal examination (prostatomegaly,
     bleeding)

6. BACK
   Tenderness
   Oedema

7. CHEST
   Heart—pericarditis, failure
   Lungs—infection, pulmonary oedema

8. LEGS
   Oedema—nephrotic syndrome, cardiac
     failure
   Bruising
   Pigmentation
   Scratch marks
   Neuropathy
   Vascular access

9. URINE ANALYSIS
   Specific gravity, pH
   Glucose—diabetes mellitus
   Blood—'nephritis', infection, stone
   Protein—'nephritis', etc.

OTHER
   Blood pressure—lying and standing
   Fundoscopy—hypertensive and diabetic
     changes, etc.

Sit the patient up and palpate the back for tenderness and sacral oedema.

Look at the jugular venous pressure with the patient at 45 degrees. Examine the heart for signs of pericarditis or cardiac failure and the lungs for pulmonary oedema.

Lie the patient down again. Look at the legs for oedema (due to the nephrotic syndrome or cardiac failure), bruising, pigmentation, scratch marks or the presence of gout. Examine for peripheral neuropathy (decreased sensation, loss of the more distal reflexes).

Examination ends with measurement of the blood pressure, lying and standing (for orthostatic hypotension), and fundoscopy to look for hypertensive and diabetic changes. Finally urinalysis is performed testing for specific gravity, pH, glucose, blood protein or leucocytes.

Suggested Reading

Original and Review Articles

Deneke M, Wheeler L, Wagner G, Ling FW, Buxton BH. An approach to relearning the pelvic examination. *J Fam Pract* 1982; 14: 782–783.

Marazzi P, Gabriel R. The haematuria clinic. *BMJ* 1994; 308: 356.

Rabinowitz R, Hulbert WC Jr, Acute scrotal swelling. *Urol Clin Nth Am* 1995; 22: 101–5.

Schroder FH, Detection of prostate cancer. *BMJ* 1995; 310: 140–1.

Zornow DH, Landes RR. Scrotal palpation. *Am Fam Physician* 1981; 23: 150–154.

Textbooks

Becker GJ, Whitworth JA, Kincaid Smith P. Clinical nephrology in medical practice. London: Blackwell, 1992.

Llach F. Papper's clinical nephrology. 3rd ed. Boston: Little Brown, 1993.

Chapter 7

THE HAEMATOLOGICAL SYSTEM

... the blood is the generative part, the fountain of life, the first to live, the last to die and the primary seat to the soul.

William Harvey (1578–1657)

The Haematological History

Presenting Symptoms (Table 7.1)

Patients with anaemia may present with weakness, tiredness, dyspnoea, fatigue or postural dizziness. Anaemia due to iron deficiency is often the result of gastrointestinal blood loss, or sometimes recurrent heavy menstrual blood loss, and so these symptoms should be sought. Disorders of platelet function or blood clotting may present with easy bruising or bleeding problems. Recurrent infection may be the first symptom of a disorder of the immune system, including leukaemia or AIDS. The patient may have noticed lymph node enlargement which can occur with lymphoma or leukaemia.

Past History

A history of gastric surgery or malabsorption may give a clue regarding the underlying cause of an anaemia. Anaemia in patients with systemic disease such as rheumatoid arthritis or uraemia can be multifactorial. Previous blood transfusions may have been required to treat the anaemia. On the other hand, patients with polycythaemia may have had many venesections (page 241).

Treatment

Anaemia may have been treated with iron supplements or B_{12} injections. Anti-inflammatory drugs or anticoagulants may be the cause of bleeding. Treatment for leukaemia or lymphoma may have involved chemotherapy, radiotherapy or both.

Social History

A patient's racial origin is relevant. Thalassaemia is common in people of Mediterranean or southern Asian origin. Rarely, very strict vegetarian diets can result in vitamin B_{12} deficiency.

Table 7.1   *Haematological History*

Major Symptoms
Symptoms of anaemia: weakness, tiredness, dyspnoea, fatigue, postural dizziness
Bleeding (menstrual, gastrointestinal)
Easy bruising, purpura, thrombotic tendency
Infection, fever or jaundice
Lymph gland enlargement
Bone pain
Paraesthesiae (e.g., B_{12} deficiency)
Skin rash
Weight loss

Family History

There may be a history of thalassaemia or sickle cell anaemia in the family. Haemophilia is a sex-linked recessive disease while von Willebrand's* disease is autosomal dominant with incomplete penetrance (Table 7.3).

The Haematological Examination

Haematological assessment does not only depend on the microscopic examination of the blood constituents. Physical signs, followed by examination of the blood film, can give vital clues about underlying disease. Haematological disease can affect the red blood cells, the white cells, the platelets and other haemostatic mechanisms as well as the mononuclear-phagocyte (reticuloendothelial) system.

General Appearance

Position the patient as for the gastrointestinal examination—lying on the bed with one pillow. Note the patient's *racial* origin. *Pallor* should be looked for as it may indicate anaemia. If there is any *bruising* look at its distribution and extent. *Jaundice* may be present and can indicate haemolytic anaemia. *Scratch marks* (following pruritus that sometimes occurs with lymphoma and myeloproliferative disease) should be noted.

The Hands

The detailed examination begins in the usual way with assessment of the hands. Look at the nails for *koilonychia*—these are dry, brittle, ridged, spoon-shaped nails which are rarely seen today. They are due to severe iron deficiency anaemia, although the mechanism is unknown. Occasionally koilonychia may be due to fungal infection. Pallor of the nailbeds may occur in anaemia but is an unreliable sign. Pallor of the *palmar creases* suggests that the haemoglobin level is less than 70 g/L, but this is also a rather unreliable sign.

Note any changes of rheumatoid or gouty *arthritis*, or connective tissue disease (Chapter 8). Rheumatoid arthritis when associated with splenomegaly and

---

*   E A von Willebrand (1870–1949), Swedish physician, described this in 1926.

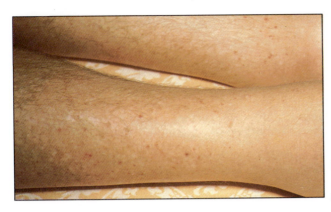

Figure 7.1
*Thrombocytopenic
purpura.*

neutropenia is called Felty's* syndrome—the mechanism of the neutropenia is unknown, but it can result in severe infection. Felty's syndrome can also be associated with thrombocytopenia, haemolytic anaemia, skin pigmentation and leg ulceration. Gouty tophi and arthropathy may be present in the hands. Gout may be a manifestation of a myeloproliferative disease. Connective tissue diseases can cause anaemia because of the associated chronic inflammation.

Now take the *pulse*. A tachycardia may be present. Anaemic patients have an increased cardiac output and compensating tachycardia because of the reduced oxygen-carrying capacity of their blood.

Look for *purpura*, which is really any sort of bruising, due to haemorrhage into the skin. The lesions can vary in size from pinheads called petechiae† (Table 7.2) to large bruises called ecchymoses (Table 7.3).

If the petechiae are raised (*palpable purpura*), this suggests an underlying systemic vasculitis, dysglobulinaemia (e.g., cryoglobulinaemia, where the lesions are painful), or bacteraemia.

The Forearms

If thrombocytopenia or capillary fragility is suspected, the Hess‡ test may be indicated. A blood pressure cuff, placed over the upper arm, is inflated to a point 10 mmHg above the diastolic blood pressure. Wait for five minutes, then deflate the cuff and wait for another five minutes before inspecting the arm. Look for petechiae which are usually most prominent in the cubital fossa and near the wrist where the skin is most lax. Fewer than five petechiae per cm^2 is normal and more than 20 is definitely abnormal, suggesting thrombocytopenia, abnormal platelet function or capillary fragility. This test is uncommonly performed these days.

Epitrochlear Nodes

These must always be palpated. The best method is to place the palm of the right hand under the patient's right elbow. The examiner's thumb can then be placed

---

* Augustus Roi Felty (1895–1964), American physician.

† Latin *petechia* a spot.

‡ Alfred Hess (1875–1933), Professor of Paediatrics, New York, described this in 1914.

Table 7.2   *Causes of Petechiae*

Thrombocytopenia
Platelet count <100 × 10⁹/L

Increased Destruction

Immunological:
    immune thrombocytopenic purpura (ITP)
    systemic lupus erythematosus
    drugs, e.g., quinine, sulphonamides, methyldopa
Non-immunological:
    damage, e.g., prosthetic heart valve
    consumption, e.g., disseminated intravascular coagulation (DIC)
    loss, e.g., haemorrhage

Reduced Production

Marrow aplasia, e.g., drugs, chemicals, radiation
Marrow invasion, e.g., carcinoma, myeloma, leukaemia, fibrosis

Sequestration

Hypersplenism

Platelet Dysfunction

Congenital or familial
Acquired:
    myeloproliferative disease
    dysproteinaemia
    chronic renal failure, chronic liver disease
    drugs, e.g., aspirin

Bleeding Due to Small Vessel Disease

Infection:
    infective endocarditis
    septicaemia (e.g., meningococcal)
    viral exanthemata (e.g., measles)
Drugs, e.g., steroids
Scurvy (vitamin C deficiency)—classically perifollicular purpura on the lower limbs, which
    is almost diagnostic of this condition
Cushing's syndrome
Vasculitis:
    polyarteritis nodosa
    Henoch-Schönlein* purpura
Fat embolism
Dysproteinaemia

* Eduard Henoch (1820–1910), Berlin physician and Johannes Schönlein (1793–1864), Berlin physician.

over the appropriate area which is proximal and slightly anterior to the medial epicondyle. This is repeated with the left hand for the other side (Figure 7.2). An enlarged epitrochlear node is usually pathological. It occurs with local infection, non-Hodgkin's* lymphoma or rarely syphilis. Note the features listed in Table 7.4.

---

* Thomas Hodgkin (1798–1866), famous physician at Guy's Hospital, London.

Table 7.3 *Causes of Ecchymoses*

Thrombocytopenia or Platelet Dysfunction (Table 7.2)

Coagulation Disorders

Acquired

Vitamin K deficiency (leading to factor II, VII, IX and X deficiency)
Liver disease (impaired synthesis of clotting factors)
Anticoagulants, e.g., heparin, warfarin, proteins with anticoagulant activity
Disseminated intravascular coagulation

Congenital

Rarely cause ecchymoses and usually present with haemorrhage
Haemophilia A (factor VIII deficiency)
Haemophilia B (factor IX deficiency, Christmas* disease)
Von Willebrand's disease (an inherited abnormality of the von Willebrand protein which is
    part of the factor VIII complex and causes a defect in platelet adhesion)

Senile Ecchymoses (due to loss of skin elasticity)

* One of the rarer eponymous diseases in that it is named after the first family 'Christmas' described as
  suffering from it, rather than the clinician who wrote the case up.

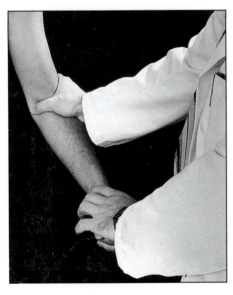

Figure 7.2
Feeling for the epitrochlear lymph node.

Axillary Nodes

These are palpated by raising the patient's arm and, using the left hand for the right side, the examiner pushes his or her fingers as high as possible into the axilla. The patient's arm is then brought down to rest on the examiner's forearm. The opposite is done for the other side (Figure 7.3).

There are five main groups of axillary nodes: (i) central; (ii) lateral (above and lateral); (iii) pectoral (medial); (iv) infraclavicular; and (v) subscapular (most inferior) (Figure 7.4). An effort should be made to feel for nodes in each of these areas of the axilla.

Table 7.4   *Characteristics of Lymph Nodes*

During the palpation of lymph nodes the following features must be considered:

Site

Palpable nodes may be localised to one region (e.g., local infection, early lymphoma) or be generalised (e.g., late lymphoma)

The palpable lymph node areas are:

   epitrochlear
   axillary
   cervical and occipital
   supraclavicular
   para-aortic (rarely palpable)
   inguinal
   popliteal

Size

Large nodes are usually abnormal (greater than 1cm)

Consistency

Hard nodes suggest carcinoma deposits, soft nodes may be normal, and rubbery nodes may be due to lymphoma

Tenderness

This implies infection or acute inflammation

Fixation

Nodes that are fixed to underlying structures are more likely to be infiltrated by carcinoma than mobile nodes

Overlying Skin

Inflammation of the overlying skin suggests infection, and tethering to the overlying skin suggests carcinoma

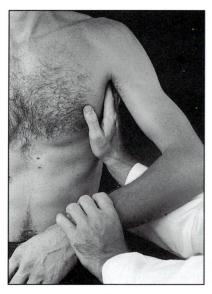

Figure 7.3
Feeling for the axillary lymph nodes.

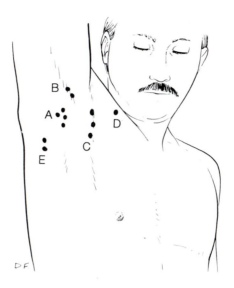

Figure 7.4   *The main groups of axillary lymph nodes: A = central; B = lateral; C = pectoral; D = infraclavicular; E = subscapular.*

The Face

The *eyes* should be examined for the presence of scleral jaundice, haemorrhage, or injection (due to increased prominence of scleral blood vessels, as in polycythaemia). Conjunctival pallor suggests anaemia and is more reliable than examination of the nailbeds or palmar creases. In Northern Europeans the combination of prematurely grey hair and blue eyes may indicate a predisposition to the autoimmune disease *pernicious anaemia*, where there is a vitamin B_{12} deficiency due to lack of intrinsic factor secretion by an atrophic gastric mucosa.

The *mouth* should be examined for hypertrophy of the gums, which may occur with infiltration by leukaemic cells especially in acute monocytic leukaemia, or with swelling in scurvy (Table 5.6). Gum bleeding must also be looked for, and ulceration, infection and haemorrhage of the buccal and pharyngeal mucosa noted. Atrophic glossitis occurs with megaloblastic anaemia or iron deficiency anaemia.

Waldeyer's* ring is a circle of lymphatic tissue in the posterior part of the oropharynx and nasopharynx and includes the tonsils and adenoids. Sometimes non-Hodgkin's lymphoma will involve Waldeyer's tonsillar ring, but Hodgkin's disease rarely does so.

Cervical and Supraclavicular Nodes

Sit the patient up and examine the cervical nodes from behind. There are eight groups. Attempt to identify each of the groups of nodes with your fingers (Figure

---

*   Heinrich Wilhelm Gottfried von Waldeyer-Hartz (b. 1836), Berlin anatomist.

7.5). Palpate first the submental node which lies directly under the chin, then the submandibular nodes which are below the angle of the jaw. Next palpate the jugular chain which lies anterior to the sternomastoid muscle and then the posterior triangle nodes which are posterior to the sternomastoid muscle. Palpate the occipital region for occipital nodes and then move to the postauricular node behind the ear and the preauricular node in front of the ear. Finally from the front, with the patient's shoulders slightly shrugged, feel in the supraclavicular fossa and at the base of the sternomastoid muscle for the supraclavicular nodes. Causes of lymphadenopathy, localised and generalised, are given in Table 7.5.

Bone Tenderness

While the patient is sitting up tap over the spine with the fist for bony tenderness. This may be caused by an enlarging marrow due to infiltration by myeloma, lymphoma or carcinoma, or due to malignant disease of the bony skeleton. Also gently press the sternum and both clavicles with the heel of the hand and then test both shoulders by pushing them towards each other with your hands.

The Abdominal Examination

Lie the patient flat again. Examine the abdomen carefully (page 160), especially for splenomegaly (Table 7.6), hepatomegaly, para-aortic nodes, inguinal nodes and testicular masses. Remember that a central deep abdominal mass may occa-

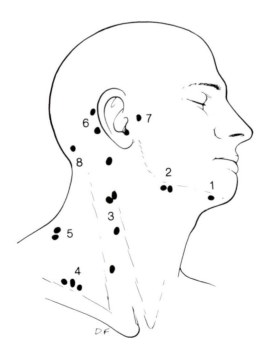

Figure 7.5 *Cervical and supraclavicular lymph nodes. 1-submental, 2-submandibular, 3-jugular chain, 4-supraclavicular, 5-posterior triangle, 6-postauricular, 7-preauricular, 8-occipital.*

Table 7.5 *Causes of Lymphadenopathy*

Generalised Lymphadenopathy
Lymphoma (rubbery and firm)
Leukaemia (e.g., chronic lymphocytic leukaemia, acute lymphocytic leukaemia)
Infections: viral (e.g., infectious mononucleosis, cytomegalovirus, HIV), bacterial (e.g., tuberculosis, brucellosis, syphilis), protozoal (e.g., toxoplasmosis)
Connective tissue diseases: e.g., rheumatoid arthritis, systemic lupus erythematosus
Infiltration: e.g., sarcoid
Drugs: e.g., phenytoin (pseudolymphoma)
Localised Lymphadenopathy
Local acute or chronic infection
Metastases from carcinoma or other solid tumours
Lymphoma, especially Hodgkin's disease

sionally be due to enlarged para-aortic nodes. Para-aortic adenopathy strongly suggests lymphoma or lymphatic leukaemia. The rectal examination may reveal evidence of bleeding or a carcinoma. (Assessment of the patient with suspected malignancy is presented in Table 7.7.)

Inguinal Nodes

There are two groups—one along the inguinal ligament and the other along the femoral vessels. Small, firm mobile nodes are commonly found in otherwise normal subjects.

The Legs

Inspect for any bruising, pigmentation or scratch marks. Palpable purpura over the buttocks and legs are present in Henoch-Schönlein* purpura. Leg ulcers may occur above the medial or lateral malleolus in association with haemolytic anaemia (including sickle cell anaemia and hereditary spherocytosis), probably as a result of tissue infarction due to abnormal blood viscosity. Leg ulcers can also occur with thalassaemia, macroglobulinaemia, thrombotic thrombocytopenic purpura, and polycythaemia, as well as in Felty's syndrome.

Very occasionally, popliteal nodes may be felt in the popliteal fossa.

The legs should also be examined for evidence of the neurological abnormalities caused by vitamin B_{12} deficiency: peripheral neuropathy and subacute combined degeneration of the spinal cord (page 398). Vitamin B_{12} is an essential cofactor in the conversion of homocysteine to methionine; in B_{12} deficiency, the lack of methionine impairs methylation of myelin basic protein. Deficiency of vitamin B_{12} can also result in optic atrophy and mental changes. Lead poisoning causes anaemia and foot (or wrist) drop.

The Fundi

Examine the fundi. An increase in blood viscosity, which occurs in diseases such as macroglobulinaemia, myeloproliferative disease or chronic granulocytic leukae-

---

* Henoch-Schönlein purpura is also characterised by glomerulonephritis (manifested by haematuria and proteinuria), arthralgias and abdominal pain.

Table 7.6 *Causes of Splenomegaly*

Massive

Common

Chronic myeloid leukaemia
Myelofibrosis

Rare

Malaria
Kala azar
Primary lymphoma of spleen

Moderate

The above causes
Portal hypertension
Lymphoma
Leukaemia (acute or chronic)
Thalassaemia
Storage diseases, e.g., Gaucher's* disease

Small

The above causes
Other myeloproliferative disorders:
  polycythaemia rubra vera
  essential thrombocythaemia
Haemolytic anaemia
Megaloblastic anaemia (rarely)
Infection:
  viral (e.g., infectious mononucleosis, hepatitis)
  bacterial (e.g., infective endocarditis)
  protozoal (e.g., malaria)
Connective tissue diseases:
  e.g., rheumatoid arthritis
  systemic lupus erythematosus
  polyarteritis nodosa
Infiltrations:
  e.g., amyloid, sarcoid

NB: Secondary carcinomatosis is a *rare* cause of splenomegaly.

*   Phillipe Charles Ernest Gaucher (b. 1854), Paris physician.

Table 7.7 *Assessing the Patient with Suspected Malignancy*

1. Palpate all draining lymph nodes
2. Examine all remaining lymph node groups
3. Examine the abdomen, particularly for hepatomegaly and ascites
4. Feel the testes
5. Perform a rectal examination and pelvic examination
6. Examine the lungs
7. Examine the breasts
8. Examine the skin and nails for melanoma

mia, can cause engorged retinal vessels and later papilloedema (page 345). Haemorrhages may occur because of a haemostatic disorder. Retinal lesions (multiple yellow-white patches) may be present in toxoplasmosis (Figure 13.1) and cytomegalovirus infections (Figure 13.2).

Examination of the Peripheral Blood Film

This is a simple and useful clinical investigation.

A properly made peripheral blood film is one of the simplest, least invasive and most readily accessible forms of 'tissue biopsy', and can be a very useful diagnostic tool in clinical medicine. An examination of the patient's blood film can (i) assess whether the morphology of red cells, white cells and platelets is normal; (ii) help to characterise the type of anaemia; (iii) detect the presence of abnormal cells and provide clues about quantitative changes in plasma proteins—e.g., paraproteinaemia; (iv) help to make the diagnosis of an underlying infection, malignant infiltration of the bone marrow, or primary proliferative haematological disorder. In the following pages are presented illustrated examples of some clinical problems diagnosed by examination of the blood film (Figures 7.6 to 7.19).

Correlation of Physical Signs and Haematological Disease

Anaemia

Anaemia is a reduction in the concentration of haemoglobin below 135g/L in an adult male and 115g/L in an adult female. Anaemia is not a disease itself, but results from an underlying pathological process (Table 7.8). It can be classified according to the blood film. Red blood cells with a low mean cell volume (MCV) appear small (microcytic) and pale (hypochromic). Those with a high MCV appear large and round or oval shaped (macrocytic). Alternatively, the red blood cells may be normal in shape and size (normochromic, normocytic) but reduced in number.

Signs of a severe anaemia of any cause include pallor, tachycardia, wide pulse pressure, systolic ejection murmurs due to a compensatory rise in cardiac output, and cardiac failure if myocardial reserve is reduced. There may be signs of the underlying cause.

Pancytopenia

Signs

There may be clinical evidence of anaemia, leucopenia (reduced numbers of white blood cells resulting in susceptibility to infection) and thrombocytopenia (petechiae and bleeding)—a deficiency in all three bone marrow cell lines. If confirmed on a blood count this condition is called pancytopenia.

Causes

Aplastic anaemia: severe hypoplasia of the erythroid, myeloid and platelet precursor cell lines in the bone marrow resulting in a bone marrow which is fatty and empty of cells. The causes are listed in Table 7.8; 50% have no cause identified.

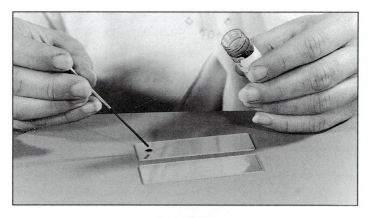

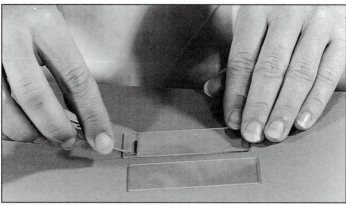

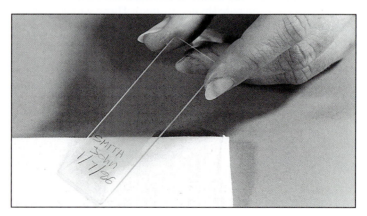

Figure 7.6 *Preparation of a peripheral blood film. After the film is made it is labelled, allowed to dry and then stained with May-Gruenwald-Giemsa stain before examination. If protected with a coverslip, the film can be stored for many years for future review.*

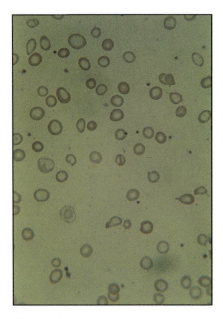

Figure 7.7

Iron deficiency anaemia. Red cells show varying shape and size and are generally hypochromic.

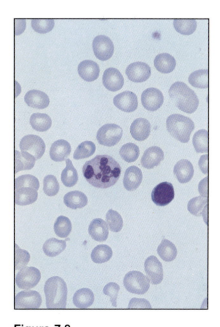

Figure 7.8

Megaloblastic anaemia. Red cells are macrocytic with many oval forms and the neutrophil is hypersegmented.

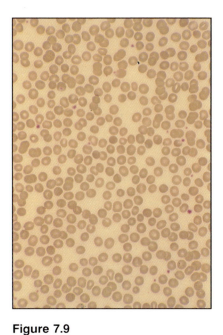

Figure 7.9

Spherocytic anaemia (hereditary spherocytosis or autoimmune haemolytic anaemia). The numerous red blood cells which are small, round and lack central pallor are spherocytes (the big red blood cells are probably reticulocytes).

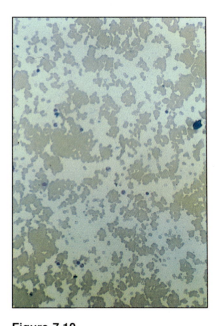

Figure 7.10

Autoagglutination (cold haemagglutinin disease). Film shows clumping of red cells (low power).

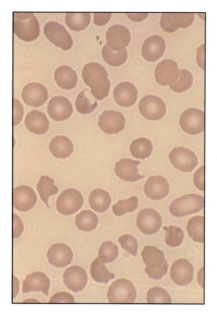

Figure 7.11

Microangiopathic haemolysis (e.g., disseminated intravascular coagulation). Frequent fragmented (bitten) red cells.

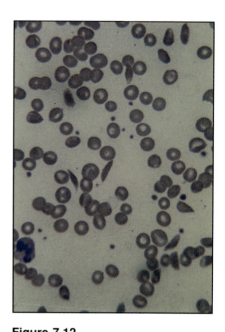

Figure 7.12

Sickle cell anaemia. Film shows several sickle-shaped cells with target cells probably secondary to the 'autosplenectomy' which occurs in this disease.

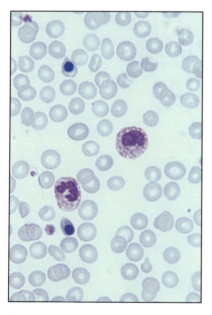

Figure 7.13

Leucoerythroblastic picture, indicative of bone marrow infiltration. Film shows circulating nucleated red blood cells and immature white cells.

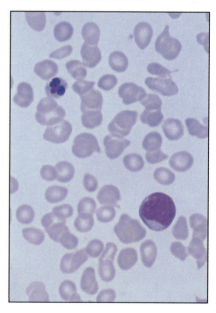

Figure 7.14   *Myelofibrosis. Film shows a dysplastic nucleated red blood cell, frequent tear-drop poikilocytes and a primitive granulocyte.*

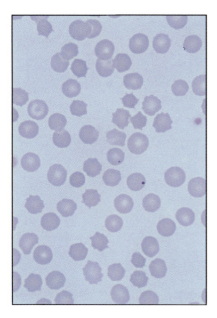

Figure 7.15

Postsplenectomy picture. Film shows several Howell-Jolly bodies, target cells and crenated cells.

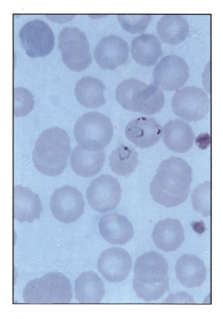

Figure 7.16

Malaria. The two red cells in the centre show the trophozoite.

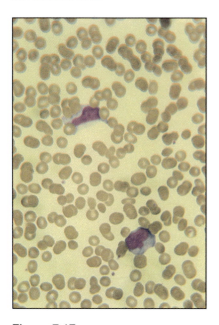

Figure 7.17

Viral illness (e.g., infectious mononucleosis). Film shows two atypical or 'switched-on' lymphocytes.

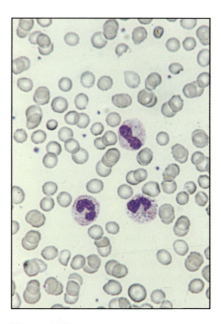

Figure 7.18

Bacterial infection (e.g., pneumonia, infective endocarditis). The white cell in the centre is a band form with prominent 'toxic' granules.

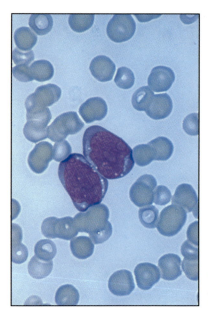

Figure 7.19

Acute leukaemia. The film shows two very primitive white cells with prominent nucleoli.

Table 7.8   *Causes of Anaemia*

Microcytic Anaemia

Iron deficiency anaemia (iron is essential for haem production)
   Chronic bleeding (commonest cause, usually from gastrointestinal or menstrual loss)
   Malabsorption, e.g., gastrectomy, coeliac disease
   Hookworm (blood loss)
   Pregnancy (increased demand)
   NB: Dietary inadequacy alone is rarely the sole cause
Thalassaemia minor (an abnormal haemoglobin)
Sideroblastic anaemia (iron incorporation into haem is abnormal)
Long-standing anaemia of chronic disease

Macrocytic Anaemia

Megaloblastic bone marrow (oval macrocytes on the blood film)
   Vitamin B_{12} deficiency due to:
     Pernicious anaemia
     Gastrectomy
     Tropical sprue or bacterial overgrowth
     Ileal disease, e.g., Crohn's disease, ileal resection (>60 cm)
     Fish tapeworm (*Diphyllobothrium latum*) in Scandinavia especially
     Poor diet (vegans, very rare)
   Folate deficiency due to:
     Dietary deficiency, especially alcoholics
     Malabsorption, especially coeliac disease
     Increased cell turnover, e.g., pregnancy, leukaemia, chronic haemolysis, chronic
       inflammation
     Antifolate drugs—phenytoin, methotrexate

—continued

Table 7.8 *Causes of Anaemia (continued)*

Non-megaloblastic bone marrow (round macrocytes on the blood film)
  Alcohol
  Cirrhosis of the liver
  Reticulocytosis, e.g., haemolysis, haemorrhage
  Hypothyroidism
  Marrow infiltration
  Myelodysplastic syndrome
  Myeloproliferative disease

Normocytic Anaemia

Bone marrow failure:
  Aplastic anaemia (bone marrow fatty or empty), e.g., drugs (such as chloramphenicol,
    indomethacin, phenytoin, gold, sulphonamides, anti-neoplastics), radiation,
    systemic lupus erythematosus, viral hepatitis, pregnancy, Fanconi syndrome,
    idiopathic
  Ineffective haematopoiesis (normal or increased bone marrow cellularity), e.g.,
    myelodysplastic syndrome, paroxysmal nocturnal haemoglobinuria
  Infiltration, e.g., leukaemia, lymphoma, myeloma, granuloma, myelofibrosis
Anaemia of chronic disease:
  Chronic inflammation
    e.g., Infection—abscess, tuberculosis
        Connective tissue disease
  Malignancy
  Endocrine deficiencies
    e.g., Hypothyroidism
        Hypopituitarism
        Addison's disease
  Liver disease
  Chronic renal failure
  Malnutrition
Haemolytic anaemia:
  Intracorpuscular defects
    e.g., Hereditary spherocytosis, elliptocytosis
        Haemoglobinopathies—sickle cell anaemia, thalassaemia
        Paroxysmal nocturnal haemoglobinura (PNH)
  Extracorpuscular defects:
    e.g., Immune: autoimmune (warm or cold antibody)
          incompatible blood transfusion
        Hypersplenism
        Trauma: marathon runners, prosthetic heart valves
        Microangiopathic: disseminated intravascular coagulation
        Toxic: malaria

Marrow infiltration by leukaemia, lymphoma, carcinoma, myeloma, myelofibrosis or granulomata.

Other: acute leukaemia (subleukaemic phase), pernicious anaemia, hypersplenism, systemic lupus erythematosus, folate deficiency.

Acute Leukaemia

Leukaemia is a neoplastic proliferation of one of the blood forming cells. Acute leukaemia presents with marrow failure from progressive infiltration of the marrow with immature cells. The course is rapidly fatal without treatment. Acute leukaemias can be divided into two main types: acute lymphoblastic leukaemia and acute myeloid leukaemia.

General Signs of Acute Leukaemia

Pallor (anaemia), fever (which usually indicates infection secondary to neutropenia), and petechiae (thrombocytopenia) are all due to bone marrow failure. Weight loss, muscle wasting (hypercatabolic state), and localised infections (e.g., of the tonsils or perirectal region, due to leucopenia) also occur.

Signs of Infiltration of the Haemopoietic System

These include: (i) bony tenderness, due to infiltration or infarction; (ii) lymphadenopathy (slight to moderate, especially in acute lymphoblastic leukaemia); (iii) splenomegaly (slight to moderate, occurs especially in acute lymphoblastic leukaemia; the spleen may be tender due to splenic infarction); and (iv) hepatomegaly (slight to moderate).

Signs of Infiltration of Other Areas

There may be (i) tonsillar enlargement (especially in acute lymphoblastic leukaemia); (ii) swelling or bleeding of the gums, especially in monocytic leukaemia; (iii) pleural effusions; (iv) nerve palsies, involving the spinal nerve roots or the cranial nerves; or (v) meningism (page 334) due to infiltration of the meninges, especially in acute lymphoblastic leukaemia.

Chronic Leukaemia

This is a haematological malignancy in which the leukaemic cell is at first well differentiated. These have a better prognosis untreated than acute leukaemia. There are two main types: chronic myeloid leukaemia and chronic lymphocytic leukaemia.

Signs of Chronic Myeloid Leukaemia

This is one of the myeloproliferative disorders. There is an expanded granulocytic mass in the bone marrow, liver and spleen.

General signs may include pallor (anaemia due to bone marrow infiltration) and secondary gout (common).

Haemopoietic system signs include massive splenomegaly and moderate hepatomegaly. NB: Lymphadenopathy is usually a sign of blast transformation.

Signs of Chronic Lymphocytic Leukaemia

There may be tiredness and pallor. Recurrent acute infections occur.

Haemopoietic system signs include marked or moderate lymphadenopathy and moderate hepatosplenomegaly.

Other signs include a Coombs* test-positive haemolytic anaemia, herpes zoster skin infections and nodular infiltrates.

---

* Robin Coombs (b. 1921), Cambridge pathologist.

Myeloproliferative Disease

This is a group of disorders of the stem cell. These include polycythaemia rubra vera, myelofibrosis, chronic myeloid leukaemia and essential thrombocythaemia. Overlapping clinical and pathological features occur in these disorders. Therefore, patients may have signs of one or more of the conditions. Any of them may progress to acute myeloid leukaemia.

Polycythaemia

This is an elevated haemoglobin concentration and can result from an increased red blood cell mass or a decreased plasma volume. Polycythaemia rubra vera results from an autonomous increase in the red blood cell production. Patients with polycythaemia often have a striking ruddy, plethoric appearance. To examine a patient with suspected polycythaemia, assess for both the manifestations of polycythaemia rubra vera and for other possible underlying causes of polycythaemia (Table 7.9).

Table 7.9 *Polycythaemia*

Signs of Polycythaemia Rubra Vera
Plethoric appearance including engorged conjunctival and retinal vessels (not specific)
Scratch marks (generalised pruritus)
Splenomegaly (80%)
Bleeding tendency (platelet dysfunction)
Peripheral vascular and ischaemic heart disease (thrombosis, slow circulation)
Gout
Mild hypertension
Causes of Polycythaemia
Absolute Polycythaemia (increased red cell mass)
Idiopathic: polycythaemia rubra vera
Secondary polycythaemia
Increased erythropoietin:
Renal disease—polycystic disease, hydronephrosis, tumour
Hepatocellular carcinoma
Cerebellar haemangioblastoma
Uterine fibroma
Virilising syndromes
Cushing's syndrome
Phaeochromocytoma
Hypoxic states (erythropoietin secondarily increased)
Chronic lung disease
Sleep apnoea
Cyanotic congenital heart disease
Abnormal haemoglobins
Carbon monoxide poisoning
Relative Polycythaemia (decreased plasma volume)
Dehydration
Stress polycythaemia: Gaisböck's* disease

* Felix Gaisböck (1868–1955), German physician, described this in 1905.

Look at the patient and estimate the state of hydration (dehydration alone can cause an elevated haemoglobin due to haemoconcentration). Note if there is a Cushingoid (page 310) or virilised (page 318) appearance. Cyanosis may be present because of an underlying condition such as cyanotic congenital heart disease or chronic lung disease. All these diseases can result in secondary polycythaemia.

The arms should be inspected for scratch marks; pruritus occurs in polycythaemia rubra vera, possibly due to basophil histamine release. Take the blood pressure: very rarely a phaeochromocytoma will cause secondary polycythaemia and hypertension.

Examine the eyes. Look for injected conjunctivae. Fundal hyperviscosity changes, including engorged, dilated retinal veins and haemorrhages may be present. Inspect the tongue for central cyanosis.

Examine the cardiovascular system for signs of cyanotic congenital heart disease and the respiratory system for signs of chronic lung disease. The abdomen must be carefully assessed for splenomegaly, which occurs in 80% of cases of polycythaemia rubra vera, but does not usually occur with the other causes of polycythaemia. There may be evidence of chronic liver disease or hepatocellular carcinoma, which may cause secondary polycythaemia. Palpate for the kidneys and perform a urinalysis. In women palpate the uterus. Polycystic kidney disease, hydronephrosis, renal carcinoma and uterine fibromata can all rarely cause secondary polycythaemia.

The legs must be inspected for scratch marks, gouty tophi and arthropathy, as well as for signs of peripheral vascular disease. In polycythaemia rubra vera, secondary gout occurs due to the increased cellular turnover resulting in hyperuricaemia. Peripheral vascular disease occurs in polycythaemia rubra vera because of thrombosis (as there is increased platelet adhesiveness and accelerated atherosclerosis) and slowed circulation due to hyperviscosity.

Look for cerebellar signs (page 407), which may be due to the presence of a cerebellar haemangioblastoma, a very rare cause of secondary polycythaemia. Examine the central nervous system for signs of a stroke due to thrombosis (page 391).

Myelofibrosis

This is a clonal haemopoietic stem cell disorder with fibrosis as a secondary phenomenon. Gradual replacement of the marrow by fibrosis and progressive splenomegaly characterise the disease.

General signs include pallor (anaemia occurs in most patients eventually) and petechiae (in 20% of patients, due to thrombocytopenia).

Haemopoietic system signs include splenomegaly (in almost all cases, and often to a massive degree—there may also be a splenic rub due to splenic infarction), hepatomegaly (occurs in 50% and can be massive), and lymphadenopathy (very uncommon).

Other signs are bony tenderness (uncommon) and gout (occurs in 5%).

Chronic Myeloid Leukaemia (see page 240)

Essential Thrombocythaemia

This is a sustained elevation of the platelet count above normal without any primary cause.

Table 7.10   *Staging of Lymphoma: Ann Arbor Classification*

Stage I
Disease confined to a single lymph node region or a single extra-lymphatic site (Ie).

Stage II
Disease confined to two or more lymph node regions on one side of the diaphragm.

Stage III
Disease confined to lymph nodes on both sides of the diaphragm with or without localised involvement of the spleen (IIIs), other extra-lymphatic organ or site (IIIe), or both.

Stage IV
Diffuse disease of one or more extra-lymphatic organs (with or without lymph node disease)

For any stage
a = no symptoms
b = fever, weight loss greater than 10% in 6 months, night sweats

General signs include spontaneous bleeding and thrombosis.
Haemopoietic system signs include splenomegaly.
Causes of thrombocytosis (platelet count more than $400 \times 10^9/L$) include: (i) following haemorrhage or surgery; (ii) postsplenectomy; (iii) iron deficiency; (iv) chronic inflammatory disease; (v) malignancy.
Causes of thrombocytosis (platelet count more than $800 \times 10^9/L$) include: (i) myeloproliferative disease; (ii) secondary to recent splenectomy or malignancy occasionally.

Lymphoma

This is a malignant disease of the lymphoid system. There are two main clinicopathological types: Hodgkin's disease (with the characteristic Reed-Sternberg* cell) and non-Hodgkin's lymphoma. Signs of lymphoma depend on the stages of the disease (Table 7.10).

Hodgkin's disease often presents in stage I or II, while non-Hodgkin's lymphoma usually presents in stage III or IV.

Signs of Hodgkin's Disease

1.   Lymph node enlargement: discrete, rubbery, painless, large and superficial nodes, often confined to one side and one lymph node group.
2.   Weight loss and fever with or without infection (reduced cell-mediated immunity) suggest a poor prognosis.
3.   Splenomegaly and hepatomegaly. Splenomegaly does not always indicate extensive disease.
4.   Organ infiltration occurs with late disease. Look especially for signs of (i) lung disease, such as a pleural effusion; (ii) bone pain or pathological fractures

---

*   Dorothy Reed (b. 1874), pathologist at Johns Hopkins Hospital, Baltimore, described these in 1902, and Karl Sternberg (1872–1935), pathologist, described giant cells in 1898.

(rare); (iii) spinal cord or nerve compression (rare); and (iv) nodular skin infiltrates (rare).

Signs of Non-Hodgkin's Lymphoma

1. Lymph node enlargement: often more than one site is involved and Waldeyer's ring is more commonly affected.
2. Hepatosplenomegaly is common.
3. Systemic signs, for example weight loss or fever, are less common.
4. Signs of extranodal spread are more common.
5. The disease may sometimes arise at an extranodal site e.g., the gastrointestinal tract.

Multiple Myeloma

This is a disseminated malignant disease of plasma cells.

General Signs

There may be signs of anaemia (due to bone marrow infiltration or as a result of renal failure), purpura (due to bone marrow infiltration and thrombocytopenia), or infection (particularly pneumonia).

Bony tenderness and pathological fractures may be present. Weight loss may be a feature. Skin changes include hypertrichosis, erythema annulare, yellow skin, and secondary amyloid deposits. There may be signs of spinal cord compression (page 397), or mental changes (due to hypercalcaemia).

Signs of chronic renal failure (page 203) which may be due to tubular damage from filtered light chains, uric acid nephropathy, hypercalcaemia, urinary tract infection, secondary amyloidosis or plasma cell infiltration.

Summary

The Haematological Examination: A Suggested Method
(Figure 7.20)

Position the patient as for a gastrointestinal examination. Make sure he or she is fully undressed. Look for bruising, pigmentation, cyanosis, jaundice and scratch marks (due to myeloproliferative disease or lymphoma). Also note the presence of frontal bossing and the racial origin of the patient.

Pick up the patient's hands. Look at the nails for koilonychia (spoon-shaped nails which are rarely seen today and indicate iron deficiency) and the changes of vasculitis. Pale palmar creases may indicate anaemia (usually the haemoglobin level has to be lower than 70 g/L). Evidence of arthropathy may be important (e.g., rheumatoid arthritis and Felty's syndrome, recurrent haemarthroses in bleeding disorders, secondary gout in myeloproliferative disorders).

Examine the epitrochlear nodes. Note any bruising. Remember petechiae are pinhead haemorrhages, while ecchymoses are larger bruises.

Go to the axillae and palpate the axillary nodes. There are five main areas: central, lateral (above and lateral), pectoral (most medial), infraclavicular and subscapular (most inferior).

Figure 7.20 *Haematological System*

Lying flat (1 pillow)

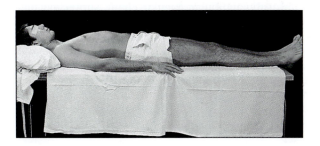

1. GENERAL INSPECTION
    Bruising (thrombocytopenia, scurvy, etc.)
    —Petechiae (pinhead bleeding)
    —Ecchymoses (large bruises)
    Pigmentation (lymphoma)
    Rashes and infiltrative lesions (lymphoma)
    Ulceration (neutropenia)
    Cyanosis (polycythaemia)
    Plethora (polycythaemia)
    Jaundice (haemolysis)
    Scratch marks (myeloproliferative diseases, lymphoma)
    Racial origin

2. HANDS
    Nails—koilonychia, pallor
    Palmar crease pallor (anaemia)
    Arthropathy (haemophilia, secondary gout, drug treatment, etc.)
    Pulse

3. EPITROCHLEAR NODES

    AXILLARY NODES

4. FACE
    Sclera—jaundice, pallor, conjunctival suffusion (polycythaemia)
    Mouth—gum hypertrophy (monocytic leukaemia, etc.), ulceration, infection, haemorrhage (marrow

aplasia, etc.); atrophic glossitis, angular stomatitis (iron, vitamin deficiencies)

5. CERVICAL NODES (sitting up)
    Palpate from behind

6. BONY TENDERNESS
    Spine
    Sternum
    Clavicles
    Shoulders

7. ABDOMEN (lying flat) and GENITALIA
    Detailed examination

8. LEGS
    Vasculitis (Henoch-Schönlein purpura—buttocks, thighs)
    Bruising
    Pigmentation
    Ulceration (e.g., haemoglobinopathies)
    Neurological signs (subacute combined degeneration, peripheral neuropathy)

9. OTHER
    Fundi (haemorrhages, infection, etc.)
    Temperature chart (infection)
    Urine analysis (haematuria, bile, etc.)
    Rectal and pelvic examination (blood loss)
    Hess test

Look at the face. Inspecting the eyes, note jaundice, pallor or haemorrhage of the sclerae, and the injected sclerae of polycythaemia. Examine the mouth. Note gum hypertrophy (e.g., from acute monocytic leukaemia or scurvy), ulceration, infection, haemorrhage, atrophic glossitis (e.g., from iron deficiency, or vitamin B_{12}

or folate deficiency) and angular stomatitis. Look for tonsillar and adenoid enlargement (Waldeyer's ring).

Sit the patient up. Examine the cervical nodes from behind. There are eight groups: submental, submandibular, jugular chain, supraclavicular, posterior triangle, postauricular, preauricular and occipital (Figure 7.5). Then feel the supraclavicular area from the front. Tap the spine with your fist for bony tenderness (caused by an enlarging marrow—e.g., in myeloma or carcinoma). Also gently press the sternum, clavicles and shoulders for bony tenderness.

Lie the patient flat again. Examine the abdomen. Don't forget to feel the testes, and to perform a rectal and pelvic examination (for tumour or bleeding). Spring the hips for pelvic tenderness. Palpate the inguinal nodes. There are two groups—along the inguinal ligament and along the femoral vessels.

Examine the legs. Note particularly leg ulcers. Examine the legs from a neurological aspect, for evidence of vitamin B_{12} deficiency or peripheral neuropathy from any other cause. Remember hypothyroidism can cause anaemia and neurological disease.

Finally, examine the fundi, look at the temperature chart, and test the urine.

Suggested Reading

Original and Review Articles

Anonymous, Cancer detection in adults by physical examination. US Public Health Service. *Am Fam Phys* 1995; 51: 871–4, 877–80, 883–5.

Beutler E. The common anemias. *JAMA* 1988; 259: 2433–2437.

Grover SA, Barkun AN, Sackett DL, Does this patient have splenomegaly? *JAMA* 1993; 270: 2218–21.

Nardone DA, Roth KM, Mazur DJ, McAfee JH. Usefulness of physical examination in detecting the presence or absence of anemia. *Arch Intern Med* 1990; 150: 201–204.

Robertson TI. Clinical diagnosis in patients with lymphadenopathy. *Med J Aust* 1979; 2: 73–76.

Textbooks

Hoffbrand AV, Pettit JE. Essential haematology. 3rd ed. London: Blackwell, 1993.

Isbister JP. Clinical haematology. A problem-oriented approach. Sydney: Williams & Wilkins. ADIS, 1986.

Jandl J. Blood. Textbook of hematology. Boston: Little Brown, 1987.

Ludlam C, editor. Clinical haematology. Edinburgh: Churchill Livingstone, 1990.

Penington D, Rush B, Castaldi P, editors. Clinical haematology in medical practice G C de Gruchy. 5th ed. Oxford: Blackwell, 1990.

Chapter 8

THE RHEUMATOLOGICAL SYSTEM

The rheumatism is a common name for many aches and pains which have yet got no peculiar appellation, though owing to very different causes.

William Herberden (1710–1801)

Rheumatology is 'the study of the Rheumatic Diseases including arthritis, rheumatic fever, fibrositis, neuralgia, myositis, bursitis, gout and other conditions producing somatic pain, stiffness and soreness' (Oxford English Dictionary supplement, 1987). The rheumatological system therefore includes diseases of the joints, tendons and muscles.

The Rheumatological History

Presenting Symptoms (Table 8.1)

Joint Pain and Swelling

The underlying aetiology of joint pain can often be determined by establishing the distribution and duration of joint involvement. Remember, arthralgia is the presence of joint pain without swelling while with arthritis there is usually pain and swelling. Determine if one or many joints are involved. Find out if the symptoms are of an acute or chronic nature and whether they are getting better or worse. The effect of rest and exercise on the joint pain should be determined. Patients with rheumatoid arthritis have joint symptoms which are worse after rest while those with osteoarthritis have pain which is worse after exercise. Ask about the sequence of onset of joint involvement. Precipitating factors such as trauma should be noted. The causes of monoarthritis and polyarthritis, and the patterns of polyarthritis in various diseases are presented in Tables 8.2, 8.3 and 8.4.

Ask about the presence of early morning stiffness and the length of time that this stiffness lasts. Morning stiffness classically occurs in rheumatoid arthritis and other inflammatory arthropathies, and the duration of stiffness is a guide to its severity.

It is vital to inquire about the functional capacity of the patient with arthritis (Table 8.5). You need to determine how independent the patient is at home and at work. If the patient needs assistance, ask if any aids and appliances are used. If the

Table 8.1 *Rheumatological History—Major Symptoms*

Joints
  Pain
  Swelling
  Morning stiffness
  Loss of function
Eyes
  Dry eyes and mouth
  Red eyes
Systemic
  Raynaud's phenomenon
  Rash, fever, fatigue, weight loss, diarrhoea, mucosal ulcers

Table 8.2 *Causes of Monoarthritis*

A Single Hot Red Swollen Joint (Acute Monoarthritis)
Septic arthritis
  Haematogenous—e.g., staphylococcal or gonococcal (latter may be polyarticular)
  Secondary to penetrating injury
Traumatic
Gout, pseudogout, or hydroxyapatite arthropathy
Haemarthrosis—e.g., haemophilia
Seronegative spondyloarthritis (occasionally)

A Single Chronic Inflamed Joint (Chronic Monoarthritis)
Chronic infection—e.g., tuberculosis
Seronegative spondyloarthritis
Pigmented villonodular synovitis

Table 8.3 *Causes of Polyarthritis*

Acute Polyarthritis
Infection—viral, bacterial
Onset of chronic polyarthritis

Chronic Polyarthritis
Rheumatoid arthritis
Seronegative spondyloarthritis
Primary osteoarthritis
Gout, pseudogout, or hydroxyapatite arthropathy
Connective tissue disease, e.g., systemic lupus erythematosus
Infection, e.g., Lyme arthritis (rare spirochaetal infection)

patient is not independent but partially dependent, you need to determine what help is needed with daily activities such as dressing and bathing.

Back Pain

This is a very common complaint. It is most often a consequence of local musculoskeletal disease. Ask where the pain is situated, whether it began suddenly

Table 8.4 *Patterns of Polyarthropathy*

Rheumatoid Arthritis

This is usually a symmetrical arthritis
Hands: proximal interphalangeal, metacarpophalangeal and wrist joints
Elbows
Small joints of the upper cervical spine
Knees
Feet: tarsal and metatarsophalangeal joints

Seronegative Spondyloarthritis

This is commonly an asymmetrical arthritis
Ankylosing Spondylitis
Sacroiliac joints and spine
Hips, knees, and shoulders
Psoriatic arthritis
Terminal interphalangeal joints
Sacroiliac joints
Rheumatoid pattern
Reiter's Syndrome
Sacroiliac joints and spine
Hips
Knees
Ankles and most of the joints of the feet

Primary Osteoarthritis

This is usually symmetrical and can affect many joints
Fingers: distal (Heberden's nodes) and proximal (Bouchard's nodes) interphalangeal
     joints, and metacarpophalangeal joints of the thumbs
Acromioclavicular joints
Small joints of the spine (lower cervical and lumbar)
Knees
Metatarsophalangeal joints of the great toes

Secondary Osteoarthritis

This is asymmetrical and affects previously injured, inflamed or infected weight-bearing
     joints
Hip
Knee
Intervertebral disc

Table 8.5 *Functional Assessment in Rheumatoid Arthritis*

Class 1:	Normal functional ability
Class 2:	Ability to carry out normal activities, despite discomfort or limited mobility of one or more joints
Class 3:	Ability to perform only a few of the tasks of the normal occupation or of self-care
Class 4:	Complete or almost complete incapacity with the patient confined to wheelchair or to bed

or gradually, whether it is localised or diffuse, whether it radiates to the limbs or elsewhere and whether the pain is aggravated by movement, coughing or straining. Musculoskeletal pain is characteristically well localised and is aggravated by movement. If there is a spinal cord lesion there may be pain that occurs in a dermatomal distribution. This helps to localise the level of the lesion (page 397). Diseases such as osteoporosis (with crush fractures), osteomalacia or infiltration of carcinoma, leukaemia or myeloma may cause progressive and unremitting back pain. The pain may be of sudden onset but is usually self-limiting if it results from the crush fracture of a vertebral body. In ankylosing spondylitis the pain is usually situated over the sacroiliac joints and lumbar spine. Pain from diseases of the abdomen and chest can also be referred to the back.

Limb Pain

This can occur from disease of the musculoskeletal system, the skin, the vascular system or the nervous system. Musculoskeletal pain may be due to trauma. Muscle disease such as polymyositis can present with an aching pain in the proximal muscles around the shoulders and hips associated with weakness (page 405). Pain and stiffness in the shoulders and hips in patients over the age of 50 years may be due to polymyalgia rheumatica. Bone disease such as osteomyelitis, osteomalacia, osteoporosis or tumours can cause limb pain. Inflammation of tendons (tenosynovitis) can produce local pain over the affected area.

Vascular disease may also produce pain in the limbs. Acute arterial occlusion causes severe pain of sudden onset (page 64). Chronic peripheral vascular disease can result in calf pain on exercise that is relieved by rest. This is called intermittent claudication (page 30). Venous thrombosis can also cause diffuse aching pain in the legs associated with swelling (page 62).

Nerve entrapment and neuropathy can both cause limb pain (page 380). Injury to peripheral nerves can result in vasomotor changes and severe limb pain. This is called *causalgia*. Even following amputation of a limb, phantom limb pain may develop and be a chronic problem.

Raynaud's Phenomenon

Raynaud's* phenomenon is an abnormal response of the fingers to cold. The fingers first turn white, then blue and finally red after exposure to cold. It is during the red phase that the pain is most severe. Patients with Raynaud's disease have Raynaud's phenomenon without an obvious underlying cause. However, it tends to be familial and females are more likely to be affected. In connective tissue diseases, Raynaud's phenomenon can occur and may lead to the formation of digital ulcers (Table 8.6).

Dry Eyes and Mouth

Dry eyes and dry mouth are characteristic of Sjögren's syndrome (Table 8.7). This syndrome may occur in isolation (primary Sjögrens) or in association with rheumatoid arthritis and other connective tissue disease. Mucus secreting glands become infiltrated with lymphocytes and plasma cells which cause atrophy and fibrosis. The dry eyes can result in conjunctivitis, keratitis and corneal ulcers. Sjögren's

---

* Maurice Raynaud (1834–1881) described this in his first work, published in Paris in 1862.

Table 8.6 *Causes of Raynaud's Phenomenon*

Reflex
Raynaud's disease (idiopathic)
Vibrating machinery injury
Cervical spondylosis

Connective Tissue Disease
Scleroderma, CREST syndrome, mixed connective tissue disease
Systemic lupus erythematosus
Polyarteritis nodosa
Rheumatoid arthritis
Polymyositis

Arterial Disease
Embolism or thrombosis
Buerger's disease (thromboangiitis obliterans)
Trauma

Haematological
Polycythaemia
Leukaemia
Dysproteinaemia
Cold agglutinin disease

Poisons
Drugs: beta-blockers, ergotamine
Vinyl chloride

Table 8.7 *Clinical Features of Sjögren's Syndrome*

In this syndrome mucus-secreting glands are infiltrated by lymphocytes and plasma cells which cause atrophy and fibrosis of glandular tissue
1. Dry eyes: conjunctivitis, keratitis, corneal ulcers (rarely vascularisation of the cornea)
2. Dry mouth
3. Chest: infection secondary to reduced mucus secretion
4. Kidneys: renal tubular acidosis or nephrogenic diabetes insipidus
5. Genital tract: atrophic vaginitis
6. Pseudolymphoma: lymphadenopathy and splenomegaly which may rarely progress to a true (usually non-Hodgkin's) lymphoma

NB: This syndrome occurs in rheumatoid arthritis and with the connective tissue diseases

syndrome can also have a secondary effect on other organs such as the lungs or kidneys.

Red Eyes

The seronegative spondyloarthropathies and Behçet's syndrome (page 286) but not rheumatoid arthritis may be complicated by iritis, as described on page 368.

Systemic Symptoms

A number of other symptoms may occur with specific rheumatological diseases. Fatigue is common with connective tissue disease. Weight loss and diarrhoea may occur with scleroderma, because of small bowel bacterial overgrowth. Mucosal ulcers are common in some connective tissue diseases such as systemic lupus erythematosus (SLE). Specific rashes can also occur. Generalised stiffness can be due to rheumatoid arthritis or scleroderma, but other causes include systemic infection (e.g., influenza). excessive exercise, polymyalgia rheumatica, neuromuscular disease (e.g., extrapyramidal disease, tetanus, myotonia, dermatomyositis) and hypothyroidism. Finally, fever may be associated with the connective tissue diseases.

Past History

It is important to inquire about any history of trauma or surgery in the past. Similarly, a history of recent infection including hepatitis, streptococcal pharyngitis, rubella, dysentery, gonorrhoea and tuberculosis may be relevant to the onset of arthralgia or arthritis. A history of tick bite may indicate that the patient has Lyme disease. Inflammatory bowel disease can result in arthritis, as described on page 191. A history of psoriasis may indicate that the arthritis is due to psoriatic arthropathy. It is also important to inquire about any history of arthritis in childhood.

Social History

Determine the patient's domestic set-up and occupation. This is particularly relevant if a chronic disabling arthritis has developed. Any history of venereal disease in the past is important but non-specific urethritis and gonorrhoea are especially relevant.

Treatment History

Document current and previous anti-arthritic medications (e.g., aspirin, other non-steroidal anti-inflammatory drugs, gold, methotrexate, penicillamine, chloroquine, steroids). Any side effects of these drugs also need to be listed. Inquire about physiotherapy and joint surgery in the past.

Family History

Some diseases associated with chronic arthritis run in families. These including rheumatoid arthritis, gout and primary osteoarthritis, the seronegative spondyloarthropathies and inflammatory bowel disease.

The Rheumatological Examination

There are certain established ways of examining the joints and related structures and it is important to be aware of the numerous systemic complications of rheumatological diseases. The actual system of examination depends on the patient's history and sometimes on the examiner's noticing an abnormality on general inspection. Formal examination of all the joints is rarely part of the routine physical examination, but students should learn how to handle each joint properly. Diseases of the extra-articular soft tissues are particularly common.

General Inspection

This is important for two reasons: first, it gives an indication of the patient's functional disability, which is essential in all rheumatological assessments, and second, certain conditions can be diagnosed by careful inspection. Look at the patient as he or she walks into the room. Does walking appear to be painful and difficult? What posture is taken, does the patient require assistance such as a stick, is there obvious deformity and what joints does it involve? Note the pattern of joint involvement, which gives a clue about the likely underlying disease (Tables 8.2 to 8.4).

For a more detailed examination the patient should be in bed undressed as far as practical. The opportunity of watching the patient remove the clothes should not be lost because arthritis can interfere with this essential daily task.

Principles of Joint Examination

Certain general rules apply to the examination of all the joints and they can be summarised as: *look*, *feel*, *move*, *measure*, and *compare with the opposite side*.

Look

The first principle is always to compare right with left. The skin is inspected for *erythema* indicating underlying inflammation and suggesting active arthritis or infection, *atrophy* suggesting chronic underlying disease, *scars* indicating previous operations such as tendon repairs or joint replacements, and *rashes*. For example, psoriasis is associated with a rash and polyarthritis (inflammation of more than one joint). The psoriatic rash consists of scaling erythematous plaques on extensor surfaces. The nails are often also affected (page 258). Also look for a vasculitic skin rash (inflammation of the blood vessels of the skin), which can range in appearance from palpable purpura or livedo reticularis (page 279) to skin necrosis.

Note any *swelling* over the joint. There are a number of possible causes: these include effusion into the joint space, hypertrophy and inflammation of the synovium (e.g., rheumatoid arthritis) or bony overgrowths at the joint margins (e.g., osteoarthritis). It may also occur when tissues around the joints become involved, as with the tendonitis or bursitis of rheumatoid arthritis.

Deformity is the sign of a chronic, usually destructive arthritis, and ranges from mild ulnar deviation of the metacarpophalangeal joints in early rheumatoid arthritis to the gross destruction and disorganisation of a denervated (Charcot's*) joint (rare) (Figure 9.17, page 323).

Look for abnormal bone alignment. *Subluxation* is said to be present when displaced parts of the joint surfaces remain partly in contact. *Dislocation* is used to describe displacement where there is loss of contact between the joint surfaces.

Muscle wasting results from a combination of disuse of the joint, inflammation of the surrounding tissues and sometimes nerve entrapment. It tends to affect muscle groups adjacent to the diseased joint (e.g., quadriceps wasting with active arthritis of the knee) and is a sign of chronicity.

---

* Jean Martin Charcot (1824–1893), Parisian physician and neurologist.

Feel

Palpate for skin *warmth*. This is done traditionally with the backs of the fingers where temperature appreciation is said to be better. A cool joint is unlikely to be involved in an acute inflammatory process. A swollen and warm joint may be affected by active synovitis (see below), infection (e.g., *Staphylococcus*) or crystal arthritis (e.g., gout). *Tenderness* is a guide to the acuteness of the inflammation. It can be graded as follows: grade I, patient complains of pain; grade II, patient complains of pain and winces; grade III, patient complains of pain, winces, and withdraws the joint; grade IV, patient does not allow palpation. This may result from joint inflammation or from lesions outside the joints (periarticular tissues). The infected joint is extremely tender and patients will often not let the examiner move the joint at all.

Palpate the joint deliberately now for evidence of *synovitis* which is a soft and spongy (boggy) swelling. This must be distinguished from an *effusion* which tends to affect large joints, but can occur in any joint. Here the swelling is fluctuant and can be made to shift within the joint (page 268). *Bony swelling* feels hard and immobile, and suggests osteophyte formation or subchondral bone thickening.

Move

More information about a joint is gained by testing the range of *passive* movement than by getting the patient to move it actively. The patient is asked to relax and let the examiner move the joint. This must be attempted gently and will be limited if the joint is painful (secondary to muscle spasm), if a tense effusion is present or if there is a fixed deformity. The joints may have limited extension (called fixed flexion deformity) or limited flexion (fixed extension deformity). Passive movement of the spine is not a practical manoeuvre (unless the examiner is very strong) and active movement is tested here. *Active* movement is more helpful in assessing integrated joint function. Hand function (page 261) and gait are usually applied as tests of *function*.

Stability of the joint is important and depends largely on the surrounding ligaments. This is tested by attempting to move the joint gently in abnormal directions.

Joint crepitus, which is a grating sensation or noise from the joint, indicates irregularity of the articular surfaces. Its presence suggests chronicity.

Measure

Accurate measurement of the range of movement of a joint is possible with a goniometer, which is a hinged rod with a protractor in the centre. The jaws are opened and lined up with the joint. Measurement of joint movements is performed from the zero starting position. For most joints this is the anatomical position in extension—e.g., the straightened knee. Movement is then recorded as the number of degrees of flexion from this position. A knee with a fixed flexion deformity may be recorded as 30° to 60°, which indicates that there is 30° of fixed flexion deformity and that flexion is limited to 60°. At some joints both flexion and extension from the anatomical position can be measured, as at the wrists. The goniometer is not routinely used by non-rheumatologists and there is a wide range of normal values for joint movement. Most clinicians estimate the approximate joint angles.

A tape measure is useful for measuring and following serially the quadriceps muscle bulk and in examination of spinal movements (page 265).

Table 8.8 *Differential Diagnosis of a Deforming Polyarthropathy*

Rheumatoid arthritis
Seronegative spondyloarthropathy, particularly psoriatic arthritis, ankylosing spondylitis or
    Reiter's disease
Chronic tophaceous gout (rarely symmetrical)
Primary generalised osteoarthritis
Infection, e.g., Lyme arthritis

Examination of Individual Joints

The Hands and Wrists (Figure 8.1)

First sit the patient over the side of the bed and place the hands on the pillow with palms down. Often examination of the hands alone will give enough information for the examiner to make a diagnosis. As a result this is quite a popular test in viva-voce examinations.

Look

Start the examination at the *wrists*. Inspect the skin for erythema, atrophy, scars and rashes. Look for swelling and its distribution. Also look for muscle wasting of the intrinsic muscles of the hand. This results in the appearance of hollow ridges between the metacarpal bones. It is especially obvious on the dorsum of the hand.

Go on to the *metacarpophalangeal joints*. Again note any skin abnormalities, swelling or deformity. Look especially for ulnar deviation and volar (palmar) subluxation of the fingers. Ulnar deviation is deviation of the phalanges at the metacarpophalangeal joints towards the medial (ulnar) side of the hand. It is usually associated with anterior subluxation of the fingers (Figure 8.2). These deformities are characteristic but not pathognomonic of rheumatoid arthritis (Table 8.8).

Next inspect the *proximal interphalangeal* and *distal interphalangeal* joints. Again note any skin changes and joint swelling. Look for the characteristic deformities of *rheumatoid arthritis*. These include *swan neck* and *boutonniére* deformity of the fingers and *Z deformity* of the thumb (Figure 8.2). They are due to joint destruction and tendon dysfunction. The swan neck deformity is hyperextension at the proximal interphalangeal joint and fixed flexion deformity at the distal interphalangeal joint. It is due to subluxation at the proximal interphalangeal joint and tendon shortening at the distal interphalangeal joint. The boutonniére (buttonhole) deformity consists of fixed flexion of the proximal interphalangeal joint and extension of the distal interphalangeal joints. This is due to protrusion of the proximal interphalangeal joint through its ruptured extensor tendon. The Z deformity of the thumb consists of hyperextension of the interphalangeal joint and fixed flexion and subluxation of the metacarpophalangeal joint.

Now look for the characteristic changes of *osteoarthritis* (Figure 8.3). Here the distal interphalangeal and first carpometacarpal joints are usually involved. *Heberden's* * *nodes* are a common deformity caused by marginal osteophytes which

---

*   William Heberden (1710–1801), London physician, and doctor to George III and Samuel Johnson.

Figure 8.1 *Examination of the Hands and Wrists*

Sitting up (hands on a pillow)

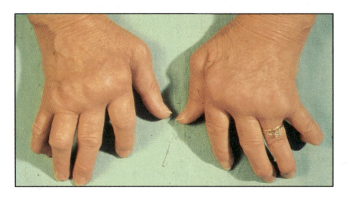

GENERAL INSPECTION
  Cushingoid
  Weight
  Iritis, scleritis, etc.
  Obvious other joint disease

LOOK
  Dorsal aspect
  Wrists
    Skin—scars, redness, atrophy, rash
    Swelling—distribution
    Deformity
    Muscle wasting
  Metacarpophalangeal joints
    Skin
    Swelling—distribution
    Deformity—ulnar deviation, volar
      subluxation, etc.
  Proximal and distal interphalangeal
      joints
    Skin
    Swelling—distribution
    Deformity—swan necking,
      boutonniére, Z, etc.
  Nails
    Psoriatic changes—pitting, ridging,
      onycholysis, hyperkeratosis,
      discoloration

FEEL AND MOVE PASSIVELY
  Wrists
    Synovitis

Effusions
Range of movement
Crepitus
Ulnar styloid tenderness
Metacarpophalangeal joints
  Synovitis
  Effusions
  Range of movement
  Crepitus
  Subluxation
Proximal and distal interphalangeal
    joints
  As above
Palmar tendon crepitus
Carpal tunnel syndrome tests
Palmar aspect
  Skin—scars, palmar erythema, palmar
    creases (anaemia)
  Muscle wasting

HAND FUNCTION
  Grip strength
  Key grip
  Opposition strength
  Practical ability

OTHER
  Elbows—subcutaneous nodules
        —psoriatic rash
  Other joints
  Signs of systemic disease

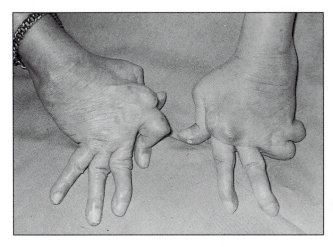

Figure 8.2
*The hands in rheumatoid
arthritis.*

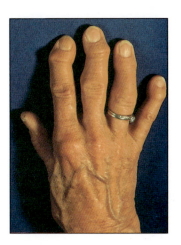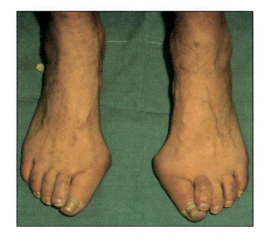

Figure 8.3   *(a) The hands and (b) the feet of a patient with osteoarthritis, showing Heberden's nodes (distal interphalangeal joints), Bouchard's nodes (proximal interphalangeal joints) and bunions.*

lie at the base of the distal phalanx. Less commonly, the proximal interphalangeal joints may be involved and osteophytes here are called *Bouchard's** nodes.

Look also to see if the phalanges appear sausage shaped. This is characteristic of psoriatic arthropathy but can also occur in patients with ankylosing spondylitis and Reiter's disease. It is due to interphalangeal arthritis and flexor tendon sheath oedema. Finger shortening due to severe destructive arthritis also occurs in psoriatic disease and is called *arthritis mutilans*. The hand may take up a *main en lorgnette* appearance due to a combination of shortening and telescoping of the digits.

---

*   Charles Jacques Bouchard (1837–1915), Parisian physician.

Now examine the *nails*. Characteristic *psoriatic* nail changes may be visible: these include pitting (small depressions in the nail), onycholysis (Figure 8.4 and page 299), hyperkeratosis (thickening of the nail), ridging and discoloration. *Vasculitic* changes around the nail folds must also be spotted when present. These consist of black to brown 1 to 2mm lesions due to skin infarction and occur typically in rheumatoid arthritis (Figure 8.5). Splinter haemorrhages may be present in patients with rheumatoid arthritis and systemic lupus erythematosus and are due to vasculitis. Periungual telangiectases occur in systemic lupus erythematosus, scleroderma or dermatomyositis.

The hands should now be turned over and the *palmar surfaces* revealed. Look at the palms for scars (from tendon repairs or transfers), palmar erythema, and muscle wasting of the thenar or hypothenar eminences (due to disuse, vasculitis or peripheral nerve entrapment).

Feel and Move

Turn the hands back again to the palm-down position. Palpate the wrists with both thumbs placed on the dorsal surface with the wrists supported underneath with the index fingers (Figure 8.6). Feel gently for synovitis (boggy swelling) and effusions. The wrist should be gently dorsiflexed (normally possible to 75°) and palmar flexed (also possible to 75°) with the examiner's thumbs. Then radial and ulnar deviation (20°) is tested (Figure 8.7). Note any tenderness or limitation of movement or joint crepitus. Palpate the ulnar styloid for tenderness which can occur in rheumatoid arthritis.

Go on now to the metacarpophalangeal joints which are palpated in a similar way with the two thumbs. Again passive movement is tested. Volar subluxation can be demonstrated by flexing the metacarpophalangeal joint with the proximal phalanx held between the thumb and forefinger. The metacarpophalangeal joint is then rocked backwards and forwards (Figure 8.8). Very little movement occurs with this manoeuvre at a normal joint. Considerable movement may be present when ligamentous laxity or subluxation is present.

Palpate the proximal and distal interphalangeal joints for tenderness, swelling and osteophytes.

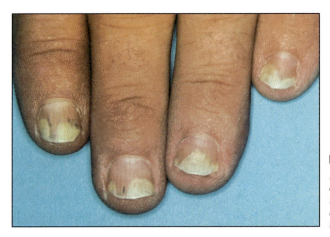

Figure 8.4

Psoriatic nails, showing onycholysis and discoloration. There is no pitting, ridging or hyperkeratosis in this case.

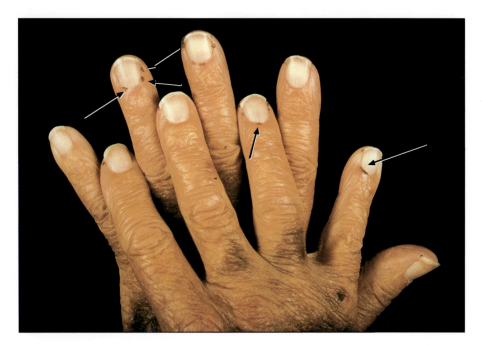

Figure 8.5   *Rheumatoid vasculitis (arrows).*

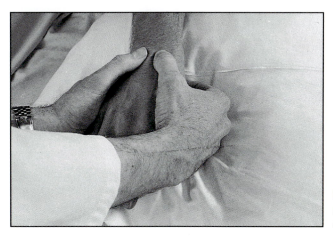

Figure 8.6
*Palpating the wrist joint—
approved method.*

Next test for *palmar tendon crepitus*. The palmar aspects of the examiner's fingers are placed against the palm of the patient's hand while he or she flexes and extends the metacarpophalangeal joints. Inflamed palmar tendons can be felt creaking in their thickened sheaths and nodules can be palpated. This indicates tenosynovitis,

A *trigger finger* may also be detected by this manoeuvre. Here the thickening of a section of digital flexor tendon is such that it tends to jam when passing through

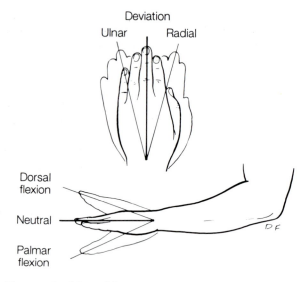

Figure 8.7 *Movements of the wrist.*

Adapted from Swash M, editor. Hutchinson's clinical methods. 19th ed. London: Ballière Tindall, 1989, with permission.

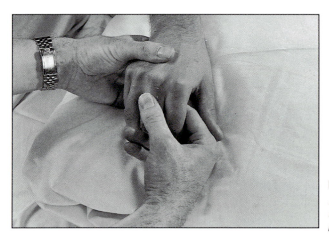

Figure 8.8

Examination for volar sub-luxation at the metacarpo-phalangeal joints.

a narrowed part of its tendon sheath. Rheumatoid arthritis is an important cause. Typically, flexion of the finger occurs freely up to a certain point where it sticks and cannot be extended (as flexors are more powerful than extensors). The application of greater force overcomes the resistance with a snap.

Tap over the flexor retinaculum (Tinel's* *sign*) which lies at the proximal part of the palm. This may cause paraesthesiae (pins and needles) in the distribution of the median nerve (page 380), when thickening of the flexor retinaculum has

---

* Jules Tinel (1879–1952), Parisian physician.

entrapped the nerve in the carpal tunnel (Table 8.9). If the carpal tunnel syndrome is suspected, ask the patient to flex both wrists for 30 seconds—paraesthesiae will often be precipitated in the affected hand if the syndrome is present *(wrist flexion test)*.

Function

It is important to test the function of the hand. *Grip strength* is tested by getting the patient to squeeze two of the examiner's fingers. Even an angry patient will rarely cause pain if given only two fingers. Serial measurements of grip strength can be made by asking the patient to squeeze a partly inflated sphygmomanometer bladder and noting the pressure developed. *Key grip* (Figure 8.9) is the grip with which a key is held between the pulps of the thumb and forefinger. Ask the patient to hold this grip tightly and try to open up his or her fingers. *Opposition strength* (Figure 8.10) is where the patient opposes the thumb and little finger and the difficulty with which these can be forced apart is assessed. Finally, *a practical test,* such as asking the patient to undo a button or write with a pen, should be performed.

Examination of the hands is not complete without feeling for the *subcutaneous nodules* of rheumatoid arthritis near the elbows (Figure 8.11). These are 0.5 to 3cm firm shotty non-tender lumps which occur typically over the olecranon. They may be attached to bone. They are found in rheumatoid factor-positive rheumatoid

Table 8.9   *Causes of Carpal Tunnel Syndrome*

Occupation related: patients who work with their wrists and hands flexed	
Rheumatoid arthritis	Obesity
Hypothyroidism	Amyloid
Acromegaly	Diabetes mellitus
Pregnancy	Idiopathic

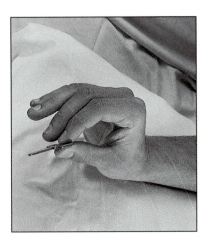

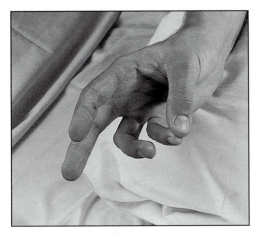

Figure 8.9   *The key grip.*   **Figure 8.10**   *Testing opposition strength.*

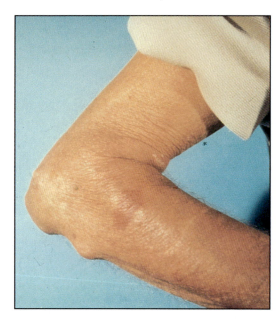

Figure 8.11
Subcutaneous nodules in rheumatoid arthritis.

arthritis. Rheumatoid nodules are areas of fibrinoid necrosis with a characteristic histological appearance and are probably initiated by a small vessel vasculitis. They are localised by trauma but can occur elsewhere, especially attached to tendons, over pressure areas in the hands or feet, in the lung, pleura, heart valves, myocardium or vocal cords. The combination of arthritis and nodules suggests the diagnostic possibilities listed in Table 8.10.

The Elbows

Look for a joint effusion, which appears as a swelling on either side of the olecranon. Discrete swellings over the olecranon or over the proximal subcutaneous border of the ulna may be due to rheumatoid nodules, gouty tophi, an enlarged olecranon bursa or rarely to other types of nodules (Table 8.10).

Feel for tenderness, particularly over the lateral and medial epicondyles, which may indicate tennis or golfer's elbow respectively. Palpate any discrete swellings. Rheumatoid nodules are quite hard, may be tender and are attached to underlying structures, while gouty tophi have a firm feeling and often appear yellow-coloured under the skin. A fluid collection in the olecranon bursa is softly fluctuant and may be tender if inflammation is present. These collections are associated with rheumatoid arthritis and gout, but often occur independently of those diseases.

Move the elbow joints. The elbow is a hinge joint. The zero position is when the arm is fully extended (0°). Normal flexion is possible to 150°. Limitation of extension is an early sign of synovitis.

The Shoulders

Movements of the shoulder are a combination of ball and socket articulation at the glenohumeral joint and motion between the scapula and the thorax. The shoulder

Table 8.10 *Causes of Arthritis Plus Nodules**

Rheumatoid arthritis
Systemic lupus erythematosus (rare)
Rheumatic fever (Jaccoud's† arthritis) (very rare)
Granulomas—e.g., sarcoid (very rare)

* Gouty tophi and xanthomata from hyperlipidaemia may cause confusion.
† Francois Jaccoud (1830–1913), Professor of Medicine, Geneva.

joint is most frequently affected by a number of non-arthritic conditions involving its bursa and surrounding tendons—e.g., 'frozen shoulder', tendonitis, bursitis. All of these disorders affect movement of the shoulder.

Look at the joint. A swelling may be visible anteriorly, but unless effusions are large these are difficult to detect. *Feel* for tenderness and swelling.

Move the joint. The zero position is with the arm hanging by the side of the body so that the palm faces forward (Figure 8.12). *Abduction* is tested with the elbow flexed. For the right shoulder the examiner stands behind the patient resting the left hand on the patient's shoulder, while the right hand abducts the elbow from the shoulder. This tests glenohumeral abduction, is done passively and is normally possible to 90°. *Elevation* is usually possible to 180° when it is performed actively since movement of the scapula is then included. *Adduction* is possible to 50°. The arm is carried forward across the front of the chest. *External rotation* is possible to 60°. With the elbow bent to 90° the arm is turned laterally as far as possible. *Internal rotation* is usually possible to 90°. It is tested actively by asking the patient to place his or her hand behind the back and then try to scratch the back as high up as possible with the thumb. *Flexion* is possible to 180°, of which the glenohumeral joint contributes about 90°. *Extension* is possible to 65°. The arm is swung backwards as in marching. During all these manoeuvres limitation with or without pain and joint crepitus are assessed.

As a general rule, intra-articular disease produces *painful* limitation of movement in *all* directions, while tendonitis produces painful limitation of movement in *one* plane only, and tendon rupture or neurological lesions produce *painless* weakness. For example, if the abnormal sign is limited shoulder abduction in the middle range (45° to 135°), this suggests 'rotator cuff' problems (i.e., the supraspinatus, infraspinatus, subscapularis and teres minor muscles) rather than arthritis. In bicipital tendonitis there is localised tenderness on palpating over the groove. Don't forget that arthritis affecting the acromioclavicular joint can be confused with glenohumeral disorders.

The Temporomandibular Joints

Look in front of the ear for swelling. *Feel* by placing a finger just in front of the ear while the patient opens and shuts the mouth. The head of the mandible is palpable as it slides forwards when the jaw is opened. Clicking and grating may be felt. This is sometimes associated with tenderness if the joint is involved in an inflammatory arthritis. Rheumatoid arthritis commonly affects the temporomandibular joint.

The Neck

Look at the cervical spine while the patient is sitting up and note particularly his or her posture (Figure 8.13). *Movement* should be tested actively. Flexion is tested

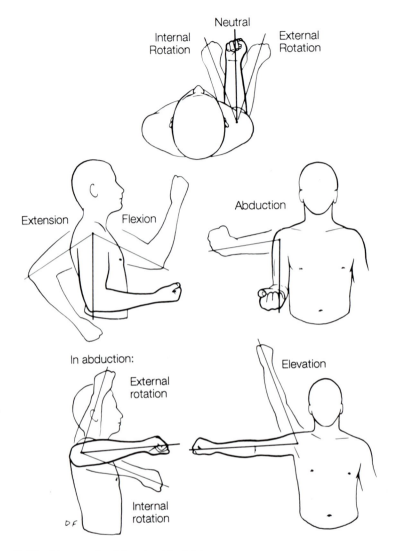

Figure 8.12 *Movements of the shoulder joint.*

Adapted from Swash M, editor. Hutchinson's clinical methods. 19th ed. London: Ballière Tindall, 1989, with permission.

by asking the patient to try to touch his or her chest with the chin (normal flexion is possible to 45°). Extension is tested by asking the patient to look up and back (normally possible to 45°). Lateral bending is tested by getting the patient to touch his or her shoulder with the ear; lateral bending is normally possible to 45°. Rotation is tested by getting the patient to look over the shoulder to the right and then to the left. This is normally possible to 70°.

The Thoracolumbar Spine and Sacroiliac Joints

The patient with bilateral sacroiliac spine arthritis usually has ankylosing spondylitis.

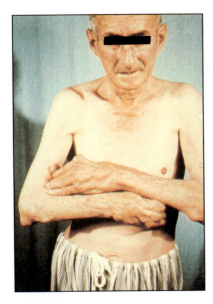

Figure 8.13

Rheumatoid arthritis. Note the head tilt due to right atlanto-axial subluxation, the rheumatoid hands and the subcutaneous rheumatoid nodules.

To start the examination have the patient standing and clothed only in underwear. *Look* for deformity, inspecting from both the back and side. Note especially loss of the normal thoracic kyphosis and lumbar lordosis, which is typical of ankylosing spondylitis. Also note any evidence of scoliosis, a lateral curvature of the spine which may be simple ('C' shaped) or compound ('S' shaped) and which can result from trauma, developmental abnormalities, vertebral body disease (e.g., rickets, tuberculosis) or muscle abnormality (e.g., polio).

Feel each vertebral body for tenderness and palpate for muscle spasm.

Movement is assessed actively. Bending movements largely take place at the lumbar spine while rotational movements occur at the thoracic spine. Range of movement is tested by observation and the use of Schober's test (see below) (Figure 8.14).

Flexion is tested by asking the patient to touch the toes with the knees straight and *extension* by asking the patient to lean backwards. *Lateral bending* is assessed by getting the patient to slide the right hand down the right leg as far as possible without bending forwards, and then the same for the left side. This movement tends to be restricted early in ankylosing spondylitis. *Rotation* is tested with the patient sitting on a stool (to fix the pelvis) and asking him or her to rotate the head and shoulders as far as possible to each side. This is best viewed from above.

Measure the lumbar flexion with *Schober's test*. A mark is made at the level of the posterior iliac spine on the vertebral column (approximately at L5). One finger is placed 5cm below and another 10cm above this mark. The patient is then asked to touch the toes. An increase of less than 5cm in the distance between the two fingers indicates limitation of lumbar flexion. The finger-to-floor distance at full flexion can be measured serially to give an objective idea of disease progression.

Assess *straight leg raising* (Lasègue's* sign) with the patient lying down by lifting the straightened leg. This will be limited by pain in lumbar disc prolapse.

---

*   Charles E Lasègue (1816–1883), Professor of Medicine in Paris.

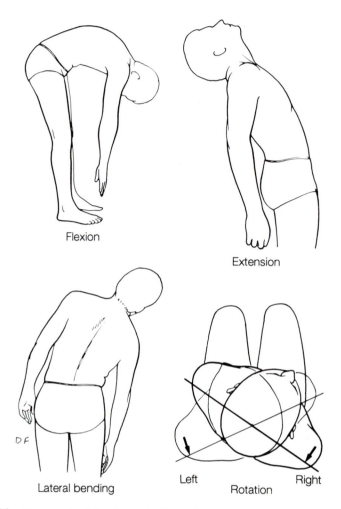

Flexion

Extension

Lateral bending

DF

Left   Right
Rotation

Figure 8.14 *Movements of the thoracolumbar spine.*

Adapted from Swash M, editor. Hutchinson's clinical methods. 19th ed. London: Ballière Tindall, 1989, with permission.

Now get the patient to lie in bed on the stomach. The sacroiliac joints lie underneath the dimples of Venus.* By tradition firm palpation with both palms overlying each other is used to elicit tenderness in patients with sacroiliitis. This is not, however, a terribly reliable sign. Test each side separately.

The Hips

Looking at the hip joint is not possible because so much muscle overlies it. *Feel* just distal to the midpoint of the inguinal ligament for joint tenderness.

---

*   Roman goddess of love—the Greek equivalent was Aphrodite.

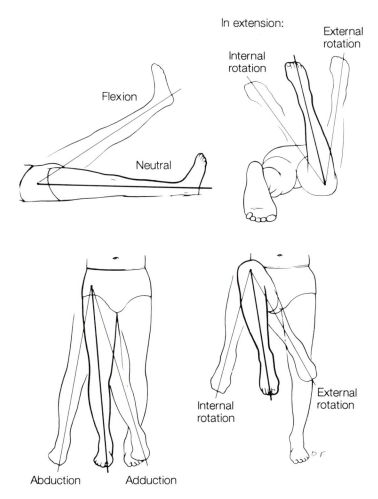

Figure 8.15 *Movements of the hip.*

Adapted from Swash M, editor. Hutchinson's clinical methods. 19th ed. London: Ballière Tindall, 1989, with permission.

Move the hip joint passively with the patient lying down, first on the back (Figure 8.15). *Flexion* is tested by flexing the patient's knee and moving the thigh towards the chest. The pelvis is kept on the bed. *Rotation* is tested with the knee and hip flexed. One hand holds the knee, the other the foot. The foot is then moved medially (*external rotation of the hip*, normally possible to 45°) then laterally (*internal rotation of the hip*, normal to 45°). *Abduction* is tested by standing on the same side of the bed as the leg to be tested. The right hand grasps the heel of the right leg while the left hand is placed over the anterior superior iliac spine to steady the pelvis. The leg is then moved outwards as far as possible. This is normally possible to 50°. *Adduction* is the opposite. The leg is carried immediately in front of the other limb and this is normally possible to 45°.

Ask the patient to roll over onto the stomach. *Extension* is then tested by placing one hand over the sacroiliac joint while the other elevates each leg. This is normally possible to about 30°. Ask the patient to stand now and perform the Trendelenburg* test. The patient stands first on one leg and then on the other. Normally the non-weight-bearing hip rises, but with proximal myopathy (page 402) or hip joint disease the non-weight-bearing side sags.

Finally, the true *leg length* (from the anterior superior iliac spine to the medial malleolus) and apparent leg length (from the umbilicus to the same lower point) for each leg should be measured. A difference in true leg length indicates hip disease on the shorter side, while apparent leg length differences are due to tilting of the pelvis.

The Knees

Look with the patient lying down on the back with both knees and thighs fully exposed. Note any quadriceps wasting and, over the knees themselves, skin changes, swelling and deformity. Swelling of the synovium is usually seen medial to the patella and in the joint's suprapatellar extension. Assess fixed flexion deformity by squatting down and looking at each knee from the side. A space under the knee will be visible if there is a permanent flexion deformity.

Feel the quadriceps for wasting. Palpate over the knees for warmth and synovial swelling.

Test carefully for a joint effusion. The *patellar tap* is used to confirm the presence of large effusions. One hand rests over the lower part of the quadriceps muscle and compresses the suprapatellar bursa. The other hand pushes the patella downwards. The sign is positive if the patella is felt to sink and then come to rest with a tap as it touches the underlying femur. The *bulge sign* is used to detect small effusions. Here the left hand compresses the suprapatellar pouch while the fingers of the right hand are run along the groove beside the patella on one side and then the other. A bulging along the groove due to a fluid wave, on the side not being compressed, is a sign of a small effusion.

Examine for patellofemoral lesions by sliding the patella sideways across the underlying femoral condyles.

Move the joint passively. Test *flexion* (normally possible to 135°) and *extension* (normal 5°) by resting one hand on the knee cap while the other moves the leg up and down. The range of movements and the presence of crepitus are noted.

Test the *ligaments* next. The lateral and medial *collateral ligaments* are assessed by having the knee slightly flexed while holding the leg, with the examiner's forearm resting along the length of the tibia; lateral and medial movements of the leg on the knee joint are tested. Meanwhile the thigh is steadied with the other hand. Movements of more than 5 to 10 degrees are abnormal. The *cruciate ligaments* are tested next by steadying the patient's foot with the examiner's elbow, again with the forearm lying along the length of the tibia. The patient's knee is flexed to 90°. One hand steadies the thigh while the other is placed behind the tibia and attempts anterior and posterior movements of the leg on the knee joint. Again, movement of more than 5 to 10 degrees is abnormal. Increased anterior movement suggests anterior cruciate ligamentous laxity and increased posterior movement suggests posterior cruciate ligamentous laxity.

---

* Friedrich Trendelenburg (1844–1924), Professor of Surgery at Rostock, Bonn and Leipzig.

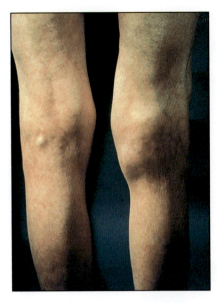

Figure 8.16
Baker's cyst of the right knee, viewed from behind.

Finally, stand the patient up. Look particularly for varus (bow-leg) and valgus (knock-knee) deformity. Look and feel the popliteal fossa for a Baker's* cyst. This is a pressure diverticulum of the synovial membrane that occurs through a hiatus in the knee capsule (Figure 8.16). It is best seen with the knee extended. Rupture of this into the calf muscle produces signs that may mimic a deep venous thrombosis (page 62).

The Ankles and Feet

This examination includes the ankle, foot and toes. *Look* at the skin. Note any swelling, deformity or muscle wasting. Deformities affecting the forefoot include hallux valgus (fixed lateral deviation of the main axis of the big toe), and clawing (fixed flexion deformity) and crowding of the toes, as occurs in rheumatoid arthritis. Sausage deformities of the toes occur with psoriatic arthropathy, ankylosing spondylitis and Reiter's disease (Figure 8.17). Look for the nail changes that suggest psoriasis. Inspect the transverse arch of the foot, which runs underneath the metatarsophalangeal joints, and the longitudinal arch which runs from the first metatarsophalangeal joint to the heel. These arches, which bear the weight of the body, may be flattened in arthritic conditions of the foot like rheumatoid arthritis. Calluses over the metatarsal heads on the plantar surface of the foot occur with subluxation of these joints (Figure 8.18).

Feel, starting with the ankle for swelling around the lateral and medial malleoli. This can be confused with pitting oedema (page 60). *Move* the *talar (ankle) joint* grasping the midfoot with one hand. *Dorsiflexion* is tested by raising the foot towards the knee—normally possible to 20°— and *plantar flexion* by performing the opposite manoeuvre, which is normally possible to 50°.

---

* William Baker (1839–1896), Surgeon at St Bartholomew's Hospital, London.

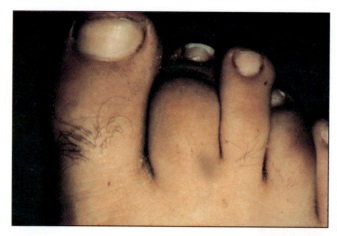

Figure 8.17
Sausage-shaped first and second toes in psoriatic arthritis.

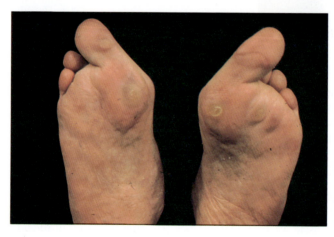

Figure 8.18
Rheumatoid feet showing bilateral hallux valgus and calluses over the metatarsal heads.

With the subtalar joint, only *inversion* and *eversion* of the foot on the ankle are tested. Tenderness on movement is more important than range at this joint. The midtarsal (midfoot) joint allows rotation of the forefoot when the hindfoot is fixed. This is done by steadying the ankle with one hand and rotating (twisting) the forefoot. Again, tenderness rather than range of movement is noted.

Squeeze the *metatarsophalangeal joints* by compressing the first and fifth metatarsals between your thumb and forefinger. Tenderness suggests inflammation, common in early rheumatoid arthritis. Each individual interphalangeal joint is then assessed by feeling and moving. These are typically affected in the seronegative spondyloarthropathies. Extremely tender involvement of the first metatarsophalangeal joint is characteristic of acute gout. In this case the joint also looks red and swollen.

Palpate the *Achilles tendon* for rheumatoid nodules (Figure 8.19) and Achilles tendonitis. Also palpate the inferior aspect of the *heel* for tenderness; this may indicate plantar fasciitis, which occurs in the seronegative spondyloarthropathies and sometimes for no apparent reason.

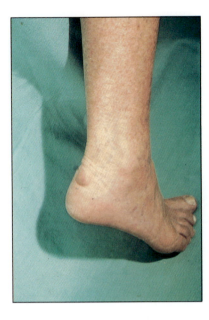

Figure 8.19
Rheumatoid nodule of the Achilles tendon.

Correlation of Physical Signs and Rheumatological Disease

Rheumatoid Arthritis (Figures 8.13 and 8.20)

This is a chronic systemic inflammatory disease of unknown aetiology which characteristically involves the joints. In the majority of cases, patients with rheumatoid arthritis have rheumatoid factor present in the serum (seropositive disease). These are heterogeneous antibodies directed against the Fc portion of altered immunoglobulin (IgG), but are not specific for rheumatoid arthritis.

To examine the patient with suspected rheumatoid arthritis sit him or her up in bed or a chair.

General Inspection

Look to see whether the patient has a Cushingoid appearance due to steroid treatment (page 310), or whether there are signs of weight loss which may indicate active disease.

The Hands

Put the hands on a pillow. Look especially for symmetrical small joint polyarthritis (the distal interphalangeal joints are usually spared). The other common abnormalities are ulnar deviation, volar subluxation of the metacarpophalangeal joints, and Z deformity of the thumb with swan neck and boutonnière deformity of the fingers. Examine the finger nails for vasculitic changes and look for wasting of the small muscles of the hand. Look at the palms for palmar erythema. Feel the palms for palmar tendon crepitus while the patient extends and flexes the fingers. Look

Figure 8.20 *Rheumatoid Arthritis*

GENERAL INSPECTION
  Cushingoid appearance
  Weight

HANDS

ARMS
  Entrapment neuropathy (e.g., carpal
    tunnel)
  Subcutaneous nodules
  Elbow joint
  Shoulder joint
  Axillary nodes

FACE
  Eyes—dry eyes (Sjögren's), scleritis,
    episcleritis, scleromalacia perforans,
    anaemia, cataracts (steroids,
    chloroquine)
  Fundi—hyperviscosity
  Face—parotids (Sjögren's)
  Mouth—dryness, ulcers, dental caries
  Temporomandibular joint (crepitus)

NECK
  Cervical spine
  Cervical nodes

CHEST
  Heart—pericarditis, valve lesions
  Lungs—effusion, fibrosis, infarction,
    infection, nodules (and Caplan's
    syndrome)

ABDOMEN
  Splenomegaly (e.g., Felty's syndrome)
  Inguinal nodes

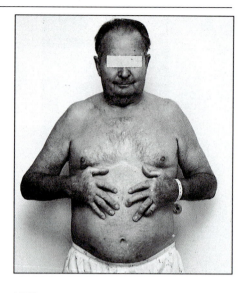

HIPS

KNEES

LOWER LIMBS
  Ulceration (vasculitis)
  Calf swelling (ruptured synovial cyst)
  Peripheral neuropathy
  Mononeuritis multiplex
  Cord compression

FEET

OTHER
  Urine: protein, blood (drugs, vasculitis,
    amyloidosis)
  Rectal examination (blood)

for signs of an ulnar nerve palsy (from ulnar nerve entrapment at the elbow) and a median nerve palsy (carpal tunnel) (page 380).

The Wrists

Look for synovial thickening and test for Tinel's sign (carpal tunnel).

The Elbows

Look around the elbows for rheumatoid nodules which suggest seropositive disease, and examine the elbow joint. Flexion contractures are common.

The Shoulders and Axillae

Here look for tenderness and limitation of movement. Also palpate the axillary nodes because enlarged nodes may indicate active disease of joints in the area which they drain.

The Eyes

Look at the eyes for redness and dryness (Sjögren's syndrome) (Table 8.7) which occurs in 10% to 15% of cases. Note also scleritis (an elevated white or purple-red lesion, which is pathologically a rheumatoid nodule and usually appears surrounded by the intense redness of the injected sclera) (Figure 8.21). These nodules occur especially in the superior parts of the sclera and are often bilateral, but affect only 1% of patients. Iritis does *not* occur.

With severe scleritis scleral thinning may occur exposing the underlying choroid. This is called scleromalacia. Look for cataracts due to steroid treatment. Conjunctival pallor may be present indicating anaemia due to iron deficiency. This can be a result blood loss from analgesic use, folate deficiency from a poor diet, hypersplenism or chronic inflammation or some combination of these.

The Parotids

Look for enlargement of the parotid glands, as occurs with Sjögren's syndrome.

The Mouth

Look for dryness of the mouth and dental caries (Sjögren's syndrome), and ulcers related to drug (e.g., gold) treatment.

The Temporomandibular Joints

Feel the temporomandibular joints for crepitus as the patient opens and shuts the mouth.

The Neck

Go on to examine the cervical spine for tenderness, muscle spasm and reduction of rotational movement. Examine for cervical lymphadenopathy.

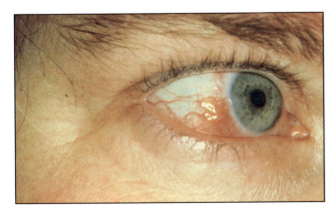

Figure 8.21
Nodular scleritis involving the sclera lateral to the iris.

The Chest

Now examine the lungs for signs of pleural effusions or pulmonary fibrosis. NB: Caplan's* syndrome is the presence of rheumatoid lung nodules in combination with pneumoconiosis.

The Heart

Listen to the heart for a pericardial rub (relatively common) and for murmurs indicating valvular regurgitation (especially the aortic valve) which may occur due to nodular involvement of a heart valve.

The Abdomen

Feel the abdomen for splenomegaly (this occurs in up to 10% of patients). Feel the inguinal lymph nodes.

The Lower Limbs

Examine the hips for limitation of joint movement, although this occurs only uncommonly. The knees, however, are more often affected and here one must note quadriceps wasting, synovial effusions and flexion contractures. Valgus deformity and ligamentous instability may occur as late complications. Look in the popliteal fossae for Baker's cysts. Go on to look at the lower parts of the legs for ulceration; this can occur as a vasculitic complication of Felty's syndrome. Examine for a stocking distribution peripheral neuropathy and for mononeuritis multiplex of the nerves of the lower limbs. There may also be signs of spinal cord compression due to anterior dislocation of the first cervical vertebra or vertical subluxation of the odontoid process.

The Ankles and Feet (Figure 8.18)

Now look for foot drop (peroneal nerve entrapment or vasculitis) and examine the ankle joint for limitation of movement. Look at the metatarsophalangeal joints for swelling and subluxation. There may also be lateral deviation and clawing of the toes. Remember that the interphalangeal joints are very rarely involved. Finally feel the Achilles tendon for nodules—a sign of seropositive disease.

Seronegative Spondyloarthropathies

Four conditions are generally accepted as belonging to this group: ankylosing spondylitis, psoriatic arthritis, Reiter's[†] disease and enteropathic arthritis. These are called the seronegative spondyloarthropathies because they were originally distinguished from rheumatoid arthritis by the absence of rheumatoid factor in the serum. However, up to 30% of patients with otherwise classical rheumatoid arthritis have no rheumatoid factor. The seronegative spondyloarthropathies overlap clinically and pathologically, and have an association with the HLA-B27 marker.

---

*   Anthony Caplan, Welsh physician, described this in 1953.

†   Hans Reiter (1881–1969), Professor of Hygiene in Berlin, described the syndrome in 1916.

Ankylosing Spondylitis

The following areas should be examined.

The back and sacroiliac joints may show: loss of lumbar lordosis and thoracic kyphosis; severe flexion deformity of the lumbar spine (rare); tenderness of the lumbar vertebrae; reduction of movement of the lumbar spine in all directions; and tenderness of the sacroiliac joints.

The legs: Achilles tendonitis; plantar fasciitis; signs of cauda equina compression (rare)—lower limb weakness, loss of sphincter control, saddle sensory loss.

The lungs: decreased chest expansion (less than 5cm); signs of apical fibrosis.

The heart: signs of aortic regurgitation.

The eyes: acute iritis (tends to recur)—painful red eye (10% to 15%) (Figure 8.22).

Rectal and stool examination: signs of inflammatory bowel disease (either ulcerative colitis or Crohn's disease). NB: Signs of secondary amyloidosis—e.g., hepatosplenomegaly, renal enlargement, proteinuria—may be present although this is a very rare complication.

Reiter's* Syndrome

Classically this disease follows urethritis or diarrhoea, with conjunctivitis and arthritis (usually asymmetrical) of the large weight-bearing joints such as the hip, knee or ankle. The following areas should be examined.

The genital region: urethral discharge; circinate balanitis—scaly superficial reddened erosions with well demarcated borders on the glans penis (Figure 8.23).

The prostate: prostatitis.

The eyes: conjunctivitis; iritis (rare).

The mouth: painless ulcers.

The back: sacroiliac joints (may be unilaterally involved).

The lower limbs (more commonly affected): knees, ankles; metatarsophalangeal joints; plantar fasciitis, Achilles tendonitis; keratoderma blennorrhagica on the sole (non-tender reddish-brown macules which become scaling papules)—this is indistinguishable from pustular psoriasis; nails thickened, opaque and brittle.

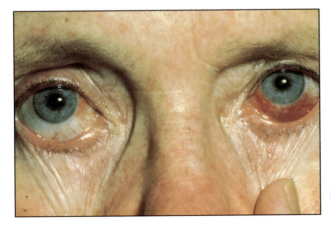

Figure 8.22
Iritis.

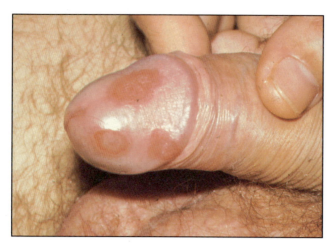

Figure 8.23
Circinate balanitis.

The hands (less commonly involved): wrists; metacarpophalangeal joints, proximal interphalangeal joints, distal interphalangeal joints; keratoderma blennorrhagica on the palms; nails.

Cardiovascular system: aortic regurgitation (rare).

Psoriatic Arthritis

Five per cent of patients with psoriasis (page 448) have arthritis.

Examine as for rheumatoid arthritis, but include the sacroiliac joints (page 264). There are five distinct groups of psoriatic arthritis.

1. Monoarticular and oligoarticular arthritis of the hands and feet (note sausage shaped digits in Figure 8.17). Most psoriatic arthritis is of this type.
2. Similar to rheumatoid arthritis (but seronegative).
3. Distal interphalangeal joint involvement with psoriatic nail changes (Figure 8.4).
4. Arthritis mutilans (destructive polyarthritis).
5. Sacroiliitis with or without peripheral joint involvement.

Enteropathic Arthritis

There are two patterns of involvement of the joints with ulcerative colitis and Crohn's disease.

1. Peripheral joint disease. This is an asymmetrical oligoarthropathy, usually affecting the lower limbs, especially the knees and ankles. It rarely causes deformity.
2. Sacroiliitis. This is indistinguishable clinically from ankylosing spondylitis.

Gouty Arthritis

Begin with the feet, as acute gouty arthritis affects the metatarsophalangeal joint of the great toe in 75% of cases. Next examine the ankles and knees, which tend

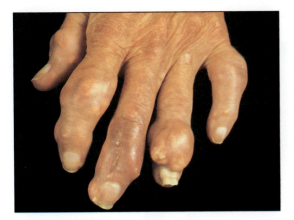

Figure 8.24
Gouty tophi of the fingers.

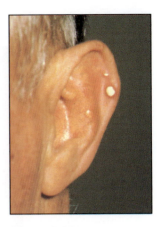

Figure 8.25
Gouty tophus of the ear.

to be involved after recurrent attacks. The fingers, wrists and elbows are affected late (Figure 8.24). Palpate for gouty tophi (these are urate deposits with inflammatory cells surrounding them) (Latin *tophus* chalk stone). The presence of tophi indicates chronic recurrent gout. They tend to occur over the joint synovia, the olecranon bursa, the extensor surface of the forearm, the helix of the ear (Figure 8.25), and in the infrapatellar and Achilles tendons.

Finally, examine for signs of the causes of secondary gout: increased purine turnover due to myeloproliferative disease (page 241), lymphoma (page 243) or leukaemia; and decreased renal urate excretion due to renal disease (page 206) or hypothyroidism (page 302). Hypertension, diabetes mellitus and ischaemic heart disease are more common amongst sufferers of gout.

Calcium Pyrophosphate Arthropathy (Pseudogout)

This may present a similar picture to that described above for true gout, but usually large joints (especially the knees) are involved. In a minority of patients there will be signs of hyperparathyroidism (page 313), haemochromatosis (page 150) or true gout.

Calcium Hydroxyapatite Arthropathy

This causes large joint arthritis (especially knee and shoulder) and is more common in elderly patients.

Systemic Lupus Erythematosus (SLE)

This is a multisystemic chronic inflammatory disease of unknown origin, named because the erosive nature of the condition was likened to the damage caused by a hungry wolf (Latin *lupus** wolf) (Figure 8.26).

---

* Lupus has been used as a name for any erosive disease of the skin, e.g., lupus vulgaris—tuberculosis of the skin.

Figure 8.26   *Systemic Lupus Erythematosus*

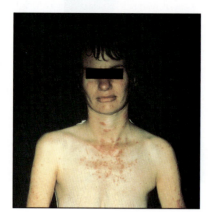

GENERAL INSPECTION
  Cushingoid
  Weight
  Mental state

HANDS
  Vasculitis
  Rash
  Arthropathy

ARMS
  Livedo reticularis
  Purpura
  Proximal myopathy (active disease or
    steroids)

HEAD
  Alopecia, lupus hairs
  Eyes—scleritis, cytoid lesions, etc.
  Mouth—ulcers, infection
  Rash—butterfly
  Cranial nerve lesions
  Cervical adenopathy

CHEST
  Cardiovascular system—endocarditis
  Respiratory system—pleural effusion,
    pleurisy, pulmonary fibrosis, collapse
    or infection

ABDOMEN
  Hepatosplenomegaly
  Tendemess

HIPS
  Aseptic necrosis

LEGS
  Feet—red soles, small joint synovitis
  Rash
  Proximal myopathy
  Cerebellar ataxia
  Neuropathy
  Hemiplegia
  Mononeuritis multiplex

OTHER
  Urine analysis (proteinuria)
  Blood pressure (hypertension)
  Temperature chart

General Inspection

Look for weight loss (due to chronic inflammation) or a Cushingoid appearance (steroid treatment, page 310). While taking the history note any abnormal mental state—psychosis may occur due to the lupus itself or to steroid therapy.

Hands

Note any vasculitis around the nail bed, particularly telangiectasia and erythema of the skin of the nail base. A rash may occur—photosensitivity is common.

Raynaud's phenomenon may occur if the examiner is lucky and the weather cold (Table 8.6). Characteristically the affected fingers become paroxysmally white followed by cyanosis and finally by a reactive hyperaemia when the fingers become red and tender (i.e., white–blue–red).

Examine for arthropathy: synovitis of the proximal and metacarpophalangeal joints, which is not destructive (non-erosive), may occur in SLE.

Forearms

Livedo reticularis may occur here; in Latin this describes skin discoloration in the form of a small net. These are connected bluish-purple streaks without discrete borders. They occur usually on the limbs and are associated with various connective tissue diseases. Look for purpura (due to vasculitis or autoimmune thrombocytopenia). Examine for a proximal myopathy (due to the disease itself or to steroid treatment). Subcutaneous nodules very rarely occur in SLE. The axillary nodes may be enlarged but will not be tender.

The Head and Neck

Alopecia (hair loss) is an important diagnostic clue, which occurs in about two-thirds of patients. Look especially for lupus hairs which are short broken hairs above the forehead. The hair as a whole may be coarse and dry as in hypothyroidism.

Examine the eyes for scleritis and episcleritis (Figure 8.21). The eyes may be red and dry (Sjögren's syndrome). Pallor of the conjunctivae occurs with anaemia, usually due to chronic disease. Occasionally jaundice due to autoimmune haemolytic anaemia may be found. Perform a fundoscopy for cytoid bodies, which are hard exudates (white spots) due to aggregates of swollen nerve fibres and are secondary to vasculitis.

A facial rash may be diagnostic (Figure 8.27). The classical rash is an erythematous 'butterfly rash' over the cheeks and bridge of the nose. Mouth ulcers on the soft or hard palate may occur and the mouth may be dry (Sjögren's syndrome).

Discoid lupus may be found in the same area or affect different parts of the body. Lesions begin as spreading red plaques which have a central area of hyperkeratosis and follicular plugging. An active lesion has an oedematous edge. The appearance may suggest psoriasis. A healed lesion may have marginal hyperpigmentation with central atrophy and depigmentation. The scalp, external ear and face are most commonly affected, but in some patients lesions may occur all over the arms and chest.

After examining the face feel for non-tender cervical lymphadenopathy.

The Chest

Signs of a pericardial rub (from pericarditis) may be found. In the respiratory examination a pleural rub (pleuritis), a pleural effusion, pulmonary fibrosis, pulmonary collapse or pulmonary hypertension may be detected. Chest disease is probably most often secondary to an interstitial pneumonitis rather than to vasculitis of the lungs.

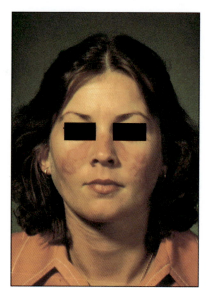

Figure 8.27
Butterfly rash of systemic lupus erythematosus.

The Abdomen

Splenomegaly, usually mild, can be detected in 10% of cases. Hepatomegaly (mild) may occur in uncomplicated cases. Chronic liver disease due to chronic active hepatitis ('lupoid hepatitis') is a separate disease rather than a variant of SLE.

The Hips

Examine the hip joint movements: in aseptic (avascular) necrosis there is tenderness on movement with preservation of hip extension, but loss of the other movements. This is due to ischaemia of the femoral head and may be related to steroid use or to the SLE itself.

The Legs

Examine for proximal myopathy (page 402) and peripheral neuropathy (mainly sensory) (page 394).

Rarely there may be signs of hemiplegia, cerebellar ataxia or chorea.

Leg ulceration over the malleoli, due to vasculitis, is important. Very occasionally the toes may be gangrenous. There may be ankle oedema from the nephrotic syndrome or fluid retention from steroids.

Urine and Blood Pressure

Perform a urine analysis (for proteinuria and haematuria) and take the blood pressure (for hypertension). Renal disease is a common complication of SLE.

Temperature

Take the temperature, as fever is common in SLE, either from secondary infection or the disease *per se.*

Scleroderma (Progressive Systemic Sclerosis)

This is a disorder of connective tissue with prominent cutaneous fibrosis. There may be occlusion of the microvasculature of the fingers, gut, lungs, heart and kidneys. The CREST syndrome (**c**alcinosis, **R**aynaud's phenomenon, o**e**sophageal motility disturbance, **s**clerodactyly and **t**elangiectasia) is a more localised form of scleroderma with a better prognosis.

General Inspection (Figure 8.28)

Look for cachexia due to dysphagia (from an oesophageal motility disturbance) or malabsorption (due to bacterial overgrowth in localised wide-mouthed diverticula resulting from atrophy of the muscularis mucosae).

Skin changes in scleroderma vary. There may be an early oedematous phase with non-tender pitting oedema of the hands which appear tightly swollen. In patients with progressive disease the oedematous skin is replaced by indurated skin which appears thickened, hard and tight. This phase usually begins in the fingers (Table 8.11).

The Hands

Examine the hands. Note particularly calcinosis (palpable nodules due to calcific deposits in the subcutaneous tissue of the fingers), Raynaud's phenomenon and sometimes atrophy of the finger pulps (due to ischaemia), sclerodactyly (tightening of the skin of the fingers leading to tapering), and multiple large telangiectasia on the fingers (Figure 8.29). This is the CRST syndrome. If telangiectasia and calcinosis are prominent, and there is no evidence of other sclerodermal changes, this makes the diagnosis of CRST syndrome most likely. In this case, there is no systemic involvement, although oesophageal motility disturbances are common (when the syndrome is called CREST).

Look for contraction deformity of the fingers, which is relatively common (Figure 8.30) and for polyarthropathy, although this is uncommon. Inspect the nail

Table 8.11   *Differential Diagnosis of Thickened Tethered Skin*

CREST syndrome
Systemic sclerosis (scleroderma)
Mixed connective tissue disease (an overlap syndrome including features of systemic sclerosis, systemic lupus erythematosus and polymyositis)
Eosinophilic fasciitis (widespread skin thickening due to inflammation of the fascia often following excessive muscle exercise. It occurs in association with eosinophilia and hypergammaglobulinaemia)
Localised morphea (heterogeneous group of disorders where there are small areas of sclerosis. The most common type is morphea which begins with large plaques of red or purple skin that evolve into sclerotic areas and may regress spontaneously over years)
Chemically induced: vinyl chloride, pentazocine, bleomycin
Pseudoscleroderma: porphyria cutanea tarda, acromegaly, carcinoid syndrome
Scleroedema: thickened skin over the shoulders and upper back in diabetes mellitus
Graft versus host disease
Silicosis
Eosinophilic myalgia syndrome (L-tryptophan)
Toxic oil syndrome

Figure 8.28   *Scleroderma*

GENERAL APPEARANCE
  'Bird like' facies
  Weight loss (malabsorption)

HANDS
  CREST—calcinosis, atrophy distal tissue
      pulp (Raynaud's), (o)esophageal
      motility disturbance, sclerodactyly,
      telangiectasia
  Dilated capillary loops (nail folds)
  Small joint arthropathy and tendon
      crepitus
  Fixed flexion deformity
  Hand function

ARMS
  Oedema (early) or skin thickening and
      tightening
  Pigmentation
  Vitiligo
  Hair loss
  Proximal myopathy

HEAD
  Alopecia
  Eyes—loss of eyebrows, anaemia,
      dryness (Sjögren's), difficulty with
      closing
  Mouth—dryness, puckered, difficulty with
      opening
  Pigmentation
  Telangiectasia
  Neck muscles—wasting and weakness

DYSPHAGIA

CHEST
  Tight skin ('Roman breast plate')
  Heart—cor pulmonale, pericarditis, failure

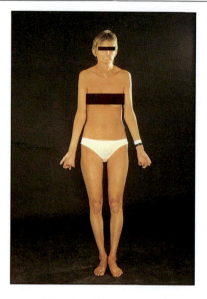

Lungs—fibrosis, reflux pneumonitis, chest
    infections, alveolar cell carcinoma,
    vasculitis

LEGS
  Skin lesions
  Vasculitis
  Small joint arthropathy
  Patellar crepitus

OTHER
  Blood pressure (hypertension with renal
      involvement)
  Urine analysis (proteinuria)
  Temperature chart (infection)
  Stool examination (steatorrhoea)

folds using a hand-held magnifying glass: in scleroderma you may see dilated capillary loops. These are best viewed on the fourth digit. Assessing hand function is important in this disease.

The Arms

Determine the extent of skin tethering in the arms. If the skin thickening extends above the wrists to the arms, legs or trunk, the diagnosis is scleroderma rather than CREST. Assess for proximal myopathy due to myositis.

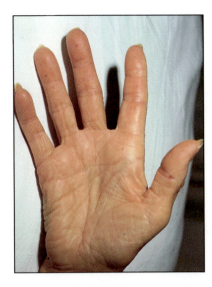

Figure 8.29
Telangiectasia of the hands in the CREST syndrome.

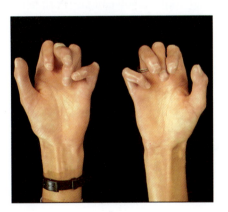 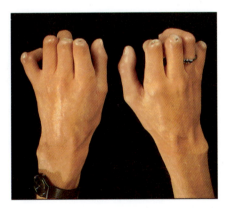

Figure 8.30   *Systemic sclerosis: signs on the hands. Sclerodactyly, tethered smooth skin, calcinosis and ulceration, atrophy of finger pulps due to Raynaud's phenomenon, and fixed flexion deformities of the fingers.*

The Face

The skin of the face is involved in progressive disease. There is loss of the normal wrinkles and skin folds as well as of the eyebrows. The face appears pinched and expressionless ('bird-like' facies). Inspect for malar telangiectasia and look for salt-and-pepper pigmentation. Ask the patient to close the eyes—skin tethering may make this incomplete. The eyes may be dry (Sjögren's syndrome), though this is uncommon, and the conjunctivae pale (there are a number of reasons for anaemia, including the presence of chronic disease, bleeding from oesophagitis, and microangiopathic haemolytic anaemia).

Ask the patient to open the mouth fully. It may appear puckered and narrow. Inability to open the mouth so that there is more than 3cm of clearance between the incisors indicates abnormal restriction.

The Chest

Inspect the skin of the chest wall, which may have acquired a tight thickened appearance, like ancient Roman breast plate armour.

Examine the lungs for pulmonary fibrosis, evidence of reflux pneumonitis, or (rarely) a pleural effusion or alveolar cell carcinoma.

Examine the heart for cor pulmonale secondary to pulmonary fibrosis or for pericarditis. Left ventricular failure may also occur due to myocardial involvement.

The Abdomen

Examine the liver. Signs of primary biliary cirrhosis may be found in patients with the CREST syndrome (especially women), but this association is very rare (page 154).

The Legs

Look for signs of vasculitis, ulceration and skin involvement. Peripheral neuropathy is rare.

Urinalysis and Blood Pressure

These are very important because renal involvement is common in scleroderma and is often associated with severe hypertension. Renal disease is one of the most common causes of death.

The Stool

Look for evidence of steatorrhoea (due to malabsorption from bacterial overgrowth).

Rheumatic Fever

This is an inflammatory disease which is a delayed sequel to infection with group A beta-haemolytic Streptococcus. It is uncommon in Western nations today. It is diagnosed by finding two major or one major and two minor criteria, plus evidence of recent streptococcal infection.

Major criteria: (i) carditis (causing tachycardia, murmurs, cardiac failure, pericarditis); (ii) polyarthritis; (iii) chorea (page 412); (iv) erythema marginatum (see below); (v) subcutaneous nodules (painless mobile swellings).

Minor criteria: (i) fever; (ii) arthralgia; (iii) previous rheumatic fever; (iv) acute phase proteins; (v) prolonged PR interval on the electrocardiogram.

Examining the Patient with Suspected Rheumatic Fever

First examine the large joints of the limbs for effusions and synovitis. Two or more joints must be involved (classically there is a transient migratory polyarthritis). Feel for subcutaneous nodules over bony prominences. Look for a rash. Erythema marginatum is a slightly raised pink or red rash which blanches with pressure. The red rings have a clear centre and round margins and occur on the trunk and proximal limbs; the rash is not found on the face. Look for choreiform movements (page 412).

Now examine the cardiovascular system for signs of pancarditis: (i) a pericardial rub due to pericarditis; (ii) congestive cardiac failure due to myocarditis; (iii) mitral or aortic regurgitation due to acute endocarditis.

Finally take the temperature.

The Vasculitides

This is a heterogeneous group of disorders characterised by inflammation and damage to blood vessels. The clinical features and major vessels involved are shown in Table 8.12.

Table 8.12   *The Vasculitides*

Clinical Syndrome	Major Vessels Inflamed or Involved	Important Clinical Features*
1. Hypersensitivity vasculitis Causes: • Connective tissue diseases—e.g., rheumatoid arthritis, SLE • Infection—e.g., hepatitis B • Drugs—(the Ps) e.g., penicillin, phenothiazines, phenylbutazone propylthiouracil (and many others) • Haematological diseases—e.g., essential cryoglobulinaemia, paraproteinaemia • Idiopathic	Capillaries and venules (leukocytoclastic vasculitis)	Very variable: • Urticaria • Palpable purpura, livedo reticularis • Henoch-Schönlein purpura • Digital infarcts • Features of underlying disease
2. Allergic granulomatosis (NB: blood eosinophilia common) Cause: unknown	Small arteries and veins	• Signs of asthma, eosinophilia • Similar to PAN (see below)
3. Wegener's† granulomatosis Cause: unknown	Arteries, capillaries and venules	• Upper respiratory tract: sinusitis, saddle nose deformity • Lungs: pneumonitis • Renal: hypertension, signs of renal failure, haematuria • Eyes: conjunctivitis, uveitis • Skin: similar to hypersensitivity vasculitis

—continued

Table 8.12   *The Vasculitides (continued)*

Clinical Syndrome	Major Vessels Inflamed or Involved	Important Clinical Features*
4. Polyarteritis nodosa (PAN) Cause: unknown Associated with hepatitis B (20%)	Medium and small arteries (fibrinoid necrosis)	• Digital gangrene, ulceration • Renal: hypertension, signs of renal failure, haematuria • GIT: haematemesis, melaena • Lung: signs of pneumonitis, effusion • CNS: mononeuritis multiplex, retinal vasculitis • Skin: similar to hypersensitivity vasculitis
5. Behçet's syndrome Cause: unknown	Medium to small arteries and veins	• Oral and genital ulcers • Eyes: uveitis • Asymmetrical large joint polyarthropathy • Thrombophlebitis • Rash • CNS: cranial or spinal cord lesions
6. Giant cell arteritis (NB: polymyalgia rheumatica a related disease) Cause: unknown	Large and medium arteries	• Tender extracranial arteries particularly the temporal • Visual disturbance, sudden blindness • Jaw claudication
7. Aortic arch (Takayasu's)‡ arteritis Cause: unknown	Aorta and its branches	• Hypertension • Loss of upper limb pulses NB: Signs have been termed 'reverse coarctation'

GIT = gastrointestinal tract   SLE = systemic lupus erythematosus
CNS = central nervous system   PAN = polyarteritis nodosa

Soft Tissue Rheumatism

This includes a number of common, painful conditions which arise in soft tissue, often around a joint. The problem may be general e.g. fibromyalgia; or restricted to a single anatomical region e.g. tendon, tenosynovium, enthesis or bursa. There are a large number of these conditions; the commoner ones are described here.

Fibromyalgia Syndrome

This syndrome is a common, frequently overlooked condition, that mostly affects women in their forties and fifties. It presents with a variable group of symptoms including widespread musculoskeletal pain, and severe and easy fatiguability. The musculoskeletal pain is mostly axial (neck and back) and diffuse. It is made worse by stress or cold. Pain maybe felt 'all over' and is unresponsive to anti-inflammatory drug treatment. The combination of pain and fatigue may cause the patient severe disability. There is usually a poor sleep pattern. The patient wakes up not feeling refreshed and more tired in the morning than later in the day.

The Examination

Look for the characteristic multiple hyperalgesic tender points (Figure 8.31). These areas are tender to finger pressure in normal people but in affected patients

Table 8.13   *Common Forms of Soft Tissue Rheumatism*

Fibromyalgia Syndrome

Shoulder Syndromes

1. Rotator cuff syndrome
2. Frozen shoulder
3. Bicipital tendonitis

Elbow Epicondylitis

1. Tennis elbow
2. Golfer's elbow

Tenosynovitis

1. De Quervain's tenosynovitis
2. Flexor tendon sheaths of the hand

Bursitis

1. Housemaid's knee
2. Olecranon bursitis
3. Trochanteric bursitis

Nerve Entrapment Syndromes

1. Carpal tunnel syndrome
2. Common peroneal nerve
3. Posterior tibial nerve (tarsal tunnel)

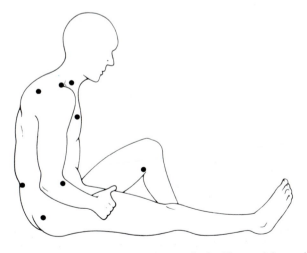

Figure 8.31   *Frequent sites of localised tenderness in the fibromyalgia syndrome.*

there is marked tenderness and a definite withdrawal response. This response should be obtained in at least ten sites in the upper and lower limbs and on both sides (i.e., it is widespread and symmetrical). Next examine for hyperalgesia at control sites such as the forehead or distal forearm, where it should be absent.

The diagnosis is based on the presence of typical symptoms and multiple hyperalgesic tender sites (with negative control sites). Inflammatory and endocrine disease must be excluded.

Shoulder Syndromes

Soft tissue disorders of the shoulder are common and have certain particular clinical features.

Rotator Cuff Syndrome

Supraspinatus tendonitis is the commonest form of rotator cuff syndrome. It is associated with degeneration and subsequent inflammation in the supraspinatus tendon as it is compressed between the acromion and humeral head when the arm is raised. It mostly affects forty to fifty year olds. Symptoms may begin following unaccustomed physical activities such as gardening.

Examination

Examine the shoulder joint. Note pain on abduction of the arm (Figure 8.32), with a painful arc of movement between 60° and 120° of abduction. Involvement of other rotator cuff tendons causes similar painful movement at those joints.

Frozen Shoulder

Capsulitis of the shoulder, or frozen shoulder, is associated with limitation of active and passive arm movements in all directions. It may follow immobilisation of the arm after a stroke. There is typically a sudden onset of shoulder pain which is worse at night and radiates to the base of the neck and down the arm. Pain is

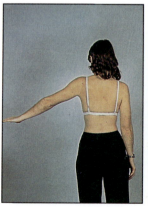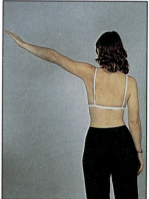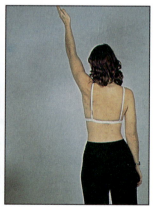

Figure 8.32 *Inflammation of the rotator cuff tendons may cause a 'painful arc' during abduction of the arm. The initial movement is painless but the next 90° of movement causes pain. When the arm reaches full abduction the pain eases as the pressure is taken off the rotator cuff apparatus.*

made worse by shoulder movement and may be bilateral. Pain and stiffness usually subside over a period of months. Complete movement may not be regained.

Examination

Examine the shoulders. There is global restriction of movement of the shoulder— i.e., it is frozen.

Elbow Epicondylitis (Tennis and Golfer's Elbow)

Many contact and non-contact sports can cause physical injury, though serious injuries are rather uncommon with certain sports (e.g., synchronised swimming). The above conditions cause pain over the epicondyles of the elbow. The lateral epicondyle is the most often affected and is called 'tennis elbow'. Pain arises from the site of insertion of the extensor muscle tendons into the lateral epicondyle (enthesis). Involvement of the medial epicondyle at the site of insertion of the flexor tendons of the forearm causes medial epicondylitis—'golfer's elbow'.

Examination

Examine for local tenderness over the lateral (Figure 8.33) or medial epicondyle (Figure 8.34). Ask the patient to extend the fingers against resistance. This will make the pain of lateral epicondylitis worse. Ask the patient to flex the fingers against resistance. This will exacerbate the pain of medial epicondylitis.

Tenosynovitis

Inflammation of the synovial tubes in which tendons run can occur in patients with rheumatoid arthritis but also in otherwise healthy people. The cause is often unaccustomed repetitive movement. A common site for tenosynovitis is at the wrist where it involves the long extensor and abductor tendons of the thumb (De Quervain's tenosynovitis) (Figure 8.35).

Examination

This reveals tenderness and swelling on the radial side of the wrist. There is pain on active or passive movement of the thumb. Examine also the other common sites of tendon involvement; the flexor tendons of the fingers and the Achilles tendon.

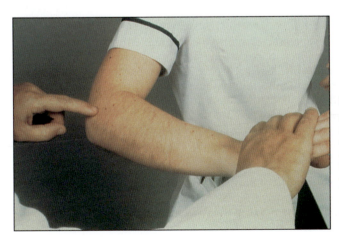

Figure 8.33

Examination of the elbow looking for signs of lateral epicondylitis. Palpation over the forearm extensor muscle origin elicits pain. Straining the muscles by resisted extension of the wrist exacerbates the symptoms.

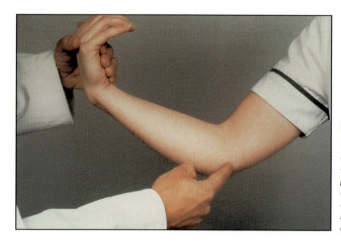

Figure 8.34

Examination to elicit signs of medial epicondylitis. Local pressure over the medial epicondyle elicits pain. Symptoms are exacerbated by resisted flexion of the wrist and fingers.

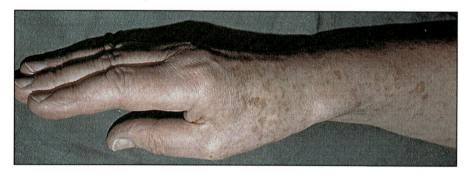

Figure 8.35 *A patient with de Quervain's tenosynovitis with characteristic swelling of the tendon sheath of the abductor pollicis longus and extensor pollicis brevis over the styloid process of the radius.*

Bursitis

Bursae are found in areas exposed to mechanical strain, either at the site where muscle or tendon glides over bone or muscle, or superficially where bony prominences are exposed to mechanical stress. Bursitis usually occurs as a local soft tissue inflammatory reaction to unusual mechanical stress. It may be associated with rheumatoid arthritis, gout or sepsis. Common sites include the prepatellar area (housemaid's knee) (Figure 8.36), over the olecranon (olecranon bursitis), and over the greater trochanter (trochanteric bursitis).

Nerve Entrapment Syndromes

These are caused by compression of peripheral nerves at vulnerable sites and are associated with pain, paraesthesiae and numbness in a particular nerve distribution. Compression of the median nerve at the wrist (carpal tunnel syndrome) is the most frequent form. The commonest cause is an overuse tenosynovitis of the flexor

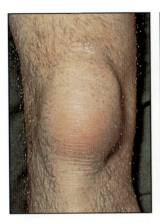
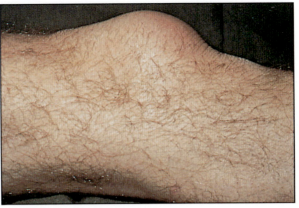

Figure 8.36 *Prepatellar bursitis. Anterior and lateral view of a red swollen and painful prepatellar bursa.*

tendon sheaths at the wrist. Fluid retention during pregnancy or from use of the oral contraceptive pill can also produce carpal tunnel symptoms. In addition, median nerve compression can occur in rheumatoid arthritis, hypothyroidism, acromegaly and amyloidosis.

Examination

Symptoms can be reproduced by gentle percussion over the carpal tunnel (Tinel's sign) or by prolonged wrist flexion (Phalen's test). Look for wasting in the median nerve distribution, and loss of motor and sensory function. These signs occur only in advanced cases.

Suggested Reading

Original and Review Articles

Deyo RA, Rainville J, Kent DL. What can the history and physical examination tell us about low back pain? *JAMA* 1992; 268: 760–765.

Frymoyer JW. Back pain and sciatica. *N Engl J Med* 1988; 318: 291–300.

Fuchs HA, Joint counts and physical measures. *Rheumc Dis Clin Nth Am* 1995; 21: 429–44.

Glockner SM, Shoulder pain: a diagnostic dilemma. *Am Fam Phys* 1995; 51: 1677–87, 1690–2.

Katz JN, Dalgas M, Stucki G, Katz NP, Bayley J, Fossel AH, Chang LC, Lipson SJ, Degenerative lumbar spinal stenosis. Diagnostic value of the history and physical examination. *Arth Rheum* 1995; 38: 1236–41.

Textbooks

Apley AG, Solomon L. Apley's system of orthopaedics and fractures. 7th ed. London: Butterworths, 1993.

Boyle AC. Color atlas of rheumatology. Chicago: Year Book Medical Publishers, 1980.

Edmonds J, Hughes G. Lecture notes on rheumatology. Oxford: Blackwell, 1985.

Kelley WN, Harris ED Jr, Ruddy S, Sledge CB, editors. Textbook of rheumatology. Vol. 1, 4th ed. Philadelphia: Saunders, 1993.

Klippel JH, Dieppe P. Rheumatology. London: Gower Medical, 1994.

Chapter 9

THE ENDOCRINE SYSTEM

A physician is obligated to consider more than a diseased organ,
more even than the whole man—he must view the man in his world.

Harvey Cushing (1869–1939)

The Endocrine History

Presenting Symptoms (Table 9.1)

Hormones control so many aspects of body function that the manifestations of endocrine disease are protean. Symptoms can include changes in body weight, appetite, bowel habit, hair distribution, pigmentation, sweating, height and menstruation, as well as polydipsia, polyuria, lethargy, headaches and impotence. Many of these symptoms have other causes as well and must be carefully evaluated. On the other hand, the patient may know which endocrine organ or group of endocrine organs has been causing a problem. In particular, there may be a history of a thyroid condition or diabetes mellitus. A list of common symptoms associated with various endocrine diseases is presented in Table 9.1. In this section some of the important symptoms associated with endocrine disease will be discussed.

Changes in Appetite and Weight

An increased appetite associated with weight loss classically occurs in thyrotoxicosis or uncontrolled diabetes mellitus. An increased appetite with weight gain may occur in Cushing's syndrome, hypoglycaemia or in hypothalamic disease. A loss of appetite with weight loss can occur with adrenal insufficiency but is also seen in anorexia nervosa and with gastrointestinal disease (particularly malignancy). A loss of appetite with weight gain can occur in hypothyroidism.

Changes in Bowel Habit

Diarrhoea is associated with hyperthyroidism and adrenal insufficiency, while constipation may occur in hypothyroidism and hypercalcaemia.

Changes in Sweating

Increased sweating is characteristic of hyperthyroidism, phaeochromocytoma, hypoglycaemia and acromegaly, but may also occur in anxiety states and at the menopause (page 453).

Table 9.1 *Endocrine History*

Major Symptoms

Appetite and weight changes
Disturbed defaecation
Sweating
Hair distribution
Lethargy
Skin changes
Pigmentation
Stature
Impotence
Menstruation
Polyuria
Lump in the neck (goitre)

Syndromes

Thyrotoxicosis: preference for cooler weather, weight loss, increased appetite
    (polyphagia), palpitations, increased sweating, nervousness, irritability, diarrhoea,
    amenorrhoea, muscle weakness, exertional dyspnoea
Hypothyroidism (myxoedema): preference for warmer weather, lethargy, swelling of
    eyelids (oedema), hoarse voice, constipation, coarse skin, hypercarotenaemia
Diabetes mellitus: polyuria, polydipsia, thirst, blurred vision, weakness, infections, groin
    itch, rash (pruritus vulvae, balanitis), weight loss, tiredness, lethargy and disturbance
    of conscious state
Hypoglycaemia: morning headaches, weight gain, seizures, sweating
Primary adrenal insufficiency: pigmentation, tiredness, loss of weight, anorexia, nausea,
    diarrhoea, nocturia, mental changes, seizures (hypotension, hypoglycaemia)
Acromegaly: fatigue, weakness, increased sweating, heat intolerance, weight gain,
    enlarging hands and feet, enlarged and coarsened facial features, headaches,
    decreased vision, voice change, decreased libido, impotence

Changes in Hair Distribution

Hirsutism refers to an increased growth of body hair in women. The clinical
evaluation and differential diagnosis are presented on page 318. The absence of
facial hair in a male suggests hypogonadism, while temporal recession of the scalp
hair in women occurs with androgen excess. The decrease in adrenal androgen
production that occurs as a result of hypogonadism or adrenal insufficiency can
cause loss of axillary and pubic hair in both sexes.

Lethargy

This can be due to a number of different diseases. Patients with hypothyroidism,
Addison's disease and diabetes mellitus can present with this problem. Anaemia,
connective tissue diseases, chronic infection (e.g., HIV, infective endocarditis),
drugs (e.g., sedatives, diuretics causing electrolyte disturbances), chronic liver
disease, renal failure and occult malignancy may also result in lethargy. Importantly, depression is a common cause of this very common symptom (page 425).

Changes in the Skin

The skin becomes coarse, pale and dry in hypothyroidism, and dry and scaly in
hypoparathyroidism. Soft tissue overgrowth occurs in acromegaly. Flushing of the

skin of the face and neck occurs in the carcinoid syndrome (due to the release of vasoactive peptides from the tumour) (page 453). Soft tissue overgrowth occurs in acromegaly and skin tags may appear in the axillae. These are called molluscum fibrinosum. Acanthosis nigricans can also occur in acromegaly and in insulin-resistant states including Cushing's syndrome and polycystic ovarian syndrome. Xanthelasma can be present in patients with diabetes or hypothyroidism.

Changes in Pigmentation

Increased pigmentation may be reported in primary adrenal insufficiency, Cushing's syndrome or acromegaly. Decreased pigmentation occurs in hypopituitarism. Localised depigmentation is characteristic of vitiligo, which may be associated with certain endocrine diseases such as Hashimoto's* disease with hypothyroidism and Addison's disease with adrenal insufficiency.

Changes in Stature

Tallness may occur in children for constitutional reasons (tall parents) or, rarely, may reflect growth hormone excess (leading to gigantism), gonadotrophin deficiency, Klinefelter's† syndrome, Marfan's syndrome or generalised lipodystrophy. Short stature can also result from endocrine disease, as discussed on page 315.

Impotence

A persistent inability to attain or sustain penile erections may occasionally be due to primary hypogonadism or to secondary hypogonadism due to hyperprolactinaemia. More often, impotence is related to emotional disorders; autonomic neuropathy (e.g., diabetes mellitus or alcoholism), spinal cord disease or testicular atrophy can also cause this problem.

Menstruation

Failure to menstruate is termed *amenorrhoea*. *Primary amenorrhoea* is defined as a failure to start menstruating by 17 years of age. True primary amenorrhoea may result from ovarian failure (e.g., X chromosomal abnormalities such as Turner's syndrome) or from pituitary or hypothalamic disease (e.g., tumour, trauma or idiopathic disease). Excess androgen production or systemic disease (e.g., malabsorption, chronic renal failure, obesity) can also result in primary amenorrhoea.

Apparent primary amenorrhoea can also occur if menstrual flow cannot escape, e.g., if there is an imperforate hymen. *Secondary amenorrhoea* is defined as the cessation of menstruation for six months or more. Pregnancy and menopause are common causes. The polycystic ovarian syndrome, hyperprolactinaemia, virilising syndromes or hypothalamic or pituitary disease can also result in this problem, as can use of the contraceptive pill or psychiatric disease.

Polyuria

Polyuria is defined as a urine volume of more than 3L/day. Patients who report urinary frequency may find it difficult to tell if large volumes of urine are being

---

*   Hakaru Hashimoto (1881–1934), Japanese surgeon.

†   Harry Fitch Klinefelter (b. 1912), Baltimore physician, described the condition when he was a medical student.

passed. Causes include diabetes mellitus (due to excessive filtration of glucose, a poorly resorbed solute); diabetes insipidus (due to inadequate renal water conservation from a central deficiency of antidiuretic hormone, or a lack of renal responsiveness to this hormone); primary polydipsia, where a patient drinks excessive water (due to psychogenic or hypothalamic disease or drugs such as chlorpromazine or thioridazine); hypercalcaemia; and tubulointerstitial or cystic renal disease.

Past History

A previous history of any endocrine condition must be uncovered. This includes surgery on the neck for a goitre. A partial thyroidectomy or radio-iodine (^{131}I) treatment in the past can lead to eventual hypothyroidism. The same may apply to radiation of the thyroid for carcinoma. A woman may have been diagnosed as having diabetes mellitus after the birth of a large baby. There may only be a past history of hypertension, which is occasionally due to an endocrine condition (e.g., phaeochromocytoma, Cushing's syndrome or Conn's syndrome). Previous thyroid surgery can be associated with hypoparathyroidism because of surgical damage to the parathyroid glands.

Previous treatment of a patient's thyroid problems may have included the use of antithyroid drugs, thyroid hormone or radioactive iodine. Surgery on the adrenals or pituitary may have been performed and this may leave the patient with decreased adrenal or pituitary function.

Patients with diabetes mellitus have an important chronic condition. Treatment may be with diet, insulin or oral hypoglycaemic agents. One must determine how well the patient understands the condition and whether he or she understands the principles of the diabetic diet and adheres to it. Find out how the blood sugar levels are monitored and whether or not the patient adjusts the insulin dose. Most patients should now be able to monitor their own blood sugar levels at home using a glucometer. There is now good evidence that good control of blood sugar levels reduces the incidence of diabetic complications. The patient should be aware of the need for attention to the feet and eyes to help prevent complications.

Patients with hypopituitarism or hypoadrenalism may be on steroid replacement; some of these people also require mineralocorticoid replacement. Details of the patient's dosage schedule should be obtained.

Social History

Many of these conditions are chronic and their complications serious. How well the patient copes with various problems and the conditions at home and work will have an important effect on the success of treatment.

Family History

There may be a history in the family of thyroid conditions or diabetes mellitus. Occasionally a family history of a multiple endocrine neoplasia (MEN) syndrome may be obtained. These are rare autosomal dominant conditions. They include pituitary tumours, medullary carcinoma of the thyroid, hyperparathyroidism, phaeochromocytoma and pancreatic tumours.

The Endocrine Examination

A formal examination of the whole endocrine system is rarely performed (page 327); it is more usual to examine for signs of specific endocrine diseases. Usually there will be some clue from the history and general inspection to indicate what approach should be pursued.

The Thyroid

The Thyroid Gland

The examiner of the thyroid gland is fortunate that this gland has been placed conveniently in the front of the neck (Table 9.2).

Inspection

The normal thyroid may be just visible in a thin young person below the cricoid cartilage. Usually only the isthmus is visible as a diffuse central swelling. Enlargement of the gland, called a goitre (Latin *guttur* throat), should be apparent on inspection. Look at the front and sides of the neck and decide if there is localised or general swelling of the gland.

The temptation to begin touching a swelling as soon as it has been detected must be resisted until a glass of water has been procured. The patient takes sips from this repeatedly so that swallowing is possible without discomfort. Ask the patient to swallow and watch the neck swelling carefully. Only a goitre or a thyroglossal cyst, because of attachment to the larynx, will rise during swallowing. A thyroid gland fixed by neoplastic infiltration may not do so, but this is rare. Swallowing also allows the shape of the gland to be seen better. It should be noted whether an inferior border is visible as the gland rises.

Inspect the skin of the neck for scars. A thyroidectomy scar forms a ring around the base of the neck in the position of a high necklace. Also look for prominent veins. Dilated veins over the upper part of the chest wall, often accompanied by filling of the external jugular vein, suggest retrosternal extension of the goitre

Table 9.2 *Causes of Neck Swellings*

Midline
Goitre (moves up on swallowing)
Thyroglossal cyst (moves on poking out the tongue with the jaw stationary)
Submental lymph nodes
Parathyroid gland (very rare)
Lateral
Lymph nodes
Salivary glands (e.g., stone, tumour)
Submandibular gland
Parotid gland (lower pole)
Skin: sebaceous cyst or lipoma
Lymphatics: cystic hygroma (translucent)
Carotid artery: aneurysm or rarely tumour (pulsatile)
Pharynx: pharyngeal pouch, or brachial arch remnant (brachial cyst)

(thoracic inlet obstruction). Rarely, redness of the skin over the gland occurs in cases of suppurative thyroiditis.

Palpation

Palpation is best begun from *behind* (Figure 9.1). Both hands are placed with the pulps of the fingers over the gland. The patient's neck should be slightly flexed so as to relax the sternomastoid muscles. Feel systematically both lobes of the gland and its isthmus. Consider the following.

Size: only an approximate estimation is possible (Figures 9.2 and 9.3). Feel particularly carefully for a lower border because its absence suggests retrosternal extension.

Shape: note whether the gland is uniformly enlarged or irregular and whether the isthmus is affected. If a *nodule* that feels distinct from the remaining thyroid tissue is palpable, determine its location, size, consistency, tenderness and mobility. Also decide if the whole gland feels nodular (multinodular goitre).

Consistency: this may vary in different parts of the gland. Soft is normal; the gland is often firm in simple goitre and typically rubbery hard in Hashimoto's thyroiditis. A stony hard node suggests carcinoma, calcification in a cyst, fibrosis, or Riedel's thyroiditis.

Tenderness: is a feature of thyroiditis (subacute or rarely suppurative), or less often of a bleed into a cyst or carcinoma.

Mobility: carcinoma may tether the gland.

Repeat the assessment while the patient swallows.

Decide if a thrill is palpable over the gland, as occurs when the gland is unusually metabolically active as in thyrotoxicosis.

Palpate the cervical lymph nodes (page 229). These may be involved in carcinoma of the thyroid. Feel each carotid artery—absence of its pulsation may very occasionally indicate malignant infiltration by thyroid carcinoma.

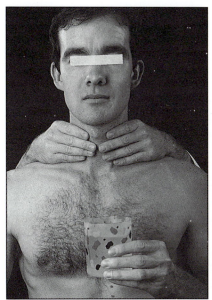

Figure 9.1

Palpating the thyroid from behind while the patient swallows sips of water.

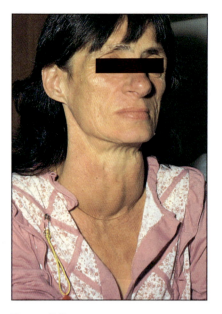

Figure 9.2 *Large goitre.*

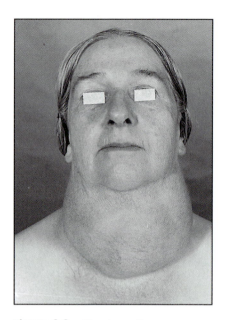

Figure 9.3 *Massive goitre.*

Move to the *front*. Palpate again using the thumbs. Localised swellings may be more easily defined here. Note the position of the trachea, which may be displaced by a retrosternal gland.

Percussion

The upper part of the manubrium can be percussed from one side to the other. A change from resonant to dull indicates a possible retrosternal goitre, but this is not a very reliable sign.

Auscultation

Listen over each lobe for a bruit. This is a sign of increased blood supply which may occur in hyperthyroidism, or occasionally from the use of antithyroid drugs. The differential diagnosis also includes a carotid bruit (louder over the carotid itself) or a venous hum (obliterated by gentle pressure over the base of the neck).

Pemberton's sign

Get the patient to lift both arms as high as possible. Wait a few moments then search the face eagerly for signs of congestion (plethora) and cyanosis. Associated respiratory distress and inspiratory stridor may occur. Look at the neck veins for distension (venous congestion). Ask the patient to take a deep breath in through the mouth and listen for stridor. This is a test for thoracic inlet obstruction due to a retrosternal goitre or any retrosternal mass (page 115).

Examination of the thyroid should be part of every routine physical examination.

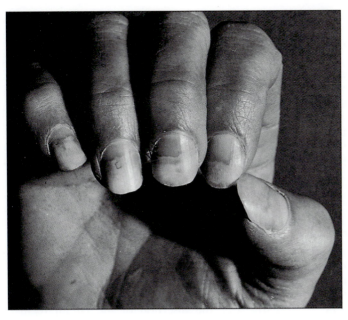

Figure 9.4
Onycholysis
(Plummer's nails).

Thyrotoxicosis

This is a disease caused by excessive concentrations of thyroid hormones. Many of the clinical features of thyrotoxicosis are characterised by signs of sympathetic overactivity, such as tremor, tachycardia and sweating. The explanation is not entirely clear. Catecholamine secretion is usually normal in hyperthyroidism; however, thyroid hormone potentiates the effects of catecholamines, possibly by increasing the number of adrenergic receptors in the tissues.

The commonest cause of thyrotoxicosis in young people is Graves'* disease, an autoimmune disease where circulating immunoglobulins stimulate TSH receptors on the surface of the thyroid follicular cells.

Examine a suspected case of thyrotoxicosis as follows.

General Inspection

Look for signs of weight loss, anxiety and the frightened facies of thyrotoxicosis.

The Hands

Ask the patient to put out the arms and look for a fine tremor (due to sympathetic overactivity). Laying a sheet of paper over the patient's fingers may more clearly demonstrate this tremor, to the amazement of less experienced colleagues.

Look at the nails for *onycholysis* (Plummer's[†] nails) (Figure 9.4). Onycholysis (where there is separation of the nail from its bed) is said to occur particularly on the ring finger, but can occur on all the fingernails, and is apparently due to

---

*   Robert Graves (1796–1853), Dublin physician.

[†]   Henry Plummer (1874–1936), physician at the Mayo Clinic, USA.

sympathetic overactivity. It is rarely seen in association with Graves' disease. Inspect now for thyroid acropachy (this looks like clubbing and is clubbing, but is not called clubbing), seen rarely in Graves' disease, but not with other causes of thyrotoxicosis.

Inspect for palmar erythema and feel the palms for warmth and sweatiness (sympathetic overactivity).

Take the pulse. Note the presence of sinus tachycardia (sympathetic overdrive) or atrial fibrillation (due to a shortened refractory period of atrial cells related to sympathetic drive and hormone–induced changes). The pulse may also have a collapsing character due to a high cardiac output.

Test for proximal myopathy and tap the arm reflexes for abnormal briskness, especially in the relaxation phase (page 374).

The Eyes

Examine the eyes for exophthalmos, which is protrusion of the eyeball out of the orbit (Figure 9.5) (Table 9.3). This may be very obvious, but if not, look carefully at the sclerae which in exophthalmos are not covered by the lower eyelid. Next look from behind over the patient's forehead for exophthalmos where the eye will be visible anterior to the superior orbital margin. Now examine for the complications of proptosis, which include: (i) chemosis (oedema of the conjunctiva and injection of the sclera, particularly over the insertion of the lateral rectus); (ii) conjunctivitis; (iii) corneal ulceration (due to inability to close the eyelids); (iv) optic atrophy (rare and possibly due to optic nerve stretching); and (v) ophthalmoplegia (the inferior rectus muscle power tends to be lost first, and later convergence is weakened).

The mechanism of exophthalmos is uncertain. It occurs only in Graves' disease. It may precede the onset of thyrotoxicosis, or may persist after the patient has become euthyroid. It is characterised by an inflammatory infiltrate of the orbital contents, but not of the globe itself. The orbital muscles are particularly affected and an increase in their size accounts for most of the increased volume of the orbital contents and therefore for protrusion of the globe. It is probably due to an autoimmune abnormality.

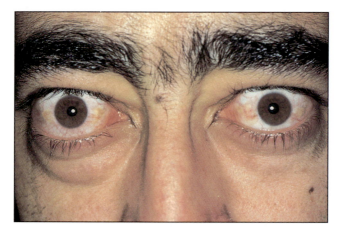

Figure 9.5   *Thyrotoxicosis: thyroid stare and exophthalmos.*

Table 9.3   *Causes of Exophthalmos*

Bilateral
Graves' disease
Unilateral
Tumours of the orbit: e.g., dermoid, optic nerve glioma, neurofibroma, granuloma
Cavernous sinus thrombosis
Graves' disease
Pseudotumours of the orbit

Next examine for the components of thyroid ophthalmopathy, which are related to sympathetic overactivity and are not specific for Graves' disease. Look for the thyroid stare (a frightened expression) and lid retraction (where there is sclera visible above the iris). Test for lid lag by asking the patient to follow your finger as it descends at a moderate rate from the upper to the lower part of the visual field. Descent of the upper lid lags behind descent of the eyeball.

If ptosis is present one should think of myasthenia gravis which can be associated with autoimmune diseases.

The Neck

Examine for thyroid enlargement, which is usually detectable. In Graves' disease the gland is classically diffusely enlarged and is smooth and firm. An associated thrill may be present. Absence of thyroid enlargement makes Graves' disease unlikely, but does not exclude it. Possible thyroid abnormalities in patients who are thyrotoxic but do not have Graves' disease include a toxic multinodular goitre, a solitary nodule (toxic adenoma), or subacute thyroiditis (De Quervain's* thyroiditis). In De Quervain's thyroiditis there is typically a moderately enlarged firm and tender gland. Thyrotoxicosis may occur without any goitre, particularly in elderly patients. Alternatively, in hyperthyroidism due to an abnormality of trophoblastic tissue (a hydatidiform mole or choriocarcinoma of the testis or uterus), or excessive thyroid hormone replacement, the thyroid gland will not usually be palpable. These causes are rare.

If a thyroidectomy scar is present, assess for hypoparathyroidism (Chvostek's† or Trousseau's‡ signs (page 315)). These signs are most often present in the first few days after operation.

The Arms

Ask the patient to raise the arms above the head and so test for proximal myopathy.

The Chest

Gynaecomastia (page 319) occurs occasionally. Examine the heart for systolic flow murmurs (due to increased cardiac output) and signs of congestive cardiac failure, which may be precipitated by thyrotoxicosis in older people.

---

* Fritz de Quervain (1868–1940), Professor of Surgery, Berne, Switzerland.

† Franz Chvostek (1835–1884), Viennese physician.

‡ Armand Trousseau (1801–1867), Parisian physician.

The Legs

Look first for pretibial myxoedema. This takes the form of bilateral firm elevated dermal nodules and plaques, which can be pink, brown or skin-coloured. They are caused by mucopolysaccharide accumulation. Despite the name this occurs only in Graves' disease and not in hypothyroidism. Test now for proximal myopathy and hyper-reflexia in the legs.

Hypothyroidism

Hypothyroidism (deficiency of thyroid hormone) is due to primary disease of the thyroid, or is secondary to pituitary or hypothalamic failure (Table 9.4). Myxoedema implies a more severe form of hypothyroidism. In myxoedema, for unknown reasons, hydrophilic mucopolysaccharides accumulate in the ground substance of tissues including the skin. This results in excessive interstitial fluid which is relatively immobile, causing skin thickening and a doughy induration.

Examine the patient with suspected hypothyroidism as follows.

General Inspection

Look for signs of obvious mental and physical sluggishness, or evidence of the very rare 'myxoedema madness'.

The Hands

Note peripheral cyanosis (due to reduced cardiac output) and swelling of the skin, which may appear cool and dry. The yellow discoloration of hypercarotenaemia (there is slowing down of hepatic metabolism of carotene) may be seen on the palms. Look for palmar crease pallor—anaemia may be due to (i) chronic disease; (ii) folate deficiency secondary to bacterial overgrowth, or vitamin B_{12} deficiency due to associated pernicious anaemia; or (iii) iron deficiency due to menorrhagia.

Take the pulse, which may be of small volume and slow. Tap over the flexor retinaculum for Tinel's sign, as the carpal tunnel is thickened in myxoedema (page 380).

The Arms

Test for proximal myopathy (rare) and a 'hung up' biceps reflex (see below).

The Face

Inspect the face (Figure 9.6). The skin, but not the sclera, may appear yellow due to hypercarotenaemia. The skin may be generally thickened, and alopecia may be present, as may vitiligo (an associated autoimmune disease).

Inspect the eyes for periorbital oedema. Loss or thinning of the outer third of the eyebrows can occur in myxoedema but is also common in healthy persons. Look for xanthelasma (due to associated hypercholesterolaemia) (page 43). Palpate for coolness and dryness of the skin and hair. There may be thinning of the scalp hair.

Look at the tongue for swelling. Ask the patient to speak and listen for coarse, croaking, slow speech. Bilateral nerve deafness may occur with endemic or congenital hypothyroidism.

Table 9.4 *Thyrotoxicosis and Hypothyroidism*

Causes of Thyrotoxicosis

Primary

Graves' disease
Toxic multinodular goitre
Toxic uninodular goitre: usually a toxic adenoma
Hashimoto's thyroiditis (early in its course; later it produces hypothyroidism)
Subacute thyroiditis (transient)
Postpartum thyroiditis (non-tender)
Iodine-induced ('Jod-Basedow* phenomenon'—iodine given after a previously deficient
    diet)

Secondary

Pituitary (very rare): TSH hypersecretion
Hydatidiform moles or choriocarcinomas: HCG secretion (rare)
Struma ovarii (rare)
Drugs, e.g., excess thyroid hormone ingestion, amiodarone

Causes of Hypothyroidism

Primary

Without a goitre (decreased or absent thyroid tissue)
    Idiopathic atrophy
    Treatment of thyrotoxicosis—e.g., ^{131}I, surgery
    Agenesis or a lingual thyroid
    Unresponsiveness to TSH
With a goitre (decreased thyroid hormone synthesis)
    Chronic autoimmune diseases—e.g., Hashimoto's thyroiditis
    Drugs, e.g., lithium, amiodarone
    Inborn errors (enzyme deficiency)
    Endemic iodine deficiency or iodine-induced hypothyroidism

Secondary

Pituitary lesions (Table 9.7)

Tertiary

Hypothalamic lesions

Transient

Thyroid hormone treatment withdrawn
Subacute thyroiditis
Postpartum thyroiditis

---

* Carl von Basedow (1799–1854), German general practitioner, described this in 1840 (*Jod*—iodine in
  German).
TSH = thyroid stimulating hormone.

The Thyroid Gland

A primary decrease in thyroid hormone results in a compensatory oversecretion of
thyroid stimulating hormone (TSH). A goitre will result if there is viable thyroid
tissue.

    Many cases of hypothyroidism are not associated with an enlarged gland as
there is little thyroid tissue. The exceptions are severe iodine deficiency, enzyme

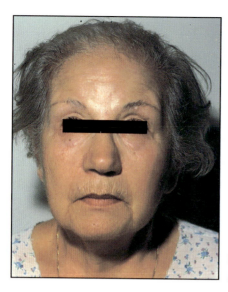

Figure 9.6
Myxoedema.

deficiency (inborn errors of metabolism), late Hashimoto's disease or treated thyrotoxicosis (Table 9.5).

The Chest

Examine the heart for a pericardial effusion and the lungs for pleural effusions.

The Legs

Ask the patient to kneel on a chair with the ankles exposed. Tap the Achilles tendon with a reflex hammer. There is normal contraction followed by delayed relaxation of the foot in hypothyroidism (the 'hung-up' reflex) (page 386). There may be non-pitting oedema. Examine for signs of peripheral neuropathy and for other uncommon neurological abnormalities associated with hypothyroidism (Table 9.6).

The Pituitary

Pituitary tumours can present in two ways—as a result of (i) local effects such as headaches, visual field loss and loss of acuity; and (ii) changes in pituitary hormone secretion. These changes include: (i) excess growth hormone, causing acromegaly; (ii) excess ACTH, causing Cushing's syndrome; and (iii) prolactin, causing secondary amenorrhoea or male infertility or deficiency (hypopituitarism).

Panhypopituitarism

This is a deficiency of most or all of the pituitary hormones and is usually due to a space–occupying lesion or destruction of the pituitary gland (Table 9.7). Hormone production is often lost in the following order: (i) growth hormone (dwarfism in children, insulin sensitivity in adults); (ii) prolactin (failure of lactation after delivery); (iii) gonadotrophins (loss of secondary sexual characteristics, secondary amenorrhoea in women, loss of libido and infertility in men); (iv) thyroid stimulat-

Table 9.5 *Goitre*

Causes of a Diffuse Goitre (patient often euthyroid)
Idiopathic (majority)
Puberty or pregnancy
Thyroiditis
  Hashimoto's
  Subacute (gland usually tender)
Simple goitre (iodine deficiency)
Goitrogens—e.g., iodine excess, drugs (e.g., lithium, phenylbutazone)
Inborn errors of thyroid hormone synthesis—e.g., Pendred's* syndrome
    (an autosomal recessive condition associated with nerve deafness)

Causes of a Solitary Thyroid Nodule
Benign:
  Dominant nodule in a multinodular goitre
  Degeneration or haemorrhage into a colloid cyst or nodule
  Follicular adenoma
  Simple cyst (rare)
Malignant:
  Carcinoma—primary or secondary (e.g., renal cell carcinoma)
  Lymphoma (rare)

* Vaughan Pendred (b. 1869), London physician.

Table 9.6 *Neurological Associations of Hypothyroidism*

Common
Entrapment: carpal tunnel, tarsal tunnel
Delayed ankle jerks
Muscle cramps

Uncommon
Peripheral neuropathy
Proximal myopathy
Hypokalaemic periodic paralysis
Cerebellar syndrome
Psychosis
Coma
Unmasking of myasthenia gravis
Cerebrovascular disease
High cerebrovascular fluid protein
Nerve deafness

ing hormone (TSH) (hypothyroidism): and (v) adrenocorticotrophic hormone (ACTH) (hypoadrenalism and hypopigmentation) with loss of secondary sexual hair due to decreased adrenal androgen production.

However, isolated single hormonal deficiencies or multiple deficiencies may occur in any combination.

General Inspection

The patient may be of short stature (failure of growth hormone secretion before growth is complete). Look for pallor of the skin (due to anaemia or occasionally

Table 9.7 *Causes of Hypopituitarism*

Space-occupying lesion
  Pituitary tumour (non-secretory or secretory)
  Other tumours: craniopharyngioma, metastatic carcinoma, sarcoma
  Granulomata: e.g., sarcoid, tuberculosis
Iatrogenic: e.g., surgery or irradiation
Head injury
Sheehan's* syndrome (postpartum pituitary haemorrhage resulting in necrosis of the
    gland)
Infarction or pituitary apoplexy
Idiopathic

* Harold Sheehan (b. 1900), Professor of Pathology, Liverpool, England, described the syndrome in 1937.

Table 9.8 *Secondary Sexual Development (Tanner Stages)*

This occurs at puberty in response to pituitary gonadotrophins

Males

1. Preadolescent
2. Enlargement of testes and scrotum
3. Lengthening of penis
4. Increase in penis breadth, glans development, and scrotal darkening
5. Adult: above plus pubic hair spread to medial surface of the thighs

Females

1. Preadolescent: papilla elevation only
2. Breast bud
3. Enlargement of breast and areola
4. Areola and papilla project above breast level
5. Adult: areola recessed and papilla projects

ACTH deficiency because of the loss of its melanocyte stimulating activity), fine wrinkled skin and lack of body hair (due to gonadotrophin deficiency). There may be complete absence of the secondary sexual characteristics (Table 9.8) if gonadotrophin failure occurred before puberty.

The Face

Look at the face more closely. Multiple skin wrinkles around the eyes are characteristic of gonadotrophin deficiency. Inspect the forehead carefully for hypophysectomy scars—transfrontal scars will be apparent (Figure 9.7) but not trans-sphenoidal ones, as this operation is performed through the base of the nose, via an incision under the upper lip.

Examine the eyes (page 366). The visual fields must be assessed for any defects, especially bitemporal hemianopia (an enlarging pituitary tumour may compress the optic chiasm) and the fundi examined for optic atrophy (optic nerve compression from a pituitary tumour). Assess the third, fourth and sixth and the first division of the fifth cranial nerves, as these may be affected by extrapituitary tumour expansion into the cavernous sinus (Figure 9.8).

Feel the facial hair over the bearded area in men for normal beard growth (which is lost with gonadotrophin deficiency).

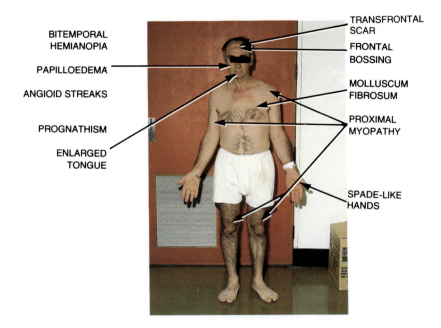

Figure 9.7 *Acromegaly.*

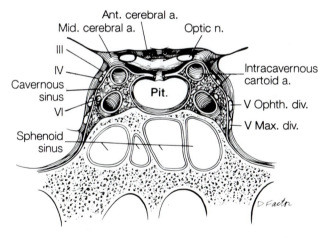

Figure 9.8 *The cavernous sinus and its relationship with the cranial nerves and pituitary gland.*

The Chest

Go on to the chest. Look for skin pallor and for a decrease in nipple pigmentation. In men, decreased body hair (axillary and chest) may be present. In women, secondary breast atrophy may be found.

The Genital Region

Loss of pubic hair occurs in both sexes. In men, testicular atrophy may be present. Atrophied testes are characteristically small and firm. The normal-sized testis is about 15 to 25mL in volume.

The Ankle Reflexes

Test for 'hung-up' jerks. These are the most reliable sign of pituitary hypothyroidism. Occasionally, pituitary hypothyroid patients may be slightly over-weight, but the classical myxoedematous appearance is usually absent.

Acromegaly*

This is excessive secretion of growth hormone, typically due to an eosinophilic pituitary adenoma. Growth hormone stimulates the liver and other tissues to produce somatomedins which in turn promote growth. Growth hormone is also a protein anabolic hormone exerting its effects at the ribosomal level, and is diabetogenic as it exerts an anti-insulin effect in muscle and increases hepatic glucose release.

Gigantism is the result of growth hormone hypersecretion occurring before puberty and fusion of the epiphyses. It results in massive skeletal, as well as soft tissue, growth. Acromegaly occurs when the growth plates have fused, so that only soft tissue and flat bone enlargement are possible.

General Inspection

The face and body habitus may be characteristic (Figure 9.7).

The Hands

Sit the patient on the side of the bed and look at the hands. Notice a wide spade-like shape (due to soft tissue and bony enlargement). Increased sweating and warmth of the palms may be noted. This is due to an increased metabolic rate. The skin may appear thickened. Changes of osteoarthritis in the hands are common and are due to skeletal overgrowth. Examine for Tinel's sign as median nerve entrapment can occur because of soft tissue overgrowth in the carpal tunnel area.

The Arms

Proximal myopathy may be present (page 402). Palpate behind the medial epicondyle (the 'funny bone') for ulnar nerve thickening.

The Axillae

Carefully inspect the axillae for skin tags (called molluscum fibrosum, which are non-tender skin-coloured protrusions). Summon up courage and feel for greasy skin. Look for acanthosis nigricans.

The Face

Look for a large supraorbital ridge which causes frontal bossing (this may also occur occasionally in Paget's disease, rickets, achondroplasia or hydrocephalus). The lips may be thickened.

---

* The acral parts are the hands and feet.

Examine the eyes for visual field defects: classically there may be bitemporal hemianopia if the pituitary tumour is large. Look in the fundi for optic atrophy (due to nerve compression) and papilloedema (due to raised intracranial pressure with an extensive tumour). The presence of angioid streaks (red, brown or grey streaks which are three to five times the diameter of a retinal vein and appear to emanate from the optic disc) should also be sought: these are due to degeneration and fibrosis of Bruch's membrane. One should also note hypertensive changes or diabetic changes in the fundus. Ocular palsies may occur with an extensive pituitary tumour (page 307).

Look in the mouth for an enlarged tongue which may not fit neatly between the teeth. The teeth themselves may be splayed and separated with malocclusion as the jaw enlarges. The lower jaw may look square and firm (as it does on some American actors). When the jaw protrudes it is called prognathism (Greek *pro* forwards, *gnathos* jaw).

The Neck

The thyroid may be diffusely enlarged or multinodular (all the internal organs may enlarge under the influence of growth hormone). Listen to the voice for hoarseness.

The Chest

Look for coarse body hair and gynaecomastia. Examine the heart for signs of arrhythmias, cardiomegaly and congestive cardiac failure, which may be due to ischaemic heart disease, hypertension or cardiomyopathy (all more common in acromegaly).

The Back

Inspect for kyphosis.

The Abdomen

Examine for hepatic, splenic and renal enlargement, and for testicular atrophy (the latter indicating gonadotrophin deficiency secondary to an enlarging pituitary tumour). Acromegaly can be associated with a mixed pituitary tumour and resultant hyperprolactinaemia can also cause testicular atrophy.

The Lower Limbs

Look for signs of osteoarthritis in the hips especially, and knees (page 266), and for pseudogout. Foot drop my be present because of common peroneal nerve entrapment (page 390).

The Urine and Blood Pressure

Test the urine for glucose, as growth hormone is diabetogenic in 25% of cases. Take the blood pressure to test for hypertension.

Finally decide if the disease is active or not. Signs of active disease include: (i) large numbers of skin tags; (ii) excessive sweating; (iii) presence of glycosuria; (iv) increasing visual field loss; (v) enlarging goitre; and (vi) hypertension. NB: headache also suggests disease activity.

The Adrenals

Cushing's Syndrome

This is due to a chronic excess of glucocorticoids. Steroids have multiple effects on the body due to stimulation of the DNA-dependent synthesis of select messenger RNAs. This leads to the formation of enzymes which alter cell function and result in increased protein catabolism and gluconeogenesis. Remember that Cushing's disease is specifically pituitary ACTH overproduction, while Cushing's syndrome is due to excessive steroid hormone production from any cause (Table 9.9).

Standing

Have the patient undress to the underpants, and if possible stand up (Figures 9.9 and 9.10). Look from the front, back and sides. Note *moon-like facies* and *central obesity*. The limbs appear thin despite sometimes very gross truncal obesity. This is the characteristic fat distribution that occurs with steroid excess. *Bruising* may be present (due to loss of perivascular supporting tissue–protein catabolism). Look for excessive *pigmentation* on the extensor surfaces (because of MSH-like activity in the ACTH molecule). Ask the patient to squat at this point to test for *proximal myopathy*, due to mobilisation of muscle tissue or excessive urinary potassium loss. Look at the back for the *'buffalo hump'* (Figure 9.11) which is due to fat deposition over the interscapular area. Palpate for bony *tenderness* of the vertebral bodies due to crush fractures from osteoporosis (a steroid anti-vitamin D effect and increased urinary calcium excretion may be responsible in part for disruption of the bone matrix).

Sitting

Ask the patient to sit on the side of the bed, but remember that he or she may be suffering from steroid psychosis and refuse to do anything you ask.

The Face and Neck

Look for plethora (this occurs in the absence of polycythaemia which, however, may also be present). The face may have a typical moon shape due to fat deposition in the upper part. Inspect for acne and hirsutism (if adrenal androgen secretion is also increased). Telangiectasia may also be present.

Examine the visual fields for signs of a pituitary tumour, and the fundi for visual field defects, optic atrophy, papilloedema and hypertensive or diabetic changes.

Look for supraclavicular fat pads.

Table 9.9 *Causes of Cushing's Syndrome*

Exogenous administration of excess steroids or ACTH (most common)
Adrenal hyperplasia
Secondary to pituitary ACTH production (Cushing's disease)
Microadenoma
Macroadenoma
Pituitary-hypothalamic dysfunction
Secondary to ACTH-producing tumours—e.g., small cell lung carcinoma
Adrenal neoplasia
Adenoma
Carcinoma (rare)

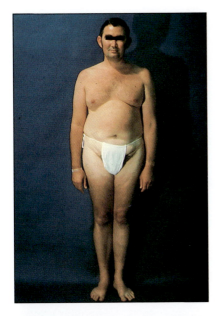

Figure 9.9
Cushing's syndrome.

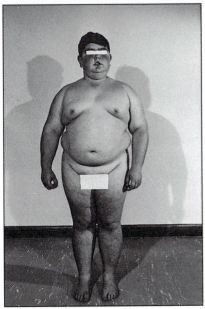

Figure 9.10   *Cushing's syndrome.*

The Abdomen

Lie the patient in bed on one pillow. Examine the abdomen for purple striae, which are due to weakening and disruption of collagen fibres in the dermis which leads to exposure of vascular subcutaneous tissues. They may also be present near

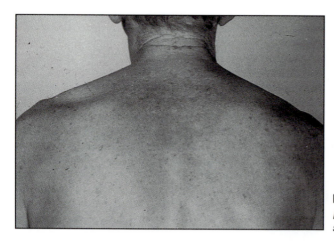

Figure 9.11
Buffalo hump in Cushing's syndrome.

the axillae on the upper arms or on the inside of the thighs. Palpate for adrenal masses (rarely a large adrenal carcinoma will be palpable over the renal area). Palpate for hepatomegaly due to fat deposition or rarely to adrenal carcinoma deposits.

The Legs

Palpate for oedema (due to salt and water retention). Look for bruising and poor wound healing.

The Urinalysis and Blood Pressure

Test the urine for sugar (as steroids are diabetogenic; this is due to an increase in hepatic gluconeogenesis and an anti-insulin effect on peripheral tissues). Hypertension is common due to salt and water retention (an aldosterone effect) and possibly to increased angiotensin secretion or a direct effect on blood vessels.

Certain signs are of particular diagnostic value in Cushing's syndrome.

Signs which suggest that adrenal carcinoma may be the underlying cause: (i) a palpable abdominal mass; (ii) signs of virilisation in the female; (iii) gynaecomastia in the male.

Signs which suggest that ectopic ACTH production may be the cause: (i) absence of the Cushingoid body habitus; (ii) more prominent oedema and hypertension; (iii) marked muscle weakness.

Significance of hyperpigmentation: this suggests an extra-adrenal tumour, or enlargement of an ACTH-secreting pituitary adenoma following adrenalectomy (Nelson's* syndrome).

Addison's[†] Disease

This is adrenocortical hypofunction with reduction in the secretion of glucocorticoids and mineralocorticoids. It is most often due to autoimmune disease of the adrenal glands. Other causes are listed in Table 9.10.

---

*   Warren Nelson (1906–1964), American endocrinologist.

[†]   Thomas Addison (1793–1860), described the disease in 1849. He, with Bright and Hodgkin, made up the famous trio of physicians at Guy's Hospital, London.

Table 9.10 *Causes of Addison's Disease*

Chronic

Primary

Autoimmune adrenal disease
Tuberculosis
Granuloma
Following heparin therapy
Malignant infiltration
HIV, AIDS and haemochromatosis and adrenoleucodystrophy

Secondary

Pituitary or hypothalamic disease

Acute

Septicaemia: meningococcal
Adrenalectomy
Any stress in a patient with chronic hypoadrenalism or abrupt cessation of prolonged
    high-dose steroid therapy

Table 9.11 *A Classification of Conditions Found in Various Combinations in Autoimmune Polyglandular Syndromes*

Type I	Type II
1. Chronic mucocutaneous candidiasis	1. Insulin-requiring diabetes (type 1)
2. Hypoparathyroidism	2. Autoimmune thyroid disease
3. Addison's disease	3. Addison's disease
	4. Myasthenia gravis

If this disease is suspected, look for cachexia. Then undress the patient and look for pigmentation in the palmar creases, elbows, gums and buccal mucosa, genital areas and in scars. This occurs because of compensatory ACTH hypersecretion in primary hypoadrenalism (when there is adrenal disease) as ACTH has melanocyte-stimulating activity. Also inspect for vitiligo (localised hypomelanosis), an autoimmune disease that is commonly associated with autoimmune adrenal failure.

Take the blood pressure and test for postural hypotension. Remember that the rest of the autoimmune disease cluster may be associated with autoimmune adrenal failure (Table 9.11).

Calcium Metabolism

Primary Hyperparathyroidism

This is due to excess parathyroid hormone (Table 9.12) which results in an increased serum calcium level, increased renal phosphate excretion and increased formation of 1,25-dihydroxycholecalciferol, by activation of adenyl cyclase in the bone and kidneys. Primary hyperparathyroidism causes problems with 'stones' (renal stones), 'bones' (osteopenia and pseudogout), 'abdominal groans' (constipation, peptic ulcer and pancreatitis) and 'psychological moans' (confusion).

Other causes of hypercalcaemia are listed in Table 9.13.

Table 9.12   *Types of Hyperparathyroidism*

Primary
Adenoma (80%)
Hyperplasia
Carcinoma (rare)

Secondary
Hyperplasia following chronic renal failure

Tertiary
The appearance of autonomous hyperparathyroidism is a complication of secondary hyperparathyroidism

Table 9.13   *Important Causes of Hypercalcaemia*

Primary hyperparathyroidism
Carcinoma (from bone metastases or humoral mediators)
Thiazide diuretics
Vitamin D excess
Excessive production of vitamin D metabolites: e.g., sarcoidosis, certain T cell lymphomas
Thyrotoxicosis
Associated with renal failure (e.g., severe secondary hyperparathyroidism)
Multiple myeloma
Prolonged immobilisation or space flight
Paget's disease and immobilisation

General Inspection

Note the mental state of the patient. Severe hypercalcaemia may cause coma or convulsions. Assess hydration (polyuria from hypercalcaemia may cause dehydration).

The Face

Look in the eyes for band keratopathy, which is rare (page 208).

The Body and Lower Limbs

Palpate the shoulders, sternum, ribs, spine and hips for bony tenderness, deformity or evidence of previous fractures. Test for proximal muscle weakness. Look for pseudogout. Take the blood pressure, as hypertension may occur.

Urinalysis

Test for blood in the urine (renal stones).

The MEN Syndromes

The multiple endocrine neoplasias (Types I and II) are autosomal dominant conditions. Hyperparathyroidism can be associated with both. MEN Type I is the association of tumours of the parathyroid, pituitary and pancreatic islet cells. MEN Type II is the association of medullary carcinoma of the thyroid, hyperparathyroidism and phaeochromocytoma.

Hypoparathyroidism

This results in hypocalcaemia with neuromuscular consequences (tetany). It is usually a postoperative complication of thyroidectomy, but can be idiopathic. Hypocalcaemia can also result from end-organ resistance to parathyroid hormone (pseudohypoparathyroidism) (Table 9.14).

Look first for Trousseau's and Chvostek's signs. *Trousseau's* sign is elicited with a blood pressure cuff placed on the arm with the pressure raised above the patient's systolic pressure. Typical contraction of the hand occurs within two minutes when hypocalcaemia has caused neuromuscular irritability. The thumb becomes strongly adducted, and the fingers are extended, except at the metacarpophalangeal joints. The appearance is that of an obstetrician about to remove the placenta manually and is called the *main d'accoucheur.*

Chvostek's sign is performed by tapping gently over the facial (seventh) cranial nerve under the ear. The nerve is hyperexcitable in hypocalcaemia and a brisk muscular twitch occurs on the same side of the face.

Next test for hyper-reflexia, again due to neuromuscular irritability.

Look at the nails for fragility and monilial infection. Note any dryness of the skin. Go to the face and look for deformity of the teeth. Examine the eyes for cataracts or papilloedema. These signs may all occur in idiopathic hypoparathyroidism, an autoimmune disease. Cataracts may also follow surgically induced hypoparathyroidism.

Pseudohypoparathyroidism

In this disease the patients have tetany (due to hypocalcaemia) as well as typical skeletal abnormalities. These include short stature, a round face, a short neck, thin stocky build and very characteristically short fourth or fifth fingers or toes (due to metacarpal or metatarsal shortening; this can be unilateral or bilateral) (Figure 9.12). Ask the patient to make a fist to demonstrate the characteristic clinical signs.

Pseudopseudohypoparathyroidism

This amusing name is given to a disease where there is no tetany (calcium concentration in the blood is normal), but the characteristic skeletal deformities are present.

Some Syndromes Associated with Short Stature

These conditions begin in childhood.

Table 9.14 *Causes of Hypocalcaemia*

Hypoparathyroidism: after thyroidectomy, idiopathic
Malabsorption
Deficiency of vitamin D
Chronic renal failure
Acute pancreatitis
Pseudohypoparathyroidism
Magnesium deficiency
Hypocalcaemia of malignant disease

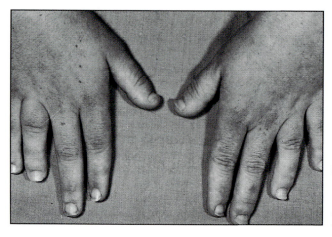

Figure 9.12

Pseudohypoparathyroidism with short fourth and fifth fingers due to metacarpal shortening.

General Inspection

First measure the height of the patient; in children this should be compared with percentile charts for age and sex. Look for the classical appearance of Turner's syndrome (Figure 9.13), Down's syndrome (Figure 9.14), achondroplasia or rickets (Figure 9.15) which may explain the short stature. One must check the height of parents and siblings as well.

Note any evidence of weight loss, including loose skin folds which may suggest a nutritional cause (starvation, malabsorption or protein loss). Look for signs of hypopituitarism or hypothyroidism, or steroid excess. Sexual precocity (early on-set of secondary sexual characteristics) causes relative tallness at first but short stature later.

The Chest

Examine for evidence of cyanotic congenital heart disease and pulmonary disease, e.g., cystic fibrosis.

The Abdomen

Look for evidence of hepatic failure or renal failure.

Turner's Syndrome (45XO) (Figure 9.13)

Sexual infantalism—female genitalia.

Upper Limbs

Lymphoedema of the hands; short fourth metacarpal bones; hyperplastic nails; increased carrying angle; hypertension.

Facies

Micrognathia (small chin); epicanthic folds, ptosis; fish-like mouth; deformed or low-set ears; hearing loss.

Neck

Webbing of the neck; low hairline; redundant skin folds on the back of the neck.

Chest

Widely spaced nipples (a shield-like chest); coarctation of the aorta.

Other

Pigmented naevi; keloid formation; lymphoedema of the legs.

Down's Syndrome (Trisomy 21) (Figure 9.14)

Facies

Oblique orbital fissures; conjunctivitis; Brushfield spots on the iris; small simple ears; flat nasal bridge; mouth hanging open; protruding tongue; narrow high arched palate.

Hands

Short broad hands; incurving fifth finger; single palmar crease; hyperflexible joints.

Chest

Congenital heart disease, especially endocardial cushion defects.

Other

Straight pubic hair; gaps between the first and second toes; mental deficiency is usually present.

Rickets (Figure 9.15)

Defective mineralisation of the *growing* skeleton, due to lack of vitamin D (e.g., nutritional or chronic renal failure), or hypophosphataemia (e.g., renal tubular disorders).

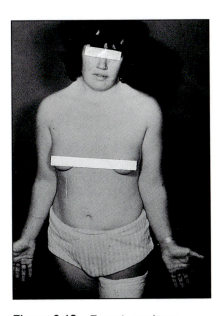

Figure 9.13   *Turner's syndrome.*

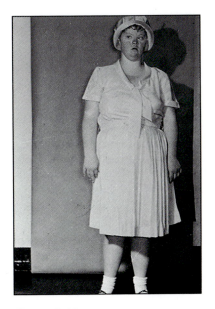

Figure 9.14   *Down's syndrome.*

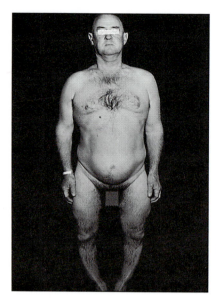

Figure 9.15

Rickets (post rachitic patient): look for frontal bossing, proximal myopathy of arms and thighs, and bowing of the ulna, femur and tibia.

Upper Limbs

Tetany; hypotonia, proximal myopathy; bowing of the radius and ulna.

Facies

Frontal bossing; parietal flattening.

Chest

'Rickety rosary'—thickening of costochondral junctions; Harrison's groove—indentation of lower ribs at the diaphragmatic attachment.

Lower Limbs

Bowing of femur and tibia; hypotonia; proximal myopathy; fractures.

Achondroplasia

This is an autosomal dominant disease of cartilage.

Short stature, short limbs, normal trunk, relatively large head, saddle-shaped nose, exaggerated lumbar lordosis, and occasionally spinal cord compression are features.

Hirsutism

This is excessive hairiness in a woman beyond what is considered normal for her race (Table 9.15). In the examination of such a patient, it is important to decide if virilisation is also present. Virilisation is the appearance of male secondary sexual characteristics (clitoromegaly, frontal hair recession, male body habitus and deepening of the voice) and indicates that excessive androgen is present.

Table 9.15 *Causes of Hirsutism*

Polycystic ovary syndrome (commonest cause)
Adrenal: Cushing's syndrome, congenital adrenal hyperplasia, virilising tumour
    (more often a carcinoma than an adenoma)
Ovarian: tumour
Drugs: phenytoin, diazoxide, streptomycin, minoxidil, anabolic steroids
Other: acromegaly, porphyria cutanea tarda

General Inspection

Ask the patient to undress to her underwear. Note the hair distribution over the face and in the midline, front and back. In general, an obvious male balding pattern (a receding hairline), hair over the beard area or on the back and chest, and hair in the escutcheon (umbilicus to groin in the middle line) is usually abnormal. Look for obvious acromegaly or Cushing's syndrome and for the skin changes of porphyria cutanea tarda (page 450).

Ask the patient to remove her underclothing and lie flat. Look for signs of virilism. These include breast atrophy and increased muscle bulk of the arms and legs, male pattern of pubic hair, and enlargement of the clitoris. Look in the axillae, the patient with polycystic ovarian syndrome may have acanthosis nigricans and associated insulin resistance.

The Abdomen

Palpate for adrenal masses, polycystic ovaries or an ovarian tumour (these are rarely palpable).

The Blood Pressure

Hypertension occurs in the rare C11-hydroxylase deficiency, which is a virilising condition.

Gynaecomastia

This is 'true' enlargement of the male breasts. Virtually no breast tissue is palpable in normal men. Remember that gynaecomastia occurs in up to 50% of adolescent boys, and also in elderly men in whom it is due to falling testosterone levels. Fat deposition ('false' enlargement) in obese men can be confused with gynaecomastia.

Examine the breasts (page 133) for evidence of localised disease (e.g., malignancy, which is rare), tenderness which indicates rapid growth, and any discharge from the nipple.

Note the general body habitus, looking especially for *Klinefelter's syndrome*. These patients are tall and thin with small, firm testes.

Look also for signs of panhypopituitarism or chronic liver disease (page 187). Thyrotoxicosis can occasionally be a cause.

Examine the genitalia now for sexual ambiguity and the testes for absence or a reduced size. Note any loss of secondary sexual characteristics.

Finally, examine the visual fields and fundi for evidence of a pituitary tumour. Causes of pathological gynaecomastia are shown in Table 9.16.

Table 9.16 *Causes of Pathological Gynaecomastia*

Increased Oestrogen Production
Leydig cell tumour (oestrogen)
Adrenal carcinoma (oestrogen)
Bronchial carcinoma (human chorionic gonadotrophin)
Liver disease (increased conversion of oestrogen from androgens)
Thyrotoxicosis (increased conversion of oestrogen from androgens)
Starvation

Decreased Androgen Production (Hypogonadal States)
Klinefelter's syndrome
Secondary testicular failure: orchitis, castration, trauma

Testicular Feminisation Syndrome

Drugs
Oestrogen receptor binders: oestrogen, digoxin, marijuana
Anti-androgens: spironolactone, cimetidine

Diabetes Mellitus*

Diabetes mellitus is characterised by hyperglycaemia due to an absolute or relative deficiency of insulin. The causes of diabetes are listed in Table 9.17. The disease can present with asymptomatic glycosuria detected on routine physical examination or with symptoms of diabetes (Table 9.1), ranging from polyuria to coma as a result of diabetic ketoacidosis.

General Inspection (Figure 9.16)

Assess for evidence of dehydration (page 20) because the osmotic diuresis caused by a glucose load in the urine can cause massive fluid loss. Note obesity (non-insulin-dependent diabetics are usually obese) or signs of recent weight loss (this can be evidence of uncontrolled glycosuria).

Look for one of the abnormal endocrine facies (e.g., Cushing's syndrome or acromegaly) and for pigmentation (e.g., haemochromatosis—bronze diabetes) as these may cause secondary diabetes.

The patient may be comatose due to dehydration, acidosis or plasma hyperosmolality. Kussmaul's breathing ('air hunger') (page 101) is present in diabetic ketoacidosis due to the acidosis (this occurs because fat metabolism is increased to compensate for the lack of availability of glucose; excess acetyl-CoA is produced which is converted in the liver to ketone bodies, and two of these are organic acids).

The Lower Limbs

Unlike most other systematic examinations, assessment of the diabetic can profitably begin with the legs as many of the major physical signs are found to be here.

---

* This disease was called diabetes by Greek and Roman physicians because the word diabetes means a siphon, referring to the large urine volume. Rather courageously, they distinguished diabetes mellitus from diabetes insipidus by the sweet taste of the urine: mellitus = sweet, insipidus = tasteless.

Table 9.17 *Causes of Diabetes Mellitus*

Criteria for diagnosis of diabetes mellitus: fasting blood sugar level of 7.8mmol/L or more, or a two-hour postprandial blood sugar level of 11.1mmol/L or more, on more than one occasion.

Primary

Type 1
Insulin-dependent diabetes mellitus (juvenile onset)

Type 2
Non-insulin-dependent diabetes mellitus:
  Non-obese
  Obese
  Maturity-onset diabetes of the young (MODY)

Secondary

Hormone-induced states (rare):
  Acromegaly
  Cushing's syndrome
  Phaeochromocytoma
  Glucagonoma

Drugs:
  Steroids
  The contraceptive pill
  Streptozotocin, diazoxide, phenytoin, thiazide diuretics

Pancreatic Disease:
  Chronic pancreatitis, carcinoma
  Haemochromatosis

Syndromes:
  Lipoatrophic diabetes (characterised by generalised lipoatrophy, hepatomegaly, hirsutism, acanthosis nigricans, hyperpigmentation and hyperlipidaemia)

Inspection

Look at the skin. The *skin* of the feet and lower legs may be hairless and atrophied due to small vessel vascular disease and resultant ischaemia (the mechanism is uncertain, but may be related to lipoprotein alterations in the vessel walls). Note any leg *ulcers*, particularly on the toes or any area of the feet exposed to pressure. These ulcers are due to a combination of ischaemia and peripheral neuropathy (the cause of the neuropathy is unknown, but may be related to small vessel ischaemia and glycosylation of neural proteins). Look for superficial skin *infection*, such as boils, cellulitis, and fungal infections. These are more common in diabetics because of a combination of high tissue glucose levels and ischaemia, which provides a favourable environment for the growth of organisms. Note any *pigmented scars* (late diabetic dermopathy). There may be small rounded plaques with raised borders lying in a linear fashion over the shins (diabetic dermopathy).

Necrobiosis lipoidica diabeticorum is a reasonably specific skin manifestation of diabetes mellitus, but is rare. It is found over the shins, where a central yellow scarred area is surrounded by a red margin when the condition is active.

Look now at the thighs for insulin injection sites. These may be associated with localised *fat atrophy* and *fat hypertrophy*, and may be related to impure insulin use

Figure 9.16 *Diabetes Mellitus*

Lying

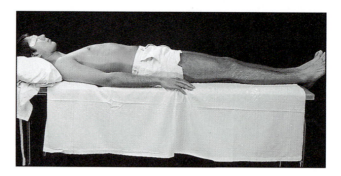

GENERAL INSPECTION
  Weight—obesity
  Hydration
  Endocrine facies
  Pigmentation—haemochromatosis, etc.

LEGS
  Inspect
    Skin—necrobiosis, hair loss, infection,
      pigmented scars, atrophy,
      ulceration, injection sites
  Muscle wasting
  Palpate
    Temperature of feet (cold, blue due to
      'small' or 'large' vessel disease)

ARMS
  Inspect
    Injection sites
    Skin lesions
  Pulse

EYES
  Fundi—cataracts, rubeosis, retinal disease
  III nerve palsy, etc.

MOUTH
  Monilia
  Infection

NECK
  Carotid arteries—palpate, auscultate

CHEST
  Signs of infection

ABDOMEN
  Liver—fat infiltration; rarely
    haemochromatosis

OTHER
  Urine analysis—glycosuria, ketones,
    proteinuria
  Blood pressure—lying and standing
  Peripheral pulses
  Femoral (auscultate)
  Popliteal
  Posterior tibial
  Dorsalis pedis
  Oedema
  Neurological assessment
    Femoral nerve mononeuritis
    Peripheral neuropathy

which causes a localised immune reaction. Note any *quadriceps muscle wasting* due to femoral nerve mononeuropathy, which is called (inaccurately) diabetic amyotrophy.

Inspect the knees for the very rare Charcot's joints (grossly deformed disorganised joints, due to loss of proprioception or pain, or both. This leads to recurrent and unnoticed injury to the joint) (Figure 9.17).

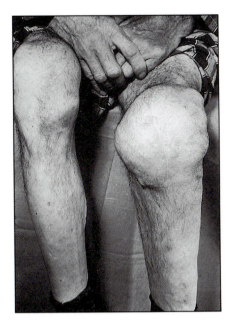

Figure 9.17
Charcot's joint of left knee. NB: This is very rare.

Palpation

Palpate any injection sites for fat atrophy or hypertrophy. Feel all the peripheral pulses and the temperature of the feet, and test the capillary return. Absent peripheral pulses, cold extremities and reduced capillary return are all evidence of peripheral vascular disease.

Neurological Examination

Assess formally for peripheral neuropathy, including dorsal column loss (diabetic pseudotabes) and tap the reflexes. Test proximal muscle power (diabetic amyotrophy) (page 420).

The Upper Limbs

Look at the nails for signs of *Candida* infection. Inspect and feel for injection sites over the upper arms. Take the blood pressure lying and standing, since diabetic autonomic neuropathy can cause postural hypotension.

The Face

The Eyes (page 366)

Test visual acuity. This may be permanently impaired because of retinal disease or temporarily disturbed because of changes in the shape of the lens associated with hyperglycaemia and water retention. Look for Argyll Robertson* pupils, which are rare in diabetes.

---

* Douglas Argyll Robertson (1837–1909), a Scottish ophthalmic surgeon and President of the Royal College of Surgeons, described these in 1869. The pupils are small, irregular and unequal, and react to accommodation but not to light. Syphilis is another cause (page 350).

Using the ophthalmoscope, begin by examining for rubeosis (new blood vessel formation over the iris which can cause glaucoma) (Figure 9.18). Then note any cataracts, which are related to sorbitol deposition in the lens (when glucose is present in high concentrations in the tissues it is converted to sorbitol by aldose reductase).

Now examine the retina where many exciting changes await the fundoscopist. There are two main types of retinal change in diabetes, non-proliferative and proliferative.

Non-proliferative changes (Figure 9.19) are directly related to ischaemia of blood vessels and include: (i) two types of haemorrhages—*dot haemorrhages* which occur in the inner retinal layers, and *blot haemorrhages* which are larger and which occur more superficially in the nerve fibre layer; (ii) *microaneurysms* which are due to vessel wall damage; and (iii) two types of exudates—*hard exudates*

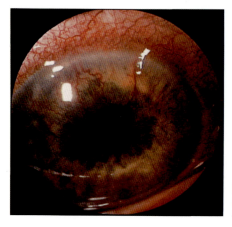

Figure 9.18 *Rubeosis iridis—new vessels on the anterior surface of the iris. These are secondary to ischaemia (often due to diabetes).*

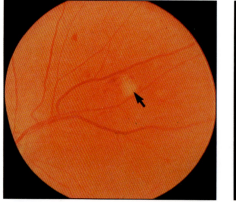

(a)

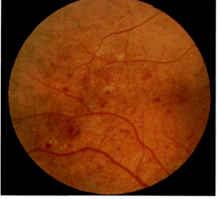

(b)

Figure 9.19 *Diabetic retinopathy: (a) soft exudate and small haemorrhages; (b) microaneurysms (dots), retinal haemorrhages (blots) and hard yellow exudates.*

which have straight edges and *soft exudates* (cotton wool spots) which have a fluffy appearance.

Proliferative changes (Figure 9.20) are changes in blood vessels in response to ischaemia of the retina. They are characterised by new vessel formation which can lead to vitreal haemorrhage, scar formation and eventually retinal detachment. The detached retina appears as an opalescent sheet which balloons forwards into the vitreous. The underlying choroid is visible through the detached retina as a bright red coloured sheet. Look also for laser scars (small brown or yellow spots) which are secondary to photocoagulation of new vessels by laser therapy.

Assess the third, fourth and sixth cranial nerves. In particular examine for a diabetic third nerve palsy from ischaemia, which usually spares the pupil (since infarction of the third nerve affects the inner pupillary fibres more than the outer fibres; in this way it differs from compressive lesions which have the opposite effect).

Other cranial nerves may be affected sometimes because of cerebrovascular accidents (large vessel atheroma). *Rhinocerebral mucormycosis* may rarely develop in very poorly controlled diabetic patients causing periorbital and perinasal swelling and cranial nerve palsies.

The Ears

Look in the ears for evidence of infection. The rare *malignant otitis externa,* usually due to *Pseudomonas aeruginosa,* causes a mound of granulation tissue in the external canal, and facial nerve palsy in 50%.

The Mouth

Look for evidence of *Candida* infection.

The Neck and Shoulders

Examine the carotid arteries for evidence of vascular disease.

There may rarely be thickening of the skin of the upper back and shoulders (scleroedema). Look for acanthosis nigricans—associated with insulin resistance.

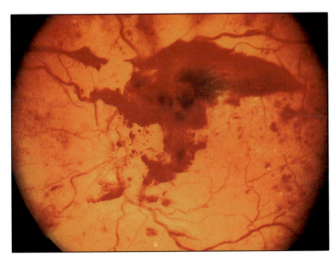

Figure 9.20
Proliferative diabetic retinopathy.

The Abdomen

Palpate for hepatomegaly (fatty infiltration, or due to haemochromatosis).

Urinalysis

Test for glucose and protein. Diabetic nephropathy (from glomerulonephritis, renal arterial disease or pyelonephritis) can cause proteinuria. The presence of nitrite and/or blood is of value as asymptomatic urinary tract infections can occur. In advanced disease there may be signs of renal failure (page 212).

Paget's* Disease (Osteitis Deformans)

This disease is characterised by excessive reabsorption of bone by osteoclasts and compensatory disorganised deposition of new bone. It may possibly be a disease of viral origin.

General Inspection

Note short stature (due to bending of the long bones of the limbs) and any obvious deformity of the head and lower limbs.

Head and Face

Inspect the scalp for enlargement in the frontal and parietal areas and measure the head circumference (greater than 55cm is usually abnormal). There may be prominent skull veins. Palpate for increased bony warmth and auscultate over the skull for systolic bruits. Both of these are due to increased vascularity of the skull vault. Oddly enough bronchial breath sounds may be audible over the Pagetic skull through the stethoscope. This is due to increased bone conduction of air. An area of very localised bony swelling and warmth may indicate development of a bony sarcoma (1% of cases of Paget's disease may develop this complication).

Examine the eyes. Assess visual acuity and visual fields, and look in the fundi for angioid streaks (page 309) and optic atrophy. Retinitis pigmentosa occurs rather more rarely (page 346). Test for hearing loss (due to bony ossicle involvement or eighth nerve compression by bony enlargement).

Examine the remaining cranial nerves (page 340); all may be involved because of bony overgrowth of the foramina or be caused by basilar invagination (platybasia) (where the posterior fossa becomes flat and the basal angle increased).

The Neck

Patients with basilar invagination have a short neck and low hairline. The head is held in extension and neck movements are decreased. Assess the jugular venous pulse, as a high output cardiac failure may be present, particularly if there is coexistent ischaemic heart disease.

The Heart

Examine for signs of cardiac failure.

---

* Sir James Paget (1814–1899), a surgeon at St Bartholomew's Hospital, was Queen Victoria's doctor.

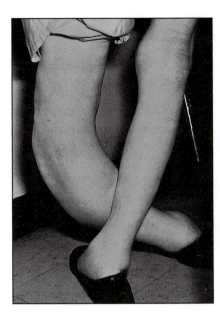

Figure 9.21
Paget's disease, showing bowing of the tibia.

The Back

Inspect for kyphosis (due to vertebral involvement causing collapse of the vertebral bodies). Tap for localised tenderness, feel for warmth and auscultate for systolic bruits over the vertebral bodies.

The Legs

Inspect for anterior bowing of the tibia and lateral bowing of the femur (Figure 9.21). Feel for bony warmth and tenderness. Note any changes of osteoarthritis in the hips and knees which often coexist with Paget's disease. Note any localised warm swelling which may indicate sarcoma.

Examine for evidence of paraplegia (page 397) which is uncommon, but can occur due to cord compression by bone or vascular shunting in the spinal cord. Cerebellar signs may rarely be present due to platybasia.

Urinalysis

Check for blood (there is an increased incidence of renal stones in Paget's disease).

Summary

The Endocrine System: A Suggested Method of Examination
(Figure 9.22)

Inspect the patient for one of the diagnostic facies or body habituses. If the diagnosis is obvious proceed with the specific examination outlined previously. If not, examine as follows.

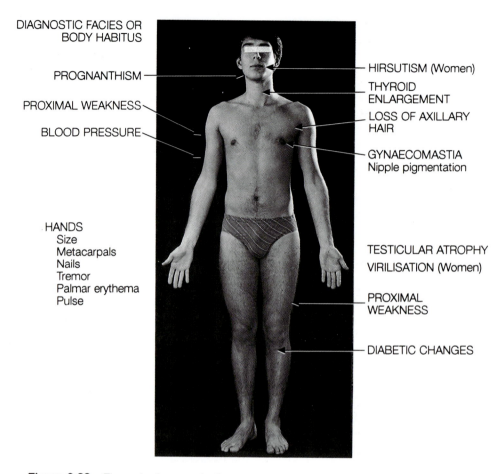

DIAGNOSTIC FACIES OR
BODY HABITUS

PROGNANTHISM

PROXIMAL WEAKNESS

BLOOD PRESSURE

HANDS
  Size
  Metacarpals
  Nails
  Tremor
  Palmar erythema
  Pulse

HIRSUTISM (Women)

THYROID
ENLARGEMENT

LOSS OF AXILLARY
HAIR

GYNAECOMASTIA
Nipple pigmentation

TESTICULAR ATROPHY
VIRILISATION (Women)

PROXIMAL
WEAKNESS

DIABETIC CHANGES

Figure 9.22   *The endocrine examination.*

Pick up the hands. Look at the overall size (acromegaly), length of the metacarpals (pseudohypoparathyroidism and pseudopseudohypoparathyroidism), for abnormalities of the nails (hyperthyroidism and hypothyroidism, and hypoparathyroidism), tremor, palmar erythema and sweating of the palms (hyperthyroidism).

Take the pulse (thyroid disease) and the blood pressure (hypertension in Cushing's syndrome, or postural hypotension in Addison's disease). Look for Trousseau's sign (tetany). Test for proximal muscle weakness (thyroid disease, Cushing's syndrome).

Go to the axillae. Look for loss of axillary hair (hypopituitarism), or acanthosis nigricans and skin tags (acromegaly).

Examine the eyes (hyperthyroidism) and the fundi (diabetes, acromegaly). Look at the face for hirsutism, or fine wrinkled hairless skin (panhypopituitarism). Note any skin greasiness, acne or plethora (Cushing's syndrome).

Look at the mouth for protrusion of the chin and enlargement of the tongue (acromegaly) or buccal pigmentation (Addison's disease).

Examine the neck for thyroid enlargement. Note any neck webbing (Turner's syndrome). Palpate for supraclavicular fat pads (Cushing's syndrome).

Inspect the chest wall for hirsutism or loss of body hair, reduction in breast size in women (panhypopituitarism) or gynaecomastia in men. Look for nipple pigmentation (Addison's disease).

Examine the abdomen for hirsutism, central fat deposition, purple striae (Cushing's syndrome) and the external genitalia for virilisation or atrophy. Look at the legs for diabetic changes.

Measure the body weight and height, and examine the urine.

Suggested Reading

Original and Review Articles

Alvi A, Johnson JT, The neck mass. A challenging differential diagnosis. *Postgrad Med* 1995; 97: 87–90, 93–94.

Bull RH, Coburn PR, Mortimer PS. Pretibial myxoedema: a manifestation of lymphoedema? *Lancet* 1993; 341: 403–404.

Braunstein GD. Gynecomastia. *N Engl J Med* 1993; 328: 490–945.

Mazzaferi EL. Management of a solitary thyroid nodule. *N Engl J Med* 1993; 328: 553–559.

Nathan DM. Long-term complications of diabetes mellitus. *N Engl J Med* 1993; 328:1676–1685.

Siminoski K, Does this patient have a goiter? *JAMA* 1995; 273: 813–17.

Utiger RD. Pathogenesis of Graves' ophthalmopathy *N Engl J Med* 1992; 326: 1772–1773.

Textbooks

Becker KL, editor. Principles and practice of endocrinology and metabolism. 2nd ed. Philadelphia: Lippincott, 1995.

Besser GM, Thorner MO. Clinical endocrinology. 2nd ed. London: Mosby-Wolfe, 1994.

Greenspan FS, Forsham PH, editors. Basic and clinical endocrinology. 3rd ed. Los Altos, California: Lange Medical; Sydney: Ramsay, 1991.

Hall R, Evered D, Greene R. A color atlas of endocrinology. 2nd ed. Chicago: Mosby-Year Book, 1990.

Chapter 10

THE NERVOUS SYSTEM

Who could have foretold, from the structure of the brain, that wine could derange its functions?

Hippocrates (460–375 BC)

The Neurological History

When obtaining the details of the neurological history (Table 10.1), it is particularly important to ascertain the *temporal course of the illness,* as this may give important information about the underlying aetiology. An acute onset of symptoms (within minutes to an hour) is suggestive of a vascular problem (e.g., the explosive severe headache of subarachnoid haemorrhage). A subacute onset (hours to days) occurs with inflammatory disorders (e.g., meningitis, cerebral abscess or the Guillain-Barré* syndrome (acute inflammatory polyradiculoneuropathy)). A more chronic symptom course suggests that the underlying disorder may be related to either a tumour (weeks to months) or a degenerative process (months to years). Metabolic or toxic disorders may present with any of these temporal profiles.

Based on the history (and physical examination), a judgement is made as to whether the disease process is *localised or diffuse,* and what *levels of the nervous system* are involved (the nervous system can be considered as having four different levels: the peripheral nervous system, the spinal cord, the posterior fossa, and the cerebral hemispheres). Consideration of the temporal course and the levels of involvement allows a logical differential diagnosis to be formulated.

Headache and Facial Pain

This is a very common symptom. It is important, as with any type of pain, to determine the character, severity, site, duration, frequency, radiation, aggravating and relieving factors and associated symptoms. For example, unilateral headache that is preceded by flashing lights and is associated with light hurting the eyes (photophobia) is likely to be a *migraine with an aura* ('classical migraine'). Pain

---

* Georges Guillain (1876–1951), Jean Alexandre Barré (1880–1967) and A Strohl described the syndrome in 1916; the last author's name was dropped because of anti-German feeling during World War I.

Table 10.1 *Neurological History*

Presenting Symptoms*

Headache, back or neck pain
Facial pain
Fits, faints or funny turns
Dizziness or vertigo
Disturbances of vision, hearing or smell
Disturbances of gait
Loss of or disturbed sensation, or weakness in a limb(s)
Disturbances of sphincter control (bladder, bowels)
Involuntary movements or tremor
Speech and swallowing disturbance
Altered cognition

Risk Factors for Cerebrovascular Disease

Hypertension
Smoking
Diabetes mellitus
Hyperlipidaemia
Atrial fibrillation, bacterial endocarditis, myocardial infarction (emboli)
Haematological disease
Family history of stroke

* Note particularly the temporal course of the illness, whether symptoms suggest focal or diffuse disease, and the likely level of involvement of the nervous system.

over one eye lasting for hours, associated with lacrimation, rhinorrhoea and flushing of the forehead, and occurring in bouts that last several weeks a few times a year is suggestive of *cluster headache*. This occurs predominantly in males. Headache over the occiput and associated with neck stiffness may be from *cervical spondylosis*. A generalised headache that is worse in the morning and is associated with drowsiness or vomiting may reflect *raised intracranial pressure*, while generalised headache associated with photophobia and fever as well as with a stiff neck of more gradual onset may be due to *meningitis*. A persistent unilateral headache over the temporal area associated with tenderness over the temporal artery and blurring of vision suggests *temporal arteritis*. Headache with pain or fullness behind the eyes or over the cheeks or forehead occurs in *acute sinusitis*. The dramatic and usually instantaneous onset of severe headache that is initially localised but becomes generalised and is associated with neck stiffness may be due to a *subarachnoid haemorrhage*. Finally, the most frequent type of headache is episodic or chronic *tension-type headache*; these are commonly bilateral, occur over the frontal, occipital or temporal areas, and may be described as a sensation of tightness that lasts for hours and recurs often. There are usually no associated symptoms such as nausea, vomiting, weakness or paraesthesiae (tingling in the limbs), and the headache does not wake the patient at night from sleep.

Pain in the face can result from trigeminal neuralgia, temporomandibular arthritis (page 263), glaucoma (page 343), cluster headache, temporal arteritis, psychiatric disease, aneurysm of the internal carotid or posterior communicating artery, or the superior orbital fissure syndrome (page 351).

Faints and Fits (see also page 29)

Transient ischaemic attacks affecting the brainstem can occasionally cause black-outs. With 'drop attacks' there is no loss of consciousness. In either case the patient falls to the ground without premonition and the attacks are of brief duration. *Hypoglycaemia* can also lead to episodes of loss of consciousness. Patients with hypoglycaemia may also report sweating, weakness and confusion before losing consciousness. Bizarre attacks of loss of consciousness occur with *hysteria*. In such attacks the patient may slump to the ground without sustaining any injury and there may be apparent fluctuations in the level of consciousness for a prolonged period.

It is important to try to differentiate syncope from *epilepsy*. However, primary syncopal events can cause a few clonic jerks in a significant number of cases. With generalised tonic-clonic seizures (grand mal epilepsy) there is abrupt loss of consciousness which may be preceded by an aura. Often the patient is incontinent of urine and faeces, and the tongue may be bitten. A witness may be able to describe the type of attack that occurred. It is important to try to determine whether any seizure is generalised or localised to one side of the body; a clonic seizure affecting part of the body may indicate a focal lesion in the central nervous system such as a tumour or abscess. If consciousness is impaired these partial seizures are de-scribed as 'complex'; if consciousness is unimpaired they are termed 'simple'. Idiopathic absence seizures ('petit mal') occur in children. These are frequent brief episodes of loss of awareness often associated with staring. Major motor move-ments are not associated with this type of epilepsy.

Dizziness

If a patient complains of dizziness, it is important to determine what is meant by this term. In true *vertigo*, there is actually a sense of motion, either of the patient or of the surroundings (page 29). When vertigo is severe it may not be possible for the patient to stand or walk, and associated symptoms of nausea, vomiting, pallor, sweating and headache may be present. 'Peripheral vestibular lesions' can cause vertigo including benign positional vertigo, vestibular neuronitis and acute labyrinthitis; there is usually no deafness or ringing in the ears (tinnitus) in such cases. Other causes include:

- those associated with deafness or tinnitus, such as ototoxic drugs (e.g., aminoglycosides);
- Ménière's* disease (which occurs in those over 50 years of age and presents with the triad of vertigo, tinnitus and deafness);
- acoustic neuroma (where patients may also have deafness and dizziness);
- central causes such as vertebrobasilar transient ischaemic attacks—these are associated with diplopia and ataxia; and
- rarely, internal auditory artery occlusion.

---

* Prosper Ménière (1799–1862), director of the Paris Institution for Deaf-Mutes, characterised this condition just before he died of post-influenzal pneumonia.

Visual Disturbances and Deafness

Problems with vision can include double vision (diplopia), blurred vision (amblyopia), light intolerance (photophobia) and visual loss (page 343). The causes of deafness are summarised on page 361.

Disturbances of Gait

Many neurological conditions can make walking difficult. These are presented on page 390. Walking may also be abnormal when orthopaedic disease affects the lower limbs or spine. Hysteria can also present with an abnormal gait.

Disturbed Sensation or Weakness in the Limbs

Pins and needles in the hands or feet may indicate nerve entrapment or a peripheral neuropathy (page 394) but can result from sensory pathway involvement at any level. The carpal tunnel syndrome is common; here there is median nerve entrapment, and patients experience pain and paraesthesiae in the hand and wrist. Sometimes pain may extend to the arm and even to the shoulder, but paraesthesiae are not felt above the wrist. These symptoms are usually worse at night and may be relieved by dangling the arm over the side of the bed or shaking the hand. Limb weakness can be caused by lesions at different levels in the motor system (page 391).

Tremor and Involuntary Movements

Action tremors are the most commonly seen. Causes include an enhanced physiological tremor, anxiety, thyrotoxicosis and benign essential tremor. Parkinson's* disease may present with a resting tremor (page 410), while in chorea there are involuntary jerky movements (page 412). Intention (or target seeking) tremor is due to cerebellar disease (page 407).

Speech and Mental Status

Speech may be disturbed by many different neurological diseases and is discussed on page 335. A number of different diseases can also result in delirium or dementia, as described on page 335.

Past Health

Inquire about a past history of meningitis or encephalitis, head or spinal injuries, a history of epilepsy or convulsions and any previous operations. Any past history of venereal disease (e.g., risk factors for AIDS or syphilis) should be obtained tactfully. Treatment with anticonvulsants, the contraceptive pill, antihypertensive agents, steroids, anticoagulants, antiplatelet agents or drugs for other disorders needs to be documented. Ask about risk factors that may predispose to the development of cerebrovascular disease (Table 10.1).

---

* James Parkinson (1755–1824), English general practitioner, published an essay on 'The Shaking Palsy' in 1817. He was nearly transported to Australia for reformist activities.

Social History

As smoking predisposes to cerebrovascular disease, the smoking history is relevant. It is useful to ask about occupation and exposure to toxins (e.g., heavy metals). Alcohol can also result in a number of neurological diseases (Table 1.3).

Family History

Any history of neurological or mental disease should be documented.

The Neurological Examination

The examination of the nervous system and the interpretation of one's findings require a lot of practice. In a viva-voce examination this more than any other system requires a polished technique. The signs need to be elicited carefully because the precise anatomical localisation of any lesions can often be determined this way. It is important, therefore, to remember some elementary neuroanatomy.

Examination can be long and difficult and it is said to take much of a day if absolutely everything which can be done (including psychometric assessment) is done. This is obviously impractical, but a screening examination that will uncover most signs takes only a relatively short time.

In brief, the following aspects of the examination must be attended to.

1. General, including examination for neck stiffness, assessment of the higher centres, speech, and abnormal movements.
2. The cranial nerves II to XII.
3. The upper limbs. Motor system: inspection, tone, power, reflexes, coordination. Sensory system: pinprick sensation, proprioception, vibration sense, light touch.
4. The lower limbs. As for the upper limbs, but including assessment of walking (gait).
5. The skull and spine for local disease.
6. The carotid arteries for bruits (page 209).

General Signs

Consciousness

Note the level of consciousness. If the patient is unconscious look for responses to various stimuli (page 414).

Neck Stiffness

Any patient with an acute neurological illness or who is febrile must be assessed for signs of meningism.

With the patient lying flat in bed the examiner slips a hand under the occiput and gently flexes the neck passively. The chin is brought up to approach the chest wall. Meningism may be caused by pyogenic or other infection of the meninges, or by blood in the subarachnoid space secondary to subarachnoid haemorrhage. There is resistance to neck flexion due to painful spasm of the extensor muscles of the neck. Painless resistance to neck flexion has a number of causes: (i) cervical spondylosis; (ii) after cervical fusion; (iii) Parkinson's disease; and (iv) raised intracranial pressure, especially if there is impending tonsillar herniation.

Kernig's* sign should also be elicited if meningitis is suspected. Flex each hip in turn, then attempt to straighten the knee while keeping the hip flexed. This is greatly limited by spasm of the hamstrings (which in turn causes pain) when there is meningism due to inflammatory exudates around the lumbar spinal roots.

Higher Centres and Speech

Handedness

Shake the patient's hand and ask if he or she is right or left handed. This is polite and allows the examiner to assess the likely dominant hemisphere. Ninety-four per cent of right-handed people and about 50% of left-handed people have a dominant left hemisphere. There is division of function between the two hemispheres, the most obvious distinction being that the dominant hemisphere controls language and mathematical functions.

Orientation

Test orientation in *person, place* and *time* by asking the patient his or her name, present location and the date (normal patients who have been in hospital for long periods often get the day wrong since one day seems very much like another in hospital). Disorientation is not a specific localising sign and may be acute and reversible (delirium) or chronic and irreversible (dementia). The mini-mental state examination (Table 11.5) is a useful way to document the progress of a confusional state or dementia over time.

Speech

At this stage dysarthria (difficulty with articulation) or dysphonia (altered quality of the voice from vocal cord disease) or dysphasia (dominant higher centre disorder in the use of symbols for communication) may be obvious. If not, before going on to compartmentalised tests one should get the patient to talk freely—propositional or free speech. In a normal clinical encounter this comes from history taking. In the viva-voce examination one should ask the patient to describe the room, his or her clothes, job or daily activities in order to get speech flowing.

For further screening, ask the patient to name two objects pointed at, and to say 'British Constitution'.

There is no need to examine further if no abnormality of speech is detected in this way.

If there is an abnormality, proceed as outlined in Table 10.2.

Dysphasia

There are four main types of dysphasia: receptive, expressive, nominal and conductive.

Receptive (posterior) dysphasia is where the patient cannot understand the spoken or written word. This condition is suggested when the patient is unable to understand any commands or questions. Speech is fluent but disorganised. It occurs with a lesion (infarction, haemorrhage or space-occupying tumour) in the

---

*   Vladimir Kernig (1840–1917), neurologist at St Petersburg, described this in 1882.

Table 10.2 *Examination of a Patient with Dysphasia*

Fluent Speech (Receptive, Conductive or Nominal Aphasia, Usually)
1. Name objects. Patients with nominal, conductive or receptive aphasia will name objects poorly.
2. Repetition. Conductive and receptive aphasic patients cannot repeat.
3. Comprehension. Only receptive aphasic patients cannot follow commands (verbal or written).
4. Reading. Conductive and receptive aphasic patients may have difficulty (dyslexia).
5. Writing. Conductive aphasic patients have impaired writing (dysgraphia) while receptive aphasic patients have abnormal content of writing. Patients with dominant frontal lobe lesions may also have dysgraphia.

Non-Fluent Speech (Expressive Aphasia, Usually)
1. Naming of objects. This is poor but may be better than spontaneous speech.
2. Repetition. May be possible with great effort. Phrase repetition (e.g., 'no ifs, ands or buts') is poor.
3. Comprehension often mildly impaired despite popular belief but written and verbal commands are followed.
4. Reading. Patients may have dyslexia.
5. Writing. Dysgraphia may be present.
6. Look for hemiparesis. The arm is more affected than the leg.
7. As patients are usually aware of their deficit they are often frustrated and depressed.

dominant hemisphere in the posterior part of the first temporal gyrus (Wernicke's* area).

Expressive (anterior) dysphasia is present when the patient understands, but cannot answer appropriately. Speech is non-fluent. This occurs with a lesion in the posterior part of the dominant third frontal gyrus (Broca's† area).

Nominal dysphasia. All types of dysphasia cause difficulty naming objects. There is also a specific type of nominal dysphasia. Here objects cannot be named (e.g., the nib of a pen) but other aspects of speech are normal. The patient may use long sentences to overcome failure to find the correct word (circumlocution). It occurs with a lesion of the dominant posterior temporoparietal area. Other causes include encephalopathy or the intracranial pressure effects of a distinct space-occupying lesion; it may also occur in the recovery phase from any dysphasia. Its localising value is therefore doubtful.

Conductive dysphasia: here patients repeat statements and name objects poorly, but can follow commands. This is thought to be caused by a lesion of the arcuate fasciculus and/or other fibres linking Wernicke's and Broca's areas.

To examine for dysphasia in more detail refer to Table 10.2. If the speech is fluent, but conveys information with paraphasic errors (e.g., 'treen' for 'train'), i.e. a word of similar sound or spelling to the one intended is used. Sometimes a word of similar meaning is used (e.g., 'go' for 'start'): this is called semantic paraphasia. The main possibilities are nominal, receptive and conductive dysphasia. Test for these by asking the patient to name an object, repeat a statement after you, and then follow commands. Then ask the patient to read and write if the above are abnormal, but remember the patient may be illiterate.

---

*   Karl Wernicke (1848–1905), Professor of Neurology at Breslau, described receptive aphasia in 1874.
†   Pierre Broca (1824–1880), Professor of Surgery at Paris, described this area in 1861.

If the speech is slow, hesitant and non-fluent, expressive dysphasia is more likely and exactly the same procedure is followed. It is important to note that many dysphasias will have mixed elements. Large lesions in the dominant hemisphere may cause global dysphasia.

Dysarthria

Here there is no disorder of the content of speech, but a difficulty with articulation. Ask the patient to say a phrase such as 'British Constitution' or 'Peter Piper picked a peck of pickled peppers.'

The commonest cause of dysarthria is alcohol intoxication. Dysarthria can also be caused by *cerebellar disease,* as there is loss of coordination which results in slow, slurred and often explosive speech, or speech broken up into syllables. This is called scanning speech (page 407). *Pseudobulbar palsy* causes a spastic dysarthria (which sounds as if the patient is trying to squeeze out words from tight lips) (page 366). *Bulbar palsies* (page 366) cause a nasal speech, while *facial muscle* weakness causes slurred speech. *Extrapyramidal disease* can be responsible for monotonous speech since it causes bradykinesia and muscular rigidity (page 410). *Mouth ulceration* or disease may occasionally mimic dysarthria. Each of these causes must be considered and examined for as appropriate.

Dysphonia

This is huskiness of the voice with decreased volume. It may be due to laryngeal disease (e.g., following a viral infection or a tumour of the vocal cord), or to recurrent laryngeal nerve palsy, but occasionally may be hysterical.

Parietal Lobe Function

Parietal, temporal and frontal lobe functions are tested if the patient is disoriented or has dysphasia, or if dementia is suspected. If the patient has a receptive aphasia, however, these tests cannot be performed. Their examination is otherwise not routine (Table 10.3). Students should now turn to page 340 and read how to examine the cranial nerves and limbs; return to this section once you have completed that task.

The parietal lobe is concerned with the reception and analysis of sensory information.

Dominant Lobe Signs

A lesion of the dominant parietal lobe in the angular gyrus causes a distinct clinical syndrome called Gerstmann's syndrome. Test for this in the following manner.

1. Ask the patient to perform simple calculations—e.g., take 7 from 100, then 7 from the answer and so forth ('serial 7s'). The inability to do this at least with partial accuracy, is called **a**calculia.
2. Ask the patient to write—inability is called **a**graphia.
3. Test for **l**eft-right disorientation by asking the patient to show you his or her right and then left hand. If this is correctly performed ask the patient to touch his or her left ear with the right hand and vice versa. Inability to do this is called left-right disorientation if the right hand is affected.
4. Ask the patient to name his or her fingers—inability to do this is called **f**inger agnosia. (The mnemonic for these four signs is **ALF.**)

Table 10.3 *Symptoms and Signs in Higher Centre Dysfunction*

Parietal Lobe

Dysphasia (dominant)

Acalculia,* agraphia,* left-right disorientation,* finger agnosia*

Sensory and visual inattention,† construction and dressing apraxia,† spatial neglect and
   inattention,† lower quadrantic hemianopia,‡ astereognosis‡

Seizures

Temporal Lobe

Memory loss

Upper quadrantic hemianopia

Dysphasia (receptive if dominant lobe)

Seizures

Frontal Lobe

Personality change

Primitive reflexes, e.g., grasp, pout

Anosmia

Optic nerve compression (optic atrophy)

Gait apraxia

Leg weakness (parasagittal)

Loss of micturition control

Dysphasia (expressive)

Seizures

Occipital Lobe

Homonymous hemianopia

Alexia

Seizures (flashing light aura)

* Gerstmann's syndrome: dominant hemisphere parietal lobe only
† Non-dominant parietal lobe
‡ Non-localising

Dominant and Non-dominant Lobe Signs

Now test for general signs of parietal lobe dysfunction which can occur with a
lesion on either side. Look for *sensory* and *visual inattention*. When one side is
tested at a time sensation is normal (page 376), but when both sides are tested
simultaneously the sensation is appreciated only on the normal side. A right-sided
parietal lesion will lead to inattention on the left side and vice versa. Formal *visual
field testing* is also important (page 343) as parietal, temporal and occipital lesions
can give distinctive defects. Examine now for *astereognosis*, which is the inability,
with eyes closed, to recognise an object placed in the hand when the ordinary
sensory modalities are intact. A parietal lobe lesion results in astereognosis on the
opposite side. *Graphaesthesia* may also be present, which is the inability to appreciate a number drawn on the hand on the opposite side to a parietal lesion.

Non-dominant Lobe Signs

Lesions here are characterised by *dressing* and *constructional apraxia.* Dressing
apraxia is tested by taking the patient's pyjama top or cardigan, turning it inside
out and asking him or her to put it back on. Patients with a non-dominant parietal
lobe lesion may find this impossible to do. Constructional apraxia is tested by

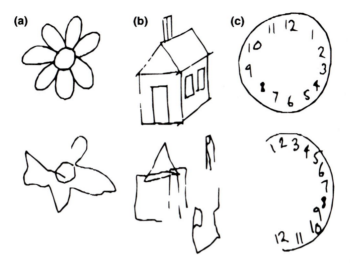

Figure 10.1 *Construction apraxia.*

asking the patient to copy an object that you have drawn (e.g., a flower or a house—Figure 10.1).

Next test *spatial neglect* by asking the patient to fill in the numbers on an empty clock face. Patients with a right parietal lesion may only fill in numbers on the left side (the other side of the clock face is ignored). Spatial neglect also occurs with dominant parietal lobe lesions but is less common.

Temporal Lobe Function

This lobe is concerned with short-term and long-term memory. Test short-term memory by the name, address, flower test—ask the patient to remember a name, address and the names of three flowers, and repeat them immediately. Then ask the patient five minutes later to repeat the names again. Test long-term memory by asking, for example, what year World War II ended. Memory may be impaired in dementia from any cause.

An alert patient with a severe memory disturbance may make up stories to fill any gaps in his or her memory. This is called confabulation, and is typical of the syndrome of Korsakoff's* psychosis (amnesic dementia).

Confabulation can be tested by asking the patient if he or she has met you before. However, be prepared for the very long, detailed and completely false story which may follow.

Korsakoff's psychosis occurs most commonly in alcoholics (where there is loss of nerve cells in the thalamic nuclei and mammillary bodies), and rarely with head injury, tumour or encephalitis. It is characterised by retrograde amnesia (memory loss for events before the onset of the illness) and an inability to memorise new information, in a patient who is alert, responsive and capable of problem-solving.

---

* Sergei Sergeyevich Korsakoff (1854–1900), Russian psychiatrist, described the syndrome in 1887.

Frontal Lobe Function

Assess first the *primitive reflexes* which are not normally present in adults but may reappear in normal old age.

1. Grasp reflex: the examiner runs his or her fingers across the palm of the patient's hand, which will grasp the examining fingers involuntarily on the side contralateral to the lesion.
2. Pout and snout reflexes: stroking or tapping with the tendon hammer over or above the upper lip induces pouting movements of the lips. This can occur with many intracranial lesions. It is not a localising sign.

Next ask the patient to *interpret a proverb*, such as 'a rolling stone gathers no moss'. Patients with frontal lobe disease give concrete explanations of proverbs. Test for loss of smell *(anosmia)* (page 341) and for *gait apraxia,* where there is marked unsteadiness in walking, which can be bizarre—the feet typically behave as if glued to the floor, causing a strange shuffling gait (page 390). Look in the *fundi;* you may rarely see optic atrophy on the side of a frontal lobe space-occupying lesion caused by compression of the optic nerve, and papilloedema on the opposite side due to secondarily raised intracranial pressure (Foster Kennedy* syndrome).

The Cranial Nerves

If possible, position the patient so that he or she is sitting over the edge of the bed. Look at the head, face and neck. If hydrocephalus has occurred in infancy—before closure of the cranial sutures—the head and face may resemble an inverted triangle. Acromegaly (page 308), Paget's disease (page 326) or basilar invagination (page 371) may be obvious. A careful *general inspection* may reveal signs easily missed when each cranial nerve is examined separately. This is particularly true of ptosis (page 368), proptosis (page 300), pupillary inequality (page 370), skew deviation of the eyes (page 352) and facial asymmetry (page 359). Inspect the whole scalp for craniotomy scars and the skin for neurofibromas (Figure 10.2). Look for any rashes, e.g., a capillary or cavernous haemangioma is seen on the face in the distribution of the trigeminal (V) nerve in the Sturge-Weber[†] syndrome. It is associated with an intracranial venous haemangioma of the leptomeninges and with seizures.

The cranial nerves are usually tested in approximately the order of their number.

The First (Olfactory) Nerve

Anatomy

This is a purely sensory nerve whose fibres arise in the mucous membrane of the nose, and pass through the cribriform plate of the ethmoid bone to synapse in the olfactory bulb. From here the olfactory tract runs under the frontal lobe and terminates in the medial temporal lobe on the same side.

---

*   Robert Foster Kennedy (1884–1952), a New York neurologist.

[†]   William Allen Sturge (b. 1850), British physician, and Frederick Parkes Weber (b. 1865), London physician.

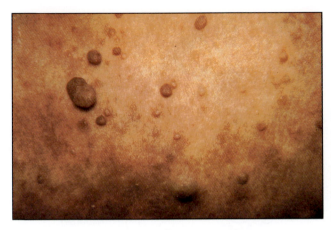

Figure 10.2

Subcutaneous neurofibromas in neurofibromatosis type I (associated with optic nerve and pontine gliomas; acoustic neuromas occur in type II).

Examination of the Nose and Sense of Smell

Note the external appearance of the nose. Look for rash or deformity. Then examine the nasal vestibule by elevating the tip of the nose (in adults a speculum is usually needed to give an adequate view).

The first nerve is not tested routinely. If the patient complains of loss of smell (anosmia) or there are other signs suggesting a frontal or temporal lobe lesion then it should be examined. Test each nostril separately with a series of bottles containing essences of familiar smells, such as coffee, vanilla and peppermint (this is traditional but not very reliable). Pungent substances such as ammonia should not be used, first because they upset the patient and second because noxious stimuli of this sort are detected by sensory fibres of the fifth (trigeminal) nerve.

Causes of Anosmia

Most cases of anosmia are bilateral. Causes include: (i) upper respiratory tract infection (commonest); (ii) meningioma of the olfactory groove; (iii) ethmoid tumours; (iv) basal skull fracture or frontal fracture, or after pituitary surgery; (v) congenital—e.g., Kallmann's syndrome (hypogonadotrophic hypogonadism); and (vi) smoking and increasing age. The main unilateral causes are head trauma without a fracture, or an early meningioma of the olfactory groove.

The Second (Optic) Nerve

Anatomy

The optic nerve is a purely sensory nerve which begins in the retina (Figure 10.3). These fibres pass through the optic foramen close to the ophthalmic artery and join the nerve from the other side at the base of the brain to form the optic chiasm. The spatial orientation of fibres from different parts of the fundus is preserved so that fibres from the lower part of the retina are found in the inferior part of the chiasm and vice versa. Fibres from the temporal visual fields (the nasal halves of the retinas) cross in the chiasm, whereas those from the nasal visual fields do not. Fibres for the light reflex from the optic chiasm finish in the superior colliculus, whence connections occur with both third nerve nuclei. The remainder of the fibres leaving the chiasm are concerned with vision and travel in the optic tract to

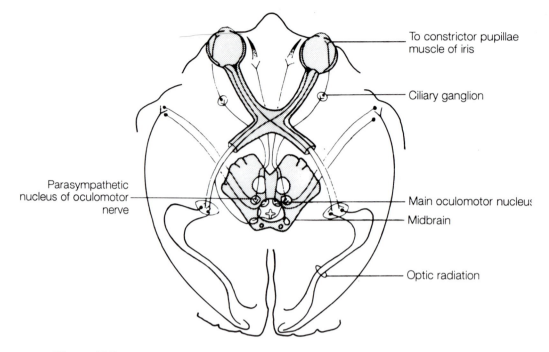

To constrictor pupillae
muscle of iris

Ciliary ganglion

Parasympathetic
nucleus of oculomotor
nerve

Main oculomotor nucleus

Midbrain

Optic radiation

Figure 10.3   *The optic pathways and visual reflexes.*

Adapted from and used with permission of Snell RS. Clinical neuroanatomy for medical students. 2nd ed.
Boston: Little Brown, 1987.

the lateral geniculate body. From here the fibres form the optic radiation and pass
through the posterior part of the internal capsule and finish in the visual cortex of
the occipital lobe. In their course they splay out so that fibres serving the lower
quadrants course through the parietal lobe while those for the upper quadrants
traverse the temporal lobe.

The result of the decussation of fibres in the optic chiasm is that fibres from the
left visual field terminate in the right occipital lobe and vice versa.

Examination

Assess visual acuity, visual fields and the fundi.

Visual acuity is tested with the patient wearing his or her spectacles, if used for
reading or driving, as refractive errors are *not* considered to be cranial nerve
abnormalities. Use a hand-held eye chart or a Snellen's* chart on the wall. Each
eye is tested separately, while the other is covered by a small card.

Formal testing with a standard Snellen's chart requires the patient to be six
metres from the chart. Unless a very large room is available, this is done using a
mirror. Normal visual acuity is present when the line marked 6 can be read
correctly with each eye (6/6 acuity). A patient who is unable to read even the
largest letter of the chart should be asked to count fingers held up in front of each

---

*   Hermann Snellen (1834–1908), Dutch ophthalmologist, invented this chart in 1862.

eye in turn, and if this is not possible then perception of hand movement is tested. Failing this, light perception only may be present.

Any abnormality of the lens, cornea, fundus or optic nerve pathway can cause reduction in visual acuity.

Causes of bilateral blindness of rapid onset include bilateral occipital lobe infarction; bilateral occipital lobe trauma; bilateral optic nerve damage, as with methyl alcohol poisoning; and hysteria.

Sudden blindness in one eye can be due to retinal artery or vein occlusion, temporal arteritis, non-arteritic ischaemic optic neuropathy and occasionally optic neuritis or migraine.

Bilateral blindness of gradual onset may be caused by cataracts; acute glaucoma; macular degeneration; diabetic retinopathy (vitreous haemorrhages); bilateral optic nerve or chiasmal compression; and bilateral optic nerve damage, for example, tobacco amblyopia.

Visual fields are examined by confrontation using a white-tipped hat pin. Always remove a patient's spectacles first. The examiner's head should be level with the patient's head. Then change to a red pin which enables detection of less obvious peripheral and central scotomata. Test each eye separately. If a patient has such poor acuity that a pin is difficult to see, the fields should be mapped with the fingers. When the right eye is being tested the patient should look straight into the examiner's left eye. The patient's head should be at arm's length and the eye not being tested should be covered. The pin should be brought into the visual field from the four main directions, diagonally towards the centre of the field of vision. Next the blind spot can be mapped out by asking about disappearance of the pin around the centre of the field of vision of each eye. Only a gross enlargement may be detectable. The following patterns of visual field loss may be detected (Figures 10.4 and 10.5).

Concentric diminution of the field (tunnel vision) may be caused by glaucoma; retinal abnormalities such as chorioretinitis or retinitis pigmentosa; papilloedema; acute ischaemia, as with migraine; and hysteria.

There is always a small area close to the centre of the visual fields where there is no vision (the *blind spot*). This is the area where the optic disc is seen on fundoscopy and is the point where the optic nerve joins the retina. The blind spot enlarges with papilloedema.

Central scotomata, or loss of central (macular) vision, may be due to demyelination of the optic nerve (multiple sclerosis causes unilateral or asymmetrical bilateral scotomata); toxic causes, such as methyl alcohol (symmetrical bilateral scotomata); nutritional causes—e.g., tobacco or alcohol amblyopia (symmetrical central or centrocecal scotomata); vascular lesions (unilateral); and gliomas of the optic nerve (unilateral).

Total unilateral visual loss is due to a lesion of the optic nerve or to unilateral eye disease.

Bitemporal hemianopia: a lesion which affects the centre of the optic chiasm will damage fibres from the nasal halves of the retinas as they decussate. This will result in loss of both temporal halves of the visual fields. Causes include a pituitary tumour, a craniopharyngioma, and a suprasellar meningioma.

Binasal hemianopia is very rare and is due to bilateral lesions affecting the uncrossed optic fibres, such as atheroma of the internal carotid siphon.

Homonymous hemianopia: a lesion which affects the optic tract or radiation damages the visual field on the right or left side. For example, left temporal and

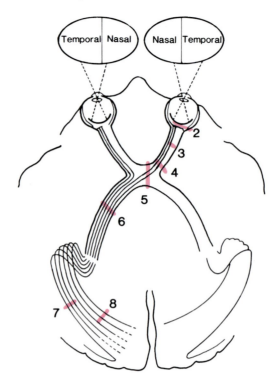

Figure 10.4 *The visual fields and optic pathways. Numbers indicate sites of lesions producing field defects shown in Figure 10.5.*

Adapted from and used with permission of Snell RS. Clinical neuroanatomy for medical students. 2nd ed. Boston: Little Brown, 1987.

right nasal field loss will occur with a right-sided lesion. The exact nature of the defect depends on the site of interruption of the fibres. In the optic tract the defect is usually complete—there is no macular sparing. In the more posterior optic radiation the macular vision is usually spared if the cause is ischaemia, but not if a destructive process such as tumour or haemorrhage is responsible. The macular cortical area is thought to have some additional blood supply from the anterior and middle cerebral arteries.

Homonymous quadrantanopia is loss of the upper or lower homonymous quadrants of the visual fields. This may be due to temporal lobe lesions (e.g., vascular lesions or tumours) which cause upper quadrantanopia, or parietal lobe lesions (e.g., vascular lesions or tumours) which cause lower quadrantanopia.

Fundoscopy does not begin with the examination of the fundus, but rather with visualisation of the cornea with the ophthalmoscope. Use the right eye to look in the patient's right eye and vice versa. This prevents contact between the noses of the patient and the examiner in the midline. Maintain your head vertical so that the patient can fix with the other eye.

Begin with the ophthalmoscope on the +20 lens setting with the patient gazing into the distance. This prevents reflex pupil contraction which occurs if the patient attempts to accommodate. Look first at the cornea and iris and then at the lens.

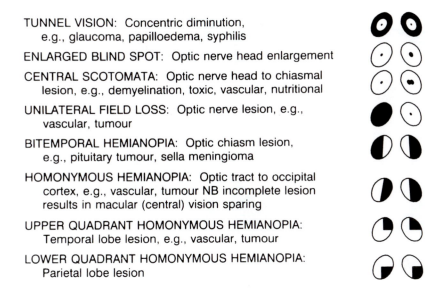

TUNNEL VISION: Concentric diminution,
e.g., glaucoma, papilloedema, syphilis

ENLARGED BLIND SPOT: Optic nerve head enlargement

CENTRAL SCOTOMATA: Optic nerve head to chiasmal
lesion, e.g., demyelination, toxic, vascular, nutritional

UNILATERAL FIELD LOSS: Optic nerve lesion, e.g.,
vascular, tumour

BITEMPORAL HEMIANOPIA: Optic chiasm lesion,
e.g., pituitary tumour, sella meningioma

HOMONYMOUS HEMIANOPIA: Optic tract to occipital
cortex, e.g., vascular, tumour NB incomplete lesion
results in macular (central) vision sparing

UPPER QUADRANT HOMONYMOUS HEMIANOPIA:
Temporal lobe lesion, e.g., vascular, tumour

LOWER QUADRANT HOMONYMOUS HEMIANOPIA:
Parietal lobe lesion

Figure 10.5   *Visual field defects with lesions at various levels along the optic pathway, at sites indicated in Figure 10.4.*

Adapted from and used with permission of Bickerstaff ER, Spillane JA. Neurological examination in clinical practice. 5th ed. Oxford: Blackwell, 1989.

Large corneal ulcers may be visible, as may undulation of the rim of the iris which is due to previous lens extraction and is called iridodonesis.

By racking the ophthalmoscope down towards O the focus can be shifted towards the fundus. Opacities in the lens (cataracts) may prevent inspection of the fundus. When the retina is in focus search first for the optic disc. This is done by following a large retinal vein back towards the disc. All these veins radiate from the optic disc.

The margins of the disc must be examined with care. The disc itself is usually a shallow cup with a clearly outlined rim. Loss of the normal depression of the optic disc will cause blurring at the margins and is called papilloedema (Figure 10.6a). If the appearance is associated with demyelination in the anterior part of the optic nerve it is called papillitis (Table 10.4). These two can be distinguished because papillitis causes visual loss but papilloedema does not.

Next note the colour of the optic disc. Normally it is a rich yellow colour in contrast to the rest of the fundus which is a rich red colour. The fundus may be pigmented in some diseases and in patients with pigmented skin. When the optic disc has a pale insipid white colour, optic atrophy is usually present (Figure 10.6b).

Each of the four quadrants of the retina should be examined systematically for abnormalities. Look especially for diabetic (page 324) and hypertensive changes (Figure 10.6c; *see also* page 69). Note haemorrhages or exudates.

There are four types of *haemorrhages*: streaky haemorrhages near the vessels (linear or flame-shaped), large ecchymoses that obliterate the vessels, petechiae which may be confused with microaneurysms, and subhyaloid haemorrhages (large effusions of blood which have a crescentic shape and well-marked borders and a fluid level may be seen). The first two types of haemorrhage occur in

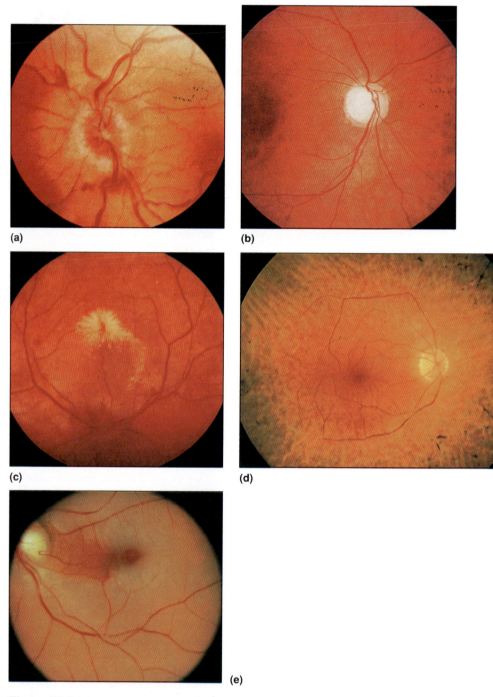

Figure 10.6   *Fundoscopy in the neurological patient: (a) papilloedema; (b) optic atrophy; (c) grade 4 hypertensive retinopathy, with papilloedema, a 'macular star' of hard exudates collecting around the fovea, and retinal oedema; (d) retinitis pigmentosa; (e) central retinal artery occlusion.*

hypertensive and diabetic retinopathy. They may also result from any cause of raised intracranial pressure or venous engorgement, or a bleeding disorder. The third type occurs in diabetes mellitus, and the fourth is characteristic of subarachnoid haemorrhage.

Look for signs of *retinal detachment*. Note the presence of *retinitis pigmentosa* where there is a scattering of black pigment in a criss-cross pattern. This will be missed if the periphery of the retina is not examined (Figure 10.6d). Retinitis pigmentosa is the most common form of retinal dystrophy; it causes loss of peripheral vision and therefore night blindness, because the periphery of the retina is concerned with night vision. In *choroidal inflammation* (page 368) there are white patches behind the retinal vessels which may be associated with discrete areas of black pigmentation.

When there is a *central retinal artery occlusion* the whole fundus appears milky-white because of retinal oedema, and the arteries become greatly reduced in diameter (Figure 10.6e).

Central retinal vein thrombosis causes tortuous retinal veins, and haemorrhages scattered over the whole retina, particularly occurring alongside the veins. The differential diagnosis is retinal vasculitis, where there is haemorrhage, new vessel formation, oedema and the presence of retinal vessels of irregular calibre.

Causes of abnormalities seen on ophthalmoscopy are summarised in Table 10.4.

Table 10.4 *Causes of Eye Abnormalities*

Cataracts
1. Old age (senile cataract)
2. Endocrine—e.g., diabetes mellitus, steroids
3. Hereditary or congenital—e.g., dystrophia myotonica, Refsum's* disease
4. Ocular disease—e.g., glaucoma
5. Radiation
6. Trauma

Papilloedema vs Papillitis

Papilloedema	Papillitis
Optic disc swollen without venous pulsation	Optic disc swollen
Acuity normal (early)	Acuity poor
Large blind spot	Large central scotoma
Peripheral constriction of visual fields	Pain on eye movement
Colour vision normal	Onset usually sudden and unilateral
Usually bilateral	Colour vision affected (particularly red desaturation)

Causes of Papilloedema
1. Space-occupying lesion (causing raised intracranial pressure) or a retro-orbital mass
2. Hydrocephalus (large cerebral ventricles)
   a) Obstructive (a block in the ventricle, aqueduct or outlet to the fourth ventricle)—e.g., tumour
   b) Communicating
      Increased formation of CSF—e.g., choroid plexus papilloma (rare)
      Decreased absorption of CSF—e.g., tumour causing venous compression, subarachnoid space obstruction from meningitis

—continued

Table 10.4 *Causes of Eye Abnormalities (continued)*

3. Benign intracranial hypertension (pseudotumour cerebri) (small or normal-sized ventricles)
   a) Idiopathic
   b) The contraceptive pill
   c) Addison's disease
   d) Drugs—e.g., nitrofurantoin, tetracycline, vitamin A, steroids
   e) Head trauma
4. Hypertension (grade 4)
5. Central retinal vein thrombosis

Causes of Optic Atrophy

1. Chronic papilloedema or optic neuritis
2. Optic nerve pressure or division
3. Glaucoma
4. Ischaemia
5. Familial—e.g., retinitis pigmentosa, Leber's[†] disease, Friedreich's ataxia

Causes of Optic Neuritis

1. Multiple sclerosis
2. Toxic—e.g., ethambutol, chloroquine, nicotine, alcohol
3. Metabolic—e.g., vitamin B_{12} deficiency
4. Ischaemia—e.g., diabetes mellitus, temporal arteritis, atheroma
5. Familial—e.g., Leber's disease
6. Infective—e.g., infectious mononucleosis

Causes of Retinitis Pigmentosa

1. Congenital (associated with cataract and deaf mutism)
2. Laurence-Moon-Biedl[‡] syndrome
3. Hereditary ataxia
4. Familial neuropathy—Refsum's disease

CSF = cerebrospinal fluid.
* Sigvald Refsum, 20th Century Norwegian physician.
† Theodor von Leber (b. 1840), Gottingen and Heidelberg ophthalmologist.
‡ John Laurence (1830–1874), London ophthalmologist, Robert Charles Moon (1844–1914), American ophthalmologist, and Arthur Biedl (1869–1933), Professor of Physiology, Prague.

The Third (Oculomotor), Fourth (Trochlear) and Sixth (Abducens) Nerves

Anatomy

The size of the pupils depends on a balance of parasympathetic and sympathetic innervation. The parasympathetic innervation to the eyes is supplied by the Edinger-Westphal* nucleus of the third nerve (stimulation of these fibres causes pupillary constriction). The sympathetic innervation to the eye is as follows: fibres from the hypothalamus go to the ciliospinal centre in the spinal cord at C8, T1 and T2, synapse, and second-order neurones exit via the anterior ramus in the thoracic trunk and synapse in the superior cervical ganglion in the neck (stimulation causes pupillary dilatation) (see page 369). Third-order neurones travel from here with the internal carotid artery to the eye. In addition, the pupillary reflexes depend for

* Ludwig Edinger (b. 1855), Frankfurt neurologist and Carl Friedrich Otto Westphal, Berlin neurologist.

their afferent limb on the optic nerve (Figure 10.3). Constriction of the pupil in response to light is relayed by the optic nerve and tract to the superior colliculus and then to the Edinger-Westphal nucleus of the third nerve in the midbrain. Efferent motor fibres from the oculomotor nucleus (Figure 10.7) travel in the wall of the cavernous sinus where they are in association with the fourth, ophthalmic division of the fifth, and the sixth cranial nerves (Figure 9.8) (page 307). These nerves leave the skull together through the superior orbital fissure. The iridoconstrictor fibres terminate in the ciliary ganglion, whence postganglionic fibres arise to innervate the iris. The rest of the third nerve supplies all the ocular muscles except the superior oblique (fourth nerve) and the lateral rectus (sixth nerve) muscles. The third nerve also supplies the levator palpebrae superioris, which elevates the eyelid (Figure 10.8).

Examination

The pupils: with the patient looking at an object at an intermediate distance, examine the pupils for size, shape, equality and regularity. Look for ptosis of the eyelids.

Test the *light reflex*. Using a pocket torch, shine the light from the side (so the patient does not focus on the light and accommodate) into one of the pupils to

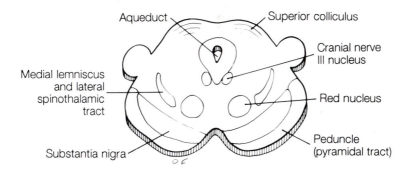

Figure 10.7   *Anatomy of the midbrain.*

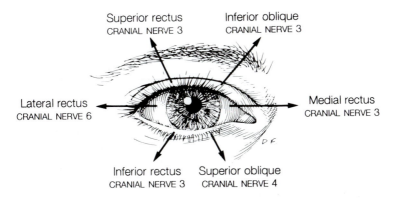

Figure 10.8   *The eye muscles and nerve innervation.*

assess its reaction to light. Inspect both pupils and repeat this procedure on the other side. Normally the pupil into which the light is shone constricts briskly—this is the *direct* response to light. Simultaneously the other pupil constricts in the same way. This is called the *consensual* response to light.

Move the torch in an arc from pupil to pupil. If an eye has optic atrophy or severely reduced visual acuity from another cause, the affected pupil will dilate paradoxically after a short time when the torch is moved from the normal eye to the abnormal eye. This is called an *afferent pupillary defect* (or the Marcus Gunn* pupillary sign).

It occurs because an eye with severely reduced acuity has reduced afferent impulses so that the light reflex is markedly decreased. When the light is shone from the normal eye to the abnormal one, the pupil dilates as reflex pupillary constriction in the abnormal eye is so reduced that relaxation after the consensual response dominates.

Now test *accommodation*. Ask the patient to look into the distance and then to focus his or her eyes on a object such as a finger or a white-topped hat pin brought to a point about 30cm in front of the nose.

There is normally constriction of both pupils—the accommodation response. It depends on a pathway from the visual association cortex descending to the third nerve nucleus. Causes of an absent light reflex with an intact accommodation reflex include a midbrain lesion (e.g., the Argyll Robertson pupil of syphilis) (page 323), a ciliary ganglion lesion (e.g., Adie's† pupil) or Parinaud's‡ syndrome. Failure of accommodation alone may occur occasionally with a midbrain lesion or with cortical blindness.

Eye movements: here failure of eye movement, double vision (diplopia) and nystagmus are assessed.

Ask the patient to look at the invaluable hat pin. The presence of these pins in the lapel of a well-cut white coat often indicates that the wearer is a neurologist. Assess voluntary eye movements in both eyes first. Ask the patient to look laterally right and left, then up and down. Remember the lateral rectus (sixth nerve) only moves the eyes horizontally outwards, while the medial rectus (third nerve) only moves the eyes horizontally inwards. The remainder of the muscle movements are a little more complicated. When the eye is abducted, the elevator is the superior rectus (third nerve) while the depressor is the inferior rectus (third nerve). When the eye is adducted, the elevator is the inferior oblique (third nerve) while the depressor is the superior oblique (fourth nerve) (Figure 10.8). The practical upshot of all this is that the testing of pure movement (that is, one muscle only) for elevation and depression is performed first with the eye adducted and then with it abducted.

Therefore, ask the patient to follow the moving hat pin in an H pattern with both eyes and tell you if double images are seen. Note failure of movement of either eye in any direction, and ask about diplopia. This indicates ocular muscle involvement. If any abnormality is detected on eye movement, then each eye must be tested separately. The other eye is covered with a card or with the examiner's hand.

Diplopia is an early sign of ocular muscle weakness because the light falls on different parts of the corresponding retinas due to slight movement differences. If

---

*   Robert Marcus Gunn (1850–1909), London ophthalmologist, described the defect in 1883.

†   William Adie (1886–1935), Australian neurologist working in Britain, described this in 1931.

‡   Henri Parinaud (1844–1905), French ophthalmologist, described this in 1889.

diplopia is present, further testing is necessary. The false image is usually paler, less distinct and more peripheral than the real one. Ask the patient whether the two images lie side by side or one above the other. If they are side by side only the lateral or medial recti can be responsible. If they lie one above the other then either of the obliques or the superior or inferior recti may be involved. To decide which pair of muscles is responsible, ask in which direction there is maximum image separation. Separation is greatest in the direction in which the weak muscle has its purest action. At the point of maximum separation cover one eye and find out which image disappears. Loss of the lateral image indicates that the covered eye is responsible. Diplopia that persists when one eye is covered can be due to astigmatism, a dislocated lens or hysteria.

Abnormal eye movement may be due to III, IV or VI nerve palsy, or to an abnormality of conjugate gaze.

Features of a Third Nerve Lesion

1. Complete ptosis (partial ptosis may occur with an incomplete lesion).
2. Divergent strabismus (eye 'down and out').
3. Dilated pupil which is unreactive to direct light (the consensual reaction in the opposite normal eye is intact) and unreactive to accommodation.

Note: always exclude a fourth (trochlear) nerve lesion when a third nerve lesion is present. Do this by tilting the head to the same side as the lesion. The affected eye will intort if the fourth nerve is intact. Alternatively ask the patient to look down and across to the opposite side from the lesion and look for intortion (remember 'SIN'— the superior oblique **in**torts the eye).

Aetiology of a Third Nerve Lesion

Third nerve lesions are most commonly related to trauma or are idiopathic. Central causes include vascular lesions in the brainstem, tumours and rarely demyelination.

Peripheral causes include: (i) compressive lesions, such as an aneurysm (usually on the posterior communicating artery), tumour, basal meningitis, nasopharyngeal carcinoma or orbital lesions—e.g., Tolosa-Hunt syndrome (superior orbital fissure syndrome—painful lesions of III, IV, VI and the first division of V); and (ii) ischaemia or infarction, as in arteritis, diabetes mellitus and migraine.

Features of a Fourth Nerve Lesion

An isolated fourth nerve palsy is rare and is usually idiopathic or related to trauma. It may occasionally occur with lesions of the cerebral peduncle. Usually it is associated with a third nerve palsy. Test this nerve by asking the patient to turn the eye in and then to try to look down: a lesion results in paralysis of the superior oblique with weakness of downwards (and outward) movement. The patient may walk around with his or her head tilted away from the lesion—that is, to the opposite shoulder (this allows the patient to maintain binocular vision).

Features of a Sixth Nerve Lesion

These are failure of lateral movement, convergent strabismus, and diplopia. These signs are maximal on looking to the affected side, and the images are horizontal and parallel to each other. The outermost image from the affected eye disappears on covering this eye (this image is usually also more blurred).

Aetiology of Sixth Nerve Lesions

Bilateral lesions may be due to trauma or Wernicke's encephalopathy (a syndrome of ophthalmoplegia, confusion and ataxia which is often associated with Korsakoff's psychosis (page 339)). Korsakoff's psychosis is due to thiamine deficiency. Mononeuritis multiplex and raised intracranial pressure are also causes of sixth nerve palsy.

Unilateral sixth nerve lesions are most commonly idiopathic or related to trauma. They may have a central (e.g., vascular lesion or tumour) or peripheral (e.g., raised intracranial pressure or diabetes mellitus) origin.

Abnormalities of Conjugate Gaze

Normal eye movements occur in an organised fashion so that the visual axes remain in the same plane throughout eye movements. There are centres for conjugate gaze in the frontal lobe for saccadic movements and in the occipital lobe for pursuit movements. Conjugate movement to the right is controlled from the left side of the brain. From these centres fibres travel to the region of the sixth nerve nucleus, from which area the medial longitudinal fasciculus coordinates movement with the contralateral third nerve (medial rectus) nucleus (Figure 10.9). A brainstem lesion causes ipsilateral paralysis of horizontal conjugate gaze and a frontal lobe lesion causes contralateral paralysis of horizontal conjugate gaze.

There are a number of possible causes for deviation of the eyes to one side. For example, *deviation of the eyes to the left* can result from: (i) a destructive lesion (usually vascular or neoplastic) which involves the pathways between the *left* frontal lobes and the oculomotor nuclei; (ii) a destructive lesion of the *right* side of the brainstem; or (iii) an irritative lesion, such as an epileptic focus, of the *right* frontal lobe which stimulates deviation of the eyes to the left.

Supranuclear palsy is loss of vertical or horizontal gaze or both (Figure 10.9). The clinical features that distinguish this from third, fourth and sixth nerve palsies include: (i) both eyes are affected; (ii) pupils may be fixed and are often unequal; (iii) there is usually no diplopia; and (iv) the reflex eye movements—e.g., on flexing and extending the neck—are usually intact.

Progressive supranuclear palsy (or Steele Richardson Olszewski* syndrome): here there is loss of vertical and later of horizontal gaze, which is associated with extrapyramidal signs (page 410), neck rigidity and dementia. Reflex eye movements on neck flexion and extension are preserved until late in the course of the disease.

Parinaud's syndrome: this is loss of vertical gaze often associated with nystagmus on attempted convergence (see below). There are pseudo-Argyll Robertson pupils. The causes of Parinaud's syndrome include a pinealoma, multiple sclerosis and vascular lesions.

Involuntary upward deviation of the eyes (*oculogyric crises*) occurs with post-encephalitic Parkinson's disease and may be seen in patients sensitive to phenothiazine derivatives or in patients on levodopa therapy.

Nystagmus

The eyes are normally maintained at rest in the middle line by the balance of tone between opposing ocular muscles. Disturbance of this tone, which depends on

---

* J Steele and J Richardson, Canadian neurologists, described this in 1964.

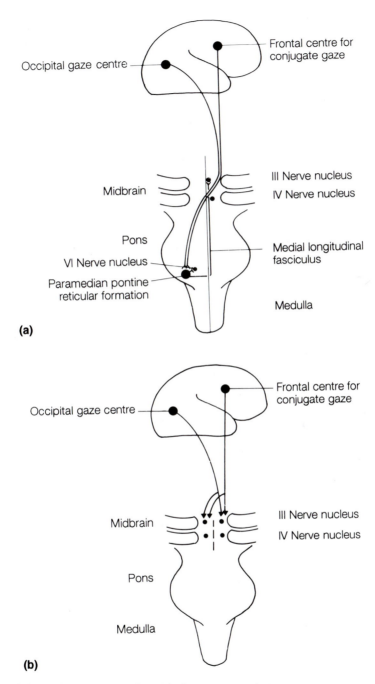

Occipital gaze centre

Frontal centre for
conjugate gaze

Midbrain

III Nerve nucleus
IV Nerve nucleus

Pons

VI Nerve nucleus

Paramedian pontine
reticular formation

Medial longitudinal
fasciculus

Medulla

(a)

Occipital gaze centre

Frontal centre for
conjugate gaze

Midbrain

III Nerve nucleus
IV Nerve nucleus

Pons

Medulla

(b)

Figure 10.9   *(a) Horizontal and (b) vertical eye movements.*

Adapted from and used with permission of Lance JW, McLeod JG. A physiological approach to clinical
neurology. 3rd ed. London: Butterworths, 1981.

impulses from the retina, the muscles of the eyes themselves and various vestibular and central connections, allows the eyes to drift in one or other direction. This drift is corrected by a quick movement (saccadic) back to the original position. When these movements occur repeatedly nystagmus is said to be present. The direction of the nystagmus is defined as that of the fast (correcting) movement, although it is the slow drift that is abnormal. Nystagmus from any cause tends to be accentuated by gaze in a direction away from the middle line. In many instances nystagmus is not present when the eyes are at rest and is only detected when the eyes are deviated (gaze-evoked nystagmus). At the extremes of gaze, fine nystagmus is normal (physiological). Therefore test for nystagmus by asking the patient to follow your pin out to 30° from the central gaze position.

Nystagmus may be jerky or pendular.

Jerky horizontal nystagmus may be due to (i) a vestibular lesion (NB: acute lesions cause nystagmus away from the side of the lesion while chronic lesions cause nystagmus to the side of the lesion); (ii) a cerebellar lesion (NB: unilateral diseases cause nystagmus to the side of the lesion); (iii) toxic causes, such as phenytoin and alcohol (may also cause vertical nystagmus but less often); and (iv) **internuclear ophthalmoplegia**. Internuclear ophthalmoplegia is present when there is nystagmus in the abducting eye and failure of adduction of the other (affected) side. This is due to a lesion of the medial longitudinal fasciculus. The most common cause in young adults with bilateral involvement is multiple sclerosis, while in the elderly, vascular disease is an important cause.

Jerky vertical nystagmus may be due to a brainstem lesion. Up-gaze nystagmus suggests a lesion in the floor of the IVth ventricle, while down-gaze nystagmus suggests a foramen magnum lesion. Phenytoin or alcohol can also cause this abnormality.

With **pendular nystagmus** the nystagmus phases are equal in duration. Its cause may be retinal (decreased macular vision—e.g., albinism) or congenital.

Note: vertical nystagmus means nystagmus where the oscillations are in a vertical direction.

A summary of how to approach the medical eye examination is given on page 366.

The Fifth (Trigeminal) Nerve

Anatomy

This nerve contains both sensory and motor fibres. Its motor nucleus and its sensory nucleus for touch lie in the pons (Figure 10.10), its proprioceptive nucleus lies in the midbrain, while its nucleus serving pain and temperature sensation descends through the medulla to reach the upper cervical cord.

The nerve itself leaves the pons from the cerebellopontine angle and runs over the temporal lobe in the middle cranial fossa. At the petrous temporal bone the nerve forms the trigeminal (Gasserian*) ganglion and from here the three sensory divisions arise. The first (ophthalmic) division runs in the cavernous sinus with the third nerve and emerges from the superior orbital fissure to supply the skin of the forehead, the cornea and conjunctiva. The second (maxillary) division emerges from the infraorbital foramen and supplies skin in the middle of the face and the mucous membranes of the upper part of the mouth, palate and nasopharynx. The

---

* Johann Laurenz Gasser (b. 1723), Viennese anatomist.

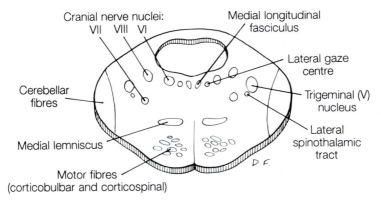

Cranial nerve nuclei:
VII   VIII   VI

Medial longitudinal
fasciculus

Lateral gaze
centre

Cerebellar
fibres

Trigeminal (V)
nucleus

Medial lemniscus

Lateral
spinothalamic
tract

Motor fibres
(corticobulbar and corticospinal)

Figure 10.10   *Anatomy of the pons.*

third (mandibular) division runs with the motor part of the nerve leaving the skull through the foramen ovale to supply the skin of the lower jaw and mucous membranes of the lower part of the mouth (Figures 10.11 and 10.12).

Pain and temperature fibres from the face run from the pons through the medulla as low as the upper cervical cord, terminating in the spinal tract nucleus as they descend. The second order neurones arise in this nucleus and ascend again as the ventral trigeminothalamic tract. Touch and proprioceptive fibres terminate in the pontine or main sensory and mesencephalic nuclei respectively to form the dorsal and ventral mesencephalic tracts. Because of this segregation in the brainstem, lesions of the medulla or upper spinal cord can cause a dissociated sensory loss of the face—loss of pain and temperature sensation, but retention of touch and proprioception.

The motor part of the nerve supplies the muscles of mastication.

Examination

Test the *corneal reflex*. Lightly touch the cornea (*not* the conjunctiva) with a wisp of cotton wool brought to the eye from the side. Reflex blinking of *both* eyes is a normal response. Ask the patient if he of she feels the touch of the cotton wool. The sensory component of the reflex is mediated by the ophthalmic division of the fifth nerve, while the reflex blink (motor) results from facial nerve innervation of the orbicularis oculi muscles.

NB: If blinking occurs only with the contralateral eye this indicates an ipsilateral seventh nerve palsy. The patient will still feel the touch of the cotton wool on the cornea.

Test *facial sensation* in the three divisions of the nerve comparing each side with the other. Test first with the sharp end of a new pin for pain sensation (never use an old pin in these days of hepatitis B, AIDS, etc.). The patient shuts his or her eyes and the pin is applied lightly to the skin. The patient is asked whether it feels sharp or dull. Loss of pain sensation will result in the pin prick feeling dull. An area of dull sensation should be mapped: testing should go *from the dull to the sharp area*. Test also above the forehead progressively back over the top of the head. If the ophthalmic division is affected sensation will return when the C2 dermatome is reached (Figure 10.12). It is important to exercise caution: too sharp a pin will

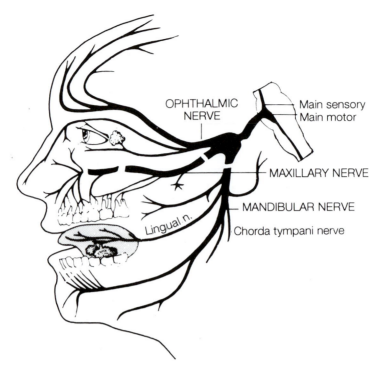

Figure 10.11   *The trigeminal nerve (cranial nerve V).*

From Chusid JG. Correlative neuroanatomy and functional neurology. 19th ed. Los Altos: Lange Medical, 1985. Published with permission.

leave a little trail of bloody spots, which is embarrassing. Temperature is not tested routinely unless syringobulbia is suspected, as temperature loss usually accompanies loss of pain sensation.

The patient keeps the eyes closed and a new piece of cotton wool is used to test light touch in the same way. The patient should be instructed to say 'yes' each time the touch of the cotton wool is felt (do *not* stroke the skin). Proprioceptive loss is not routinely tested on the face (and indeed it would be rather a difficult thing to do!).

Now examine the *motor division* of the nerve. Begin by inspecting for wasting of the temporal and masseter muscles. Ask the patient then to clench the teeth and palpate for contraction of the masseter above the mandible. Then get the patient to open the mouth (pterygoid muscles) and hold it open while the examiner attempts to force it shut. Breaking the jaw does not contribute to the urbane image of the neurologist so too much force must not be applied to the mouth. A unilateral lesion of the motor division causes the jaw to deviate towards the weak (affected) side.

Finally, test the *jaw jerk*. The patient lets the mouth fall open slightly and the examiner's finger is placed on the tip of the jaw and tapped lightly with a tendon hammer. Normally there is a slight closure of the mouth or no reaction at all. In an upper motor neurone lesion (page 391) above the pons the jaw jerk is greatly exaggerated. This is commonly seen in pseudobulbar palsy (page 366).

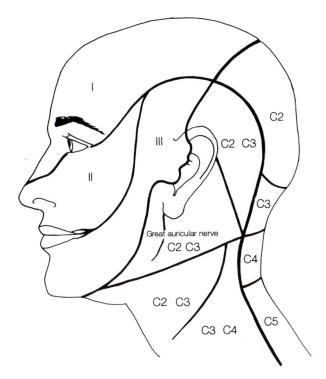

Figure 10.12   *Dermatomes of the head and neck.*

Causes of a Fifth Nerve Lesion

Central (pons, medulla and upper cervical cord) causes include a vascular lesion, tumour or syringobulbia.

Peripheral (middle fossa) causes include an aneurysm, tumour (secondary or primary) or chronic meningitis.

Trigeminal ganglion (petrous temporal bone) causes include an acoustic neuroma, a meningioma, or a fracture of the middle fossa.

Cavernous sinus causes involve the ophthalmic division only and are usually associated with third, fourth and sixth nerve palsies. They include aneurysm, tumour or thrombosis.

Remember, if there is total loss of sensation in all three divisions of the nerve, this suggests that the level of the lesion is at the ganglion or the sensory root—e.g., an acoustic neuroma (Figure 10.13). If there is total sensory loss in one division only, this suggests a postganglionic lesion. The ophthalmic division is most commonly affected because it runs in the cavernous sinus and through the orbital fissure where it is vulnerable to a number of different insults.

If there is dissociated sensory loss (loss of pain, but preservation of touch sensation) this suggests a brainstem or upper cord lesion, such as syringobulbia, foramen magnum tumour, or infarction in the territory of the posterior inferior cerebellar artery. If touch sensation is lost, but pain sensation is preserved, this is usually due to an abnormality of the pontine nuclei, such as a vascular lesion or tumour. Motor loss can also be central or peripheral.

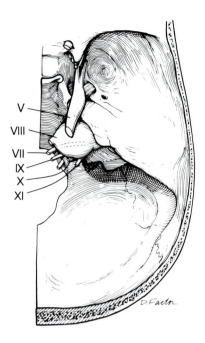

Figure 10.13   *Cerebellopontine angle tumour. A neuroma arising from the acoustic (VIII) nerve compresses adjacent structures, including the trigeminal (V) and facial (VII) nerves and the brainstem and cerebellum (removed to permit the cranial nerves to be seen).*

Adapted from Simon RP, Aminoff MJ, Greenberg DA. Clinical neurology 1989. Appleton and Lange, 1989, with permission.

The Seventh (Facial) Nerve

Anatomy

The seventh nerve nucleus lies in the pons next to the sixth cranial nerve nucleus (Figure 10.10). The nerve leaves the pons with the eighth nerve through the cerebellopontine angle (Figure 10.14). After entering the facial canal it enlarges to become the geniculate ganglion. The branch which supplies the stapedius muscle is given off from within the facial canal. The chorda tympani (containing taste fibres from the anterior two-thirds of the tongue) joins the nerve in the facial canal. The seventh nerve leaves the skull via the stylomastoid foramen. It then passes through the middle of the parotid gland and supplies the muscles of facial expression.

Examination

Inspect for *facial asymmetry*, as a seventh nerve palsy can cause unilateral drooping of the corner of the mouth, and smoothing of the wrinkled forehead and the nasolabial fold (Figure 10.15). However, with bilateral facial nerve palsies symmetry can be maintained.

Test the *muscle power*. Ask the patient to look up and wrinkle his or her forehead. Look for loss of wrinkling and feel the muscle strength by pushing down against the corrugation on each side. This movement is preserved on the side of an

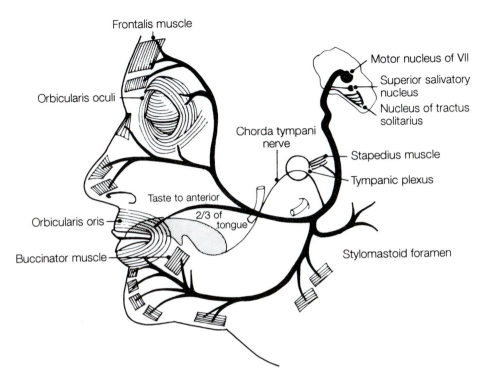

Frontalis muscle

Orbicularis oculi

Chorda tympani nerve

Motor nucleus of VII

Superior salivatory nucleus

Nucleus of tractus solitarius

Stapedius muscle

Tympanic plexus

Taste to anterior 2/3 of tongue

Orbicularis oris

Buccinator muscle

Stylomastoid foramen

Figure 10.14 *The facial nerve (cranial nerve VII). Note: The branches of the facial nerve "Two Zebras Bit My Car"—Temporal, Zygotic, Buccal, Mandibular, Cervical.*

Adapted from Chusid JG. Correlative neuroanatomy and functional neurology. 19th ed. Los Altos: Lange Medical, 1985. Published with permission.

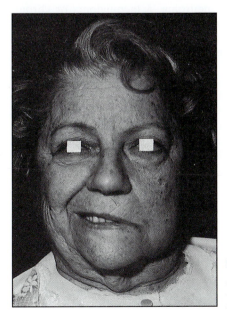

Figure 10.15

Left upper motor neurone facial weakness showing drooping of the corner of the mouth, flattened nasolabial fold, and sparing of the forehead.

upper motor neurone lesion (a lesion which occurs above the level of the brainstem nucleus) because of bilateral cortical representation of these muscles. The remaining muscles of facial expression are usually affected on the side of an upper motor neurone lesion, although occasionally the orbicularis oculi are preserved. In a lower motor neurone lesion (at the level of the nucleus or nerve root), all muscles of facial expression are affected on the side of the lesion.

Next ask the patient to shut the eyes tightly. Compare how deeply the eyelashes are buried on the two sides and then try to force open each eye. Note whether Bell's* phenomenon is evident. Note: Bell's phenomenon is just that. It is present in everyone (although not always visible unless one has a VII nerve palsy). In this case, when the patient attempts to shut the eye on the side of a lower motor neurone VII nerve palsy, there is upward movement of the eyeball and incomplete closure of the eyelid. Next ask the patient to grin and compare the nasolabial grooves, which are smooth on the weak side.

If a lower motor neurone lesion is detected, check quickly for the ear and palatal vesicles of herpes zoster of the geniculate ganglion—the Ramsay Hunt† syndrome.

Examining for taste on the anterior two-thirds of the tongue is not usually required. If necessary it can be tested by asking the patient to protrude the tongue to one side: sugar, vinegar, salt and quinine (sweet, sour, saline and bitter) are placed one at a time on each side of the tongue. The patient indicates the taste by pointing to a card with the various tastes listed on it. The mouth is rinsed with water between each sample.

Causes of a Seventh (Facial) Nerve Palsy

Upper motor neurone lesion (supranuclear): vascular lesions or tumours are the common causes. Note that lesions of the frontal lobes may cause weakness of the emotional movements of the face alone; voluntary movements are preserved.

Lower motor neurone lesion: *pontine* causes (often associated with V and VI lesions) include vascular lesions, tumours, syringobulbia or multiple sclerosis. *Posterior fossa* lesions include an acoustic neuroma, a meningioma or chronic meningitis. At the level of the *petrous temporal bone*, Bell's palsy (an idiopathic acute paralysis of the nerve), a fracture, the Ramsay Hunt syndrome or otitis media may occur, while the parotid gland may be affected by a tumour or sarcoidosis. Remember, Bell's palsy is the most common cause of a facial nerve palsy.

Causes of bilateral facial weakness: this may be due to the Guillain-Barré syndrome, sarcoid, bilateral parotid disease, Lyme disease or rarely mononeuritis multiplex. NB: myopathy and myasthenia gravis can also cause bilateral facial weakness which, however, is not due to facial nerve involvement.

Causes of loss of taste alone: unilateral loss of taste, without other abnormalities, can occur with middle ear lesions involving the chorda tympani or lingual nerve, but these are very rare.

The Eighth (Acoustic) Nerve

Anatomy

There are two components: the cochlear, with afferent fibres subserving hearing, and the vestibular containing afferent fibres subserving balance. Fibres for hearing

---

* Sir Charles Bell (1774–1842), Professor of Anatomy at the Royal College of Surgeons, later Professor of Surgery at Edinburgh, described facial nerve palsy in 1821.

† James Ramsay Hunt (1874–1937), American neurologist.

originate in the organ of Corti* and run to the cochlear nuclei in the pons. From here there is bilateral transmission to the medial geniculate bodies and thence to the superior gyrus of the temporal lobes. Fibres for balance begin in the utricle and semicircular canals, and join auditory fibres in the facial canal. They then enter the brainstem at the cerebellopontine angle. After entering the pons, vestibular fibres run widely throughout the brainstem and cerebellum.

Examination of the Ear and Hearing

Look to see if the patient is wearing a hearing aid; remove it. Examine the pinna and look for scars behind the ears. Pull on the pinna gently (it is tender if the patient has external ear disease or temporomandibular joint disease). Feel for nodes (pre- and post-auricular) that may indicate disease of the external auditory meatus.

Inspect the patient's external auditory meatus. The adult canal angulates, so in order to see the eardrum it is necessary to pull up and backwards on the auricle before inserting the otoscope. The normal eardrum (tympanic membrane) is pearly grey and concave. Look for wax or other obstructions, and inspect the eardrum for inflammation or perforation.

Next test hearing. A simple test involves covering the opposite auditory meatus with a finger, moving this about as a distraction while whispering a number in the other ear. This should be standardised by the use of set numbers for different tones. For example, the number 68 is used to test high tone and 100 to test low tone. Whispering should be performed towards the end of expiration in an attempt to standardise the volume and at about 60cm from the ear. If partial deafness is suspected perform Rinné's and Weber's tests.

Rinné's† test: a 256 Hertz vibrating tuning fork is placed on the mastoid process, behind the ear, and when the sound is no longer heard it is placed in line with the external meatus. Normally the note is audible at the external meatus. If a patient has nerve deafness the note is audible at the external meatus, as air and bone conduction are reduced equally, so that air conduction is better (as is normal). This is termed Rinné-positive. If there is a conduction (middle ear) deafness no note is audible at the external meatus. This is termed Rinné-negative.

Weber's‡ test: a vibrating 256 Hertz tuning fork is placed on the centre of the forehead. Normally the sound is heard in the centre of the forehead. Nerve deafness causes the sound to be transmitted to the normal ear. A patient with a conduction deafness finds the sound louder in the abnormal ear.

Causes of Deafness

Nerve deafness may be due to (i) environmental exposure to noise (boilermaker's deafness); (ii) tumours—e.g., an acoustic neuroma; (iii) degeneration—e.g., presbycousis; (iv) trauma—e.g., fracture of the petrous temporal bone; (iv) toxicity—e.g., aspirin, streptomycin or alcohol; (vi) infection—e.g., congenital rubella syndrome, congenital syphilis; (vii) Ménière's disease; (viii) brainstem disease (rare); or (ix) vascular disease of the internal auditory artery (rare).

Conduction deafness may be due to (i) wax; (ii) otitis media; (iii) otosclerosis; or (iv) Paget's disease of bone.

---

*   Alfonso Corti (b. 1822), Italian anatomist.

†   Heinrich Adolf Rinné (1819–1968), German ear specialist.

‡   Sir Hermann Weber (1832–1918), London physician.

Examination of Vestibular Function

If a patient complains of vertigo (an hallucination of motion—e.g., of the room spinning around) (Latin *vertere* turn), the *Hallpike* manoeuvre* should be performed. The patient sits up; having warned him or her what is about to occur, the examiner grasps the patient's head between the hands and gets him or her to lie back quickly so that the head lies 30 degrees below the horizontal. At the same time, the head is rotated 30 degrees towards the examiner. Ask the patient to keep the eyes open. If the test is positive, after a short latent period vertigo and nystagmus (rotatory) towards the affected (lowermost) ear occur for several seconds and then abate and are not reproducible for 10 to 15 minutes. This result is seen in the condition called *benign positional vertigo*. It is due to a change in the utricle and occurs for example following infection, trauma or vascular disease. The mechanisms are not well understood. If there is no latent period, no fatiguability or the nystagmus persists or is variable, this suggests that there is a lesion of the brainstem (e.g., multiple sclerosis) or cerebellum (e.g., metastatic carcinoma).

Causes of Vestibular Abnormalities

Labyrinthine causes include acute labyrinthitis, motion sickness, streptomycin toxicity or, rarely, Ménière's disease.

Vestibular causes include vestibular neuronitis as well as all the causes of nerve deafness.

In the brainstem, vascular lesions, tumours of the cerebellum or fourth ventricle, demyelination, or vasospastic conditions such as migraine may involve the central connections of the vestibular system.

Vertigo may be associated with temporal lobe dysfunction (e.g., ischaemia or complex partial seizures).

The Ninth (Glossopharyngeal) and Tenth (Vagus) Nerves

Anatomy

These nerves have motor, sensory and autonomic functions. Nerve fibres from nuclei in the medulla (Figure 10.16) form multiple nerve rootlets as they exit the medulla. These join to form the ninth and tenth nerves and also contribute to the eleventh nerve. The nerves emerge from the skull through the jugular foramen (Figure 10.17). The ninth nerve receives sensory fibres from the nasopharynx, pharynx, middle and inner ear and from the posterior third of the tongue (including taste fibres). It also carries secretory fibres to the parotid gland. The tenth nerve receives sensory fibres from the pharynx and larynx and innervates muscles of the pharynx, larynx and palate.

Examination

Get the patient to open the mouth and inspect the palate with a torch. Note any displacement of the uvula. Then ask the patient to say 'Ah!'. If the uvula is drawn to one side this indicates a unilateral tenth nerve palsy. Note that the uvula is drawn towards the normal side.

Now test gently for the *gag reflex* (ninth is the sensory component and tenth the motor component). Touch the back of the pharynx on each side with a spatula.

---

*   Charles Hallpike (1900–1979), English ear, nose and throat surgeon.

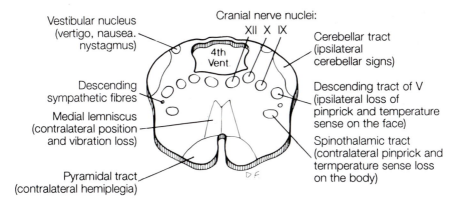

Vestibular nucleus
(vertigo, nausea.
nystagmus)

Cranial nerve nuclei:
XII X IX

4th
Vent.

Cerebellar tract
(ipsilateral
cerebellar signs)

Descending
sympathetic fibres

Descending tract of V
(ipsilateral loss of
pinprick and temperature
sense on the face)

Medial lemniscus
(contralateral position
and vibration loss)

Spinothalamic tract
(contralateral pinprick and
termperature sense loss
on the body)

Pyramidal tract
(contralateral hemiplegia)

Figure 10.16   *Anatomy of the medulla: correlation between lesions and clinical features.*

Remember to ask the patient if the touch of the spatula (ninth) is felt each time. Normally, there is reflex contraction of the soft palate. If contraction is absent and sensation is intact this suggests a tenth nerve palsy. The most common cause of a reduced gag reflex is old age. Of more concern to the examiner is the patient with an exaggerated but still normal reflex.

Ask the patient to speak in order to assess hoarseness (which may occur with a unilateral recurrent laryngeal nerve lesion), and then to cough. Listen for the characteristic bovine cough that occurs with bilateral recurrent laryngeal nerve lesions. It is not necessary routinely to test taste on the posterior third of the tongue (ninth nerve).

Test swallowing of a small amount of water.

Causes of a Ninth (Glossopharyngeal) and Tenth (Vagus) Nerve Palsy

Central causes: vascular lesions (e.g., lateral medullary infarction, due to vertebral or posterior inferior cerebellar artery disease), tumours, syringobulbia and motor neurone disease.

   Peripheral (posterior fossa) lesions: aneurysms, tumours, chronic meningitis, the Guillain-Barré syndrome.

The Eleventh (Accessory) Nerve

Anatomy

The central portion of this nerve arises in the medulla close to the nuclei of the ninth, tenth and twelfth nerves and its spinal portion arises from the upper five cervical segments. It leaves the skull with the ninth and tenth nerves through the jugular foramen (Figure 10.17). Its central division gives motor fibres to the vagus and the spinal division innervates the trapezius and sternomastoid muscles.

Examination

Ask the patient to shrug the shoulders. Feel the bulk of the trapezius muscles and attempt to push the shoulders down. Then instruct the patient to turn the head against resistance (the examiner's hand). Remember that the right sternomastoid turns the head to the left. Feel the muscle bulk of the sternomastoids.

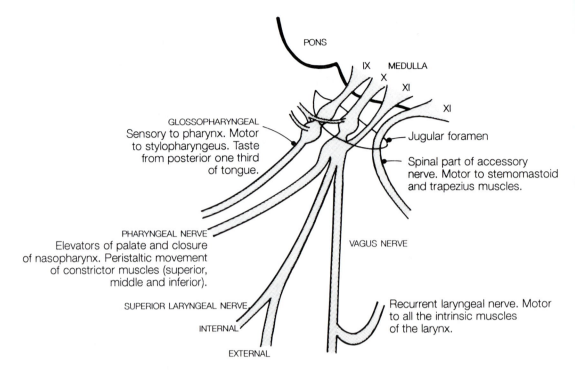

Figure 10.17   *The lower cranial nerves—glossopharyngeal (IX), vagus (X) and accessory (XI).*

From and used with permission of Walton JN. Brain's diseases of the nervous system. 9th ed. Oxford: Oxford University Press, 1985.

Causes of Eleventh Nerve Lesions

Unilateral: trauma involving the neck or the base of the skull, poliomyelitis, basilar invagination (platybasia), syringomyelia, and tumours near the jugular foramen.

   Bilateral: motor neurone disease, poliomyelitis, and the Guillain-Barré syndrome. NB: Bilateral sternomastoid and trapezius weakness also occurs in muscular dystrophy (especially dystrophia myotonica).

The Twelfth (Hypoglossal) Nerve

Anatomy

This nerve also arises from the medulla. It leaves the skull via the hypoglossal foramen. It is the motor nerve for the tongue.

Examination

Inspect the tongue at rest on the floor of the mouth. Look for wasting and fasciculations (fine irregular non-rhythmical muscle fibre contractions). These indicate a lower motor neurone lesion. Fasciculations may be unilateral or bilateral (Figure 10.18).

   Ask the patient to poke out the tongue which will deviate towards the weaker (affected) side if there is a unilateral lower motor neurone lesion (Figure 10.19).

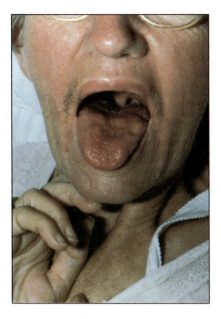

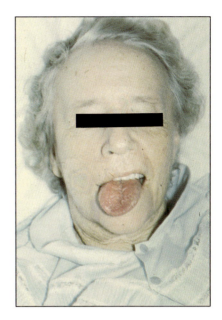

Figure 10.18
Fasciculations of the tongue in motor neurone disease.

Figure 10.19
Right hypoglossal (XII) nerve palsy—lower motor neurone lesion.

The tongue, like the face and palate, has a bilateral upper motor neurone innervation in most people, so a unilateral upper motor neurone lesion often causes no deviation.

A clinically obvious upper motor neurone lesion of the twelfth nerve is usually bilateral and results in a small immobile tongue. The combination of bilateral upper motor neurone lesions of the ninth, tenth and twelfth nerves is called pseudobulbar palsy.

A lower motor neurone lesion of the twelfth nerve causes fasciculation, wasting and weakness. If the lesion is bilateral it causes dysarthria.

Causes of Twelfth (Hypoglossal) Nerve Palsy

Bilateral upper motor neurone lesions may be due to vascular lesions, motor neurone disease or tumours e.g., metastases to the base of the skull.

Unilateral lower motor neurone lesions with a central cause include: vascular lesions, such as thrombosis of the vertebral artery; motor neurone disease; and syringobulbia. Peripheral causes include: in the posterior fossa, aneurysms or tumours, chronic meningitis and trauma; in the upper neck, tumours or lymphadenopathy; and the Arnold Chiari* malformation. The Arnold Chiari malformation is a congenital malformation of the base of the skull with herniation of a tongue of cerebellum and medulla into the spinal canal causing lower cranial nerve palsies, cerebellar limb signs (due to tonsillar compression) and upper motor neurone signs in the legs.

---

* Julius Arnold (1835–1915) and Hans Chiari (1851–1916), German pathologists.

Causes of **bilateral lower motor neurone lesions** include motor neurone disease, the Guillain-Barré syndrome, poliomyelitis, and the Arnold Chiari malformation.

Multiple Cranial Nerve Lesions

The clinical features of pseudobulbar and bulbar palsies are shown in Table 10.5, and the causes of multiple cranial nerve palsies are listed in Table 10.6.

The Head and Neck

Inspect and palpate the skull for lumps, such as a meningioma or a sarcoma. Auscultate the skull by placing the diaphragm of the stethoscope on the frontal bone, and then on the lateral occipital bones, and then the bell over each eye (with the opposite eye open). Ask the patient to hold the breath each time. Then auscultate over the carotid arteries. Bruits heard over the skull may be due to an arteriovenous malformation, advanced Paget's disease, or a vascular meningioma, or they may be conducted from the carotids.

Medical Examination of the Eyes: A Summary

Method (Figure 10.20)

The patient should sit at the edge of the bed facing the examiner while the examination begins with inspection. Ptosis is best detected at this stage while

Table 10.5 *Clinical Features of Pseudobulbar and Bulbar Palsies*

Feature	Pseudobulbar (Bilateral UMN lesions of IX, X and XII)	Bulbar (Bilateral LMN lesions of IX, X and XII)
Gag reflex	Increased or normal	Absent
Tongue	Spastic	Wasted, fasciculations
Jaw jerk	Increased	Absent or normal
Speech	Spastic dysarthria	Nasal
Other	Bilateral limb UMN (long tract) signs	Signs of the underlying cause— e.g., limb fasciculations
	Labile emotions	Normal emotions
Causes	Bilateral cerebrovascular disease (e.g., both internal capsules)	Motor neurone disease
	Multiple sclerosis	Guillain-Barré syndrome
	Motor neurone disease	Poliomyelitis
		Brainstem infarction

UMN = upper motor neurone   LMN = lower motor neurone

Table 10.6 *Causes of Multiple Cranial Nerve Palsies*

Nasopharyngeal carcinoma
Chronic meningitis—e.g., carcinoma, haematological malignancy, tuberculosis, sarcoidosis
Guillain-Barré syndrome (spares sensory nerves)
Brainstem lesions. These are usually due to vascular disease causing crossed sensory or motor paralysis (i.e., cranial nerve signs on one side and contralateral long tract signs). Patients with a brainstem tumour may also have similar signs
Arnold Chiari malformation
Trauma
Paget's disease
Mononeuritis multiplex (rarely) e.g., diabetes mellitus

Figure 10.20   *The Medical Eye Examination*

Sitting up

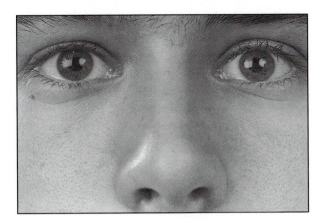

GENERAL INSPECTION
  Diagnositic facies

EYELIDS
  Xanthelasma

CORNEA
  Comeal arcus
  Band keratopathy
  Kayser-Fleischer rings

SCLERA
  Jaundice
  Pallor
  Injection

PTOSIS

EXOPHTHALMOS
  Lid lag

ORBITS AND EYEBALL
  Palpate—Tenderness
        —Brow (for loss of sweating in
         Horner's syndrome)

OTHER
  Depends on findings, e.g., other cranial
      nerves, long tract signs, urine analysis
      (e.g., diabetes mellitus)

NEUROLOGICAL EXAMINATION
  Acuity
    Eye chart—each eye separately
  Fields
    Pin confrontation—each eye
    Central vision
  Fundi
    Cornea
    Lens
    Humour
    Colour of disc and state of cup
    Retina—vessels, exudates,
          haemorrhages, pigmentation, etc.
  Pupils
    Shape, size
    Light reflex—direct and consensual
    Assess for afferent pupillary defect
    Accommodation
  Eye movements
    III, IV, VI nerves—movement, diplopia,
        nystagmus
    Gaze palsies (e.g., supranuclear
        lesions)
    Fatiguability (myasthenia)
  Corneal reflex (V and VII)

standing well back from the patient. Look then for any corneal abnormalities, such as band keratopathy (page 208) or Kayser-Fleischer rings (Wilson's disease, page 156). Look at the colour of the sclerae: yellow (jaundice), blue (in osteogenesis imperfecta, because the thin sclerae allow the choroidal pigment to show through), or red (Tables 10.7 and 10.8). Note scleral pallor or telangiectasia.

Look from behind and above the patient for exophthalmos (page 300). Proceed then as for the cranial nerve examination—that is, testing visual acuity, visual fields

Table 10.7 *Causes of a Red and Painful Eye*

Disease	Distribution of Redness	Corneal Surface	Pupil
Bacterial conjunctivitis	Peripheral conjunctiva Bilateral (central sparing)	Normal	Normal
Episcleritis	Segmental, often around cornea Unilateral	Normal	Normal
Acute iritis	Around cornea Unilateral	Dull (vision blurred)	Small, irregular shape, may be no light response
Glaucoma	Around cornea Unilateral	Dull	Mid-oval shape, no light response
Corneal ulcer	Around cornea Unilateral	Dull Fluorescein dye stains ulcer	Normal
Subconjunctival haemorrhage	Localised haemorrhage No posterior limit	Normal	Normal
Conjunctival haemorrhage	Localised haemorrhage Posterior limit present	Normal	Normal

Table 10.8 *Causes of Uveitis*

Iritis (Anterior Uveitis)
Idiopathic
Generalised disease
   Seronegative spondyloarthropathies
   Inflammatory bowel disease
   Diabetes mellitus
   Granulomatous disease—e.g., sarcoidosis
   Infections—e.g., gonococcal, syphilis, toxoplasmosis, brucellosis, tuberculosis

Choroiditis (Posterior Uveitis)
Idiopathic
Generalised disease
   Diabetes mellitus
   Granulomatous disease—e.g., sarcoidosis
   Infections—e.g., toxoplasmosis, syphilis, tuberculosis, toxocaral infection

The uveal tract consists of the anterior uvea (iris) and posterior uvea (ciliary body and choroid).

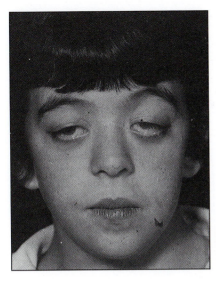

Figure 10.21
Bilateral ptosis after upward gaze in myasthenia gravis.

and pupillary responses to light and accommodation, and then performing ophthalmoscopy.

Begin ophthalmoscopy by examining the cornea and lens and then the retina. Note any abnormalities of the cornea, lens or humour. Look for retinal changes of diabetes mellitus and hypertension. Also inspect carefully for optic atrophy, papilloedema, angioid streaks, retinal detachment, central vein or artery thrombosis, and retinitis pigmentosa.

Test the eye movements. Look also for fatiguability of eye muscles by asking the patient to look up (Figure 10.21) at the hat pin for about half a minute. In myasthenia gravis (page 407) the muscles tire and the eyelids begin to droop. Test for lid lag if hyperthyroidism seems a possibility.

Test the corneal reflex.

Palpate the orbits for tenderness. Auscultate the eyes with the bell of the stethoscope—the eye being tested is shut while the other is open and the patient is asked to stop breathing. Consider the possibility that the patient may have a glass eye. This should be suspected if visual acuity is zero in one eye and no pupillary reaction is apparent. Attempts to examine and interpret the fundus of a glass eye are always unsuccessful and embarrassing.

Horner's* Syndrome

Interruption of the sympathetic innervation of the eye at any point (Figure 10.22) results in Horner's syndrome (Table 10.9). This is the presence of *partial ptosis* (as sympathetic fibres supply the smooth muscle of both eyelids) and a *constricted pupil* (unbalanced parasympathetic action) which reacts normally to light (Figure 10.23). Test for a difference (decrease) in the *sweating* over each eyebrow with the back of the finger (absence of this sign does not exclude the diagnosis).

---

* Johann Friedrich Horner (1831–1886), Professor of Ophthalmology, Zürich, described this in 1869.

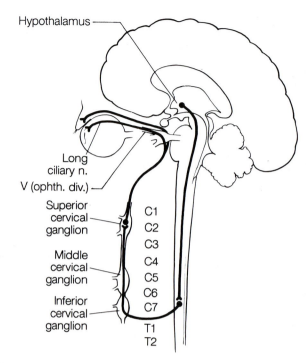

Hypothalamus

Long ciliary n.

V (ophth. div.)

Superior cervical ganglion

Middle cervical ganglion

Inferior cervical ganglion

C1
C2
C3
C4
C5
C6
C7
T1
T2

Figure 10.22 *Oculosympathetic pathway involved in Horner's syndrome. This 3-neurone pathway projects from the hypothalamus to the intermediolateral column of the cervical spinal cord, then to the superior cervical ganglion and finally to the pupil, the levator palpebrae and the sweat glands of the face. A lesion at any site along the pathway can produce Horner's syndrome.*

Adapted from Simon RP, Aminoff MJ, Greenberg DA. Clinical neurology 1989. Appleton and Lange, 1989, with permission.

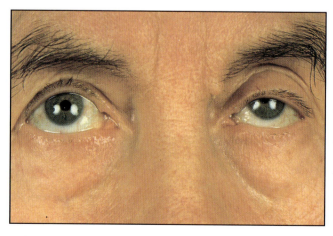

Figure 10.23

Left Horner's syndrome, with ptosis, miosis, and lack of sweating.

Table 10.9 *Causes of Horner's Syndrome*

1. Carcinoma of the apex of the lung (usually squamous cell carcinoma)
2. Neck
• Malignancy—e.g., thyroid
• Trauma or surgery
3. Lower trunk brachial plexus lesions
• Trauma
• Tumour
4. Carotid arterial lesion
• Carotid aneurysm or dissection
• Pericarotid tumours (Raeder's syndrome)*
• Cluster headache
5. Brainstem lesions
• Vascular disease (especially the lateral medullary syndrome)
• Tumour
• Syringobulbia
6. Syringomyelia (rare)

*   Sweating unaffected, as tumour localised to internal carotid artery.

NB: Enophthalmos or retraction of the eye, which is often mentioned as a feature of Horner's syndrome, probably does not occur in man. It may occur in the cat. Horner's original paper was very specific about miosis and ptosis but only casually mentioned that 'the position of the eye seemed very slightly inward'. Apparent enophthalmos results from a combination of ptosis and an elevated lower lid (upside down ptosis}.

Horner's syndrome may be part of the lateral medullary syndrome*, so that the other signs to be looked for include: nystagmus to the side of the lesion; ipsilateral fifth (pain and temperature), ninth and tenth cranial nerve lesions; ipsilateral cerebellar signs (page 407); and contralateral pain and temperature loss over the trunk and limbs (page 403).

Next ask the patient to speak and note any hoarseness of the voice which may be due to a recurrent laryngeal nerve palsy from lung carcinoma or from a lower cranial nerve lesion.

Go on now to look at the hands for clubbing and test for weakness of finger abduction (page 104). If any of these signs is present, perform a respiratory examination concentrating on the apices of the lungs for signs of lung carcinoma.

Examine the neck for lymphadenopathy, thyroid carcinoma and a carotid aneurysm or bruit. Syringomyelia may rarely be a cause of this syndrome so the examination should be completed by testing for dissociated sensory loss (page 399). Remember syringomyelia may cause a bilateral Horner's syndrome.

The Limbs and Trunk

General Examination Approach

It is most important to have a set order of examination of the limbs for neurological signs so that nothing is omitted. The following scheme is a standard approach.

---

*   Occlusion of any of the following vessels may result in this syndrome: vertebral; posterior inferior cerebellar; superior, middle or inferior lateral medullary arteries.

Motor system:	General inspection
	Posture
	Muscle bulk
	Abnormal movements
	Skin
	Fasciculations
	Tone
	Power
	Reflexes
	Coordination
Sensory system:	Pain and temperature
	Vibration and proprioception
	Light touch

General Inspection

1. Stand back and look at the patient for an *abnormal posture*—e.g., that due to hemiplegia caused by a stroke. In this case the upper limb is flexed and there is adduction and pronation of the arm, while the lower limb is extended (page 391).

2. Look for *muscle wasting* which indicates a denervated muscle, a primary muscle disease or disuse atrophy. Compare one side with the other for wasting and try to work out which muscle groups are involved (proximal, distal or generalised, symmetrical or asymmetrical).

3. Inspect for *abnormal movements,* such as tremor of the wrist or arm (page 411).

4. Inspect the *skin,* e.g., for evidence of neurofibromatosis, cutaneous angiomata in a segmental distribution (associated with syringomyelia and spinal astrocytoma) or herpes zoster.

The Upper Limbs

The Motor System

General

Shake hands with the patient and introduce yourself. A patient who cannot relax his or her hand grip has myotonia (an inability to relax muscles after voluntary contraction). The commonest cause of this is the muscle disease dystrophia myotonica (page 403). Once your hand has been extracted from the patient's, and after pausing briefly for the vitally important general inspection, ask the patient to undress so that the arms and shoulder girdles are completely exposed.

Sit the patient over the edge of the bed if this is possible. Next ask the patient to hold out both hands with the arms extended and the eyes closed. Watch the arms for evidence of drifting (movement of one or both arms from the initial neutral position). There are only three causes for drift of the arms.

1. Upper motor neurone (pyramidal) weakness. The drift of the limb here is due to muscle weakness and tends to be in a downward direction. The drifting typically starts distally with the fingers and spreads proximally.

2. Cerebellar disease. The drift here is due to hypotonia and is usually upwards.

Table 10.10   *Causes of Fasciculations*

Motor neurone disease
Motor root compression
Peripheral neuropathy—e.g., diabetic
Primary myopathy
Thyrotoxicosis

NB • Myokymia resembles coarse fasciculation of the same muscle group, and is particularly common in the orbicularis oculi muscles where it is usually benign. Focal myokymia, however, often represents brainstem disease like multiple sclerosis or glioma.
• Fibrillation is only seen on the electromyogram.

3.   Loss of proprioception. The drift here (pseudoathetosis) is due to loss of joint position sense and can be in any direction.

Ask the patient to relax the arms and rest them on his or her lap. Inspect the large muscle groups for *fasciculations* (Table 10.10). These are irregular contractions of small areas of muscle which have no rhythmical pattern. Fasciculation may be coarse or fine and is present at rest, but not during voluntary movement.* If present with weakness and wasting, fasciculation indicates degeneration of the lower motor neurone. It is usually benign if unassociated with other signs of a motor lesion. Causes of fasciculations are shown in Table 10.10.

Tone

Tone is tested at both the wrists and elbows. Rotation of the wrists with supination and pronation of the elbow joints (supporting the patient's elbow with one hand and holding the hand with the other) is performed passively and the patient should be told to relax to allow the examiner to move the joints freely. The best passive movements to demonstrate changes in tone are rotation and pronation and supination of the forearm. If the patient resists these movements the joints should be moved unpredictably and at different rates.

With experience it is possible to decide if tone is normal, increased (hypertonic, as in an upper motor neurone or extrapyramidal lesion) or decreased (hypotonic, as in a lower motor neurone lesion).

Power

Muscle strength is assessed by gauging the examiner's ability to overcome the patient's full voluntary muscle resistance. To decide whether the power is normal, the patient's age, gender and build should be taken into account. Power is graded according to the following scheme (although this lacks sensitivity at the higher grades):

0—complete paralysis

1—flicker of contraction possible

2—movement is possible when gravity is excluded

---

*   If no fasciculation is seen, tapping over the bulk of the brachioradialis and biceps muscles with the finger or with a tendon hammer, and watching again has been recommended but this is controversial. Most neurologists do not do this. The reason is that fasciculations are spontaneous. Any muscle movement from a local stimulus is not spontaneous. Even if they occur they may have nothing to do with fasciculations.

3—movement is possible against gravity but not if any further resistance is added

4—movement is possible against gravity and some resistance

5—normal power.*

If power is reduced decide whether this is symmetrical or asymmetrical, whether it involves only particular muscle groups, or whether it is proximal, distal or general. It is also important to consider whether any painful joint or muscle disease is interfering with the assessment (Chapter 8). Asymmetrical muscle weakness is most often the result of a peripheral nerve, brachial plexus or root lesion, or an upper motor neurone lesion.

Shoulder. *Abduction* (C5, C6): the patient should abduct the arms with the elbows flexed and resist the examiner's attempt to push them down. Adduction (C6, C7, C8): the patient should adduct the arms with the elbows flexed and not allow the examiner to separate them.

Elbow. *Flexion* (C5, C6): the patient should bend the elbow and pull so as not to let the examiner straighten it out. Extension (C7, C8): the patient should bend the elbow and push so as not to let the examiner bend it.

Wrist. *Flexion* (C6, C7): the patient should bend the wrist and not allow the examiner to straighten it. Extension (C7, C8): the patient should extend the wrist and not allow the examiner to bend it.

Fingers. *Extension* (C7, C8): the patient should straighten the fingers and not allow the examiner to push them down (push with the side of your hand across the patient's metacarpophalangeal joints). Flexion (C7, C8): the patient squeezes two of the examiner's fingers. Abduction (C8, T1): the patient should spread out the fingers and not allow the examiner to push them together.

Reflexes

Make sure the patient is resting comfortably with the elbows flexed and hands lying pronated on the lap and not overlapping one another.

Biceps jerk (C5, C6): place one forefinger on the biceps tendon and tap this with the tendon hammer (Figure 10.24). The hammer should be held near its end and the head allowed to fall with gravity on to the positioned forefinger. The examiner soon learns not to hit too hard. Normally, if the reflex arc is intact, there is a brisk contraction of the biceps muscle with flexion of the forearm at the elbow followed by prompt relaxation.

If a reflex appears to be absent, always test following a reinforcement manoeuvre. For example, ask the patient to clench the teeth tightly just before you let the hammer fall. Sometimes normal reflexes can only be elicited after reinforcement, but they should still be symmetrical.

An increased jerk occurs with an upper motor neurone lesion (page 391). A decreased or absent reflex occurs with a breach in any part of the reflex motor arc—the muscle itself (e.g., myopathy), the motor nerve (e.g., neuropathy), the anterior spinal cord root (e.g., spondylosis), the anterior horn cell (e.g., poliomyelitis) or the sensory arc (sensory root or sensory nerve).

Triceps jerk (C7, C8): support the elbow with one hand and tap over the triceps tendon (Figure 10.25). Normally triceps contraction results in forearm extension.

Brachioradialis (supinator) jerk (C5, C6): strike the lower end of the radius just above the wrist. To avoid hurting the patient by striking the radial nerve directly

---

* You should not be able to overcome a normal adult patient's power, at least in the legs.

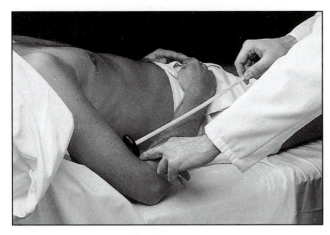

Figure 10.24
The biceps jerk.

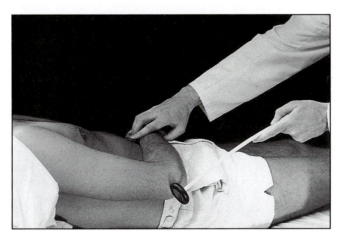

Figure 10.25
The triceps jerk.

one should place one's own first two fingers over this spot and then strike the fingers, as with the biceps jerk. Normally contraction of the brachioradialis causes flexion of the elbow.

Inverted brachioradialis (supinator) jerk: if finger flexion is the only response when the patient's wrist is tapped, the response is said to be inverted. This is associated with an absent biceps jerk and an exaggerated triceps jerk. It indicates a spinal cord lesion at the C5 or C6 level due, for example, to compression (e.g., disc prolapse), trauma or syringomyelia. It occurs because a lower motor neurone lesion at C5 or C6 is combined with an upper motor neurone lesion affecting the reflexes below this level (page 397).

Finger jerks (C8): the patient rests the hand palm upwards with the fingers slightly flexed. The examiner's hand is placed over the patient's and the hammer struck over the examiner's fingers. Normally, slight flexion of all the fingers occurs.

The reflexes can be simply recorded as follows:

0   —indicates absent reflexes
+   —indicates reduced reflexes
++   —indicates normal reflexes
+++   —indicates exaggerated reflexes
++++—indicates exaggerated reflexes and clonus.

Coordination

The cerebellum has multiple connections (afferent and efferent) to sensory pathways, brainstem nuclei, thalamus and the cerebral cortex. Via these connections the cerebellum plays an integral role in coordinating voluntary movement. A standard series of simple tests is used to test coordination. Always demonstrate these movements for the patient's benefit.

Finger-nose test: ask the patient to touch his or her nose with the index finger and then turn the finger around and touch the examiner's outstretched forefinger at nearly full extension of the shoulder and elbow. The test should be done both briskly and slowly and repeated a number of times with the patient's eyes open and later closed.

Look for the following abnormalities: (i) intention tremor, which is tremor increasing as the target is approached (there is no tremor at rest); (ii) past-pointing, where the patient's finger overshoots the target. These abnormalities occur with cerebellar disease.

Rapidly alternating movements: ask the patient to pronate and supinate his or her hand on the dorsum of the other hand as rapidly as possible. This movement is slow and clumsy in cerebellar disease and is called dysdiadochokinesis.*

Rapidly alternating movements may also be affected in extrapyramidal disorders (e.g., Parkinson's disease) and in pyramidal disorders (e.g., internal capsule infarction).

Rebound: ask the patient to lift the arms rapidly from the sides and then stop. Hypotonia due to cerebellar disease causes delay in stopping the arms. This method of demonstrating rebound is preferable to the more often used one where the patient flexes the arm at the elbow against the examiner's resistance. When the examiner suddenly lets go, violent flexion of the arm may occur and, unless prevented, the patient can strike himself or herself in the face. Therefore only medical students trained in self defence should use this method.

Muscle weakness may also cause clumsiness, but motor testing should have revealed any impairment of this sort.

The Sensory System

To test sensation, which is a difficult assessment and can be frustratingly time consuming, use the following routine.

Spinothalamic Pathway (Pain and Temperature)

Pain and temperature fibres enter the spinal cord and cross a few segments higher to the opposite spinothalamic tract (Figure 10.26). This tract ascends to the brainstem.

---

* Actually dysdiadochokinesis is the inability to perform alternating movements of both wrists with the arms and forefingers extended. Diadoche is a Greek word meaning succession. The problem here is with successive movements. The Diadochi were the successors of Alexander the Great. They divided his empire.

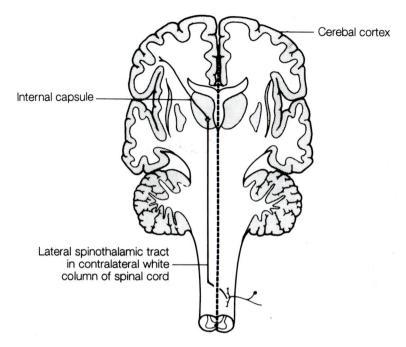

Cerebal cortex

Internal capsule

Lateral spinothalamic tract
in contralateral white
column of spinal cord

Figure 10.26   *Pain and temperature pathways.*

Adapted from and used with permission of Snell RS. Clinical neuroanatomy for medical students. 2nd ed.
Boston: Little Brown, 1987.

Pain (pinprick) testing: to test the spinothalamic pathway. Pain is the only
modality tested routinely here. Using a new pin, demonstrate to the patient that
this induces a relatively sharp sensation by touching lightly a normal area, such as
the anterior chest wall. Then ask the patient to close the eyes and say whether the
pin prick feels sharp or dull. Begin proximally on the upper arm and test in each
dermatome (Figure 10.28) (this is the area of skin supplied by a vertebral spinal
segment). Also compare right with left in the same dermatome. Map out the extent
of any area of dullness. Always do this by going from the area of dullness to the
area of normal sensation.

Temperature testing: this can be done in a similar fashion using test tubes filled
with hot and cold water. It is done only in special circumstances—e.g., for suspected syringomyelia.

Posterior Columns (Vibration and Proprioception)

These fibres enter and ascend ipsilaterally in the posterior columns of the spinal
cord to the nucleus gracilis and nucleus cuneatus in the medulla, where they
decussate (Figure 10.27).

Vibration testing: use a 128 Hertz tuning fork (not a 256 Hertz fork). Ask the
patient to close the eyes and then place the vibrating tuning fork on one of the
distal interphalangeal joints. The patient should be able to describe a feeling of
vibration. The examiner then deadens the tuning fork with the hand, and the
patient should be able to say exactly when this occurs. Compare one side with the

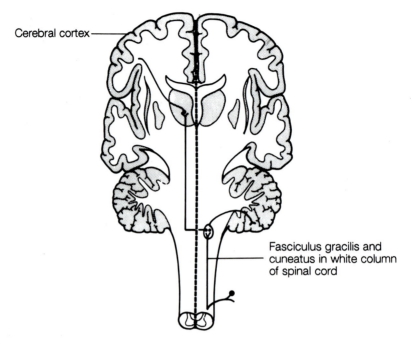

Cerebral cortex

Fasciculus gracilis and
cuneatus in white column
of spinal cord

Figure 10.27   *Vibration and joint position sense pathways.*

Adapted from and used with permission of Snell RS. Clinical neuroanatomy for medical students. 2nd ed. Boston: Little Brown, 1987.

other. If vibration sense is reduced or absent, test over the ulnar head at the wrist, then the elbows (over the olecranon) and then the shoulders to determine the level of abnormality.

Proprioception testing: use the distal interphalangeal joint of the patient's index finger. When the patient has his or her eyes open, grasp the distal phalanx from the sides and move it up and down to demonstrate these positions. Then ask the patient to close the eyes while these manoeuvres are repeated randomly. Normally, movement through even a few degrees is detectable, and should be reported correctly. If there is an abnormality, proceed to test the wrists and elbows similarly.

Light touch testing: some fibres travel in the posterior columns (i.e., ipsilaterally) and the rest cross the middle line to travel in the anterior spinothalamic tract (i.e., contralaterally). For this reason light touch is of the least discriminating value.

Test light touch by touching the skin with a wisp of cotton wool. Ask the patient to shut the eyes and say 'yes' when the touch is felt. Do not stroke the skin because this moves hair fibres. Test each dermatome comparing left and right sides.

Interpretation of Sensory Abnormalities

Try to fit the distribution of any sensory loss into a dermatome (due to a spinal cord or nerve root lesion), a single peripheral nerve territory (page 379), a peripheral neuropathy pattern (glove distribution, page 394), or a hemisensory loss (due to spinal cord or upper brainstem or thalamic lesion).

Sensory dermatomes of the upper limb (Figure 10.28) can be recognised by memorising the following rough guides: C5 supplies the shoulder tip and outer part of the upper arm; C6 supplies the lateral aspect of the forearm and thumb; C7 supplies the middle finger; C8 supplies the little finger; T1 supplies the medial aspect of the upper arm.

Examination of the Peripheral Nerves of the Upper Limb

A lesion of a peripheral nerve causes a characteristic motor and sensory loss. Peripheral nerve lesions may have local causes, such as trauma or compression, or may be part of a mononeuritis multiplex, where more than one nerve is affected by systemic disease.

The Radial Nerve (C5–C8)

This is the *motor nerve* supplying the triceps and brachioradialis and the extensor muscles of the hand. The characteristic deformity which results from radial nerve injury is *wrist drop*. To demonstrate this, if it is not already obvious, get the patient to flex the elbow, pronate the forearm and extend the wrist. If a lesion occurs above the upper third of the upper arm the triceps muscle is also affected. Therefore, test elbow extension, which will be absent if the lesion is high.

Test *sensation* using a pin over the area of the anatomical snuff box. Sensation here is lost with a radial nerve lesion at any level (Figure 10.29).

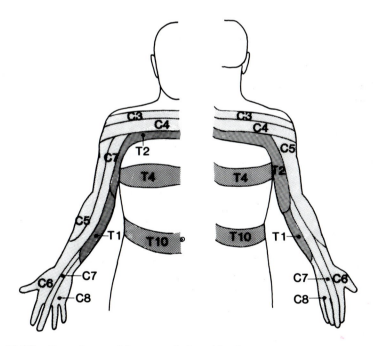

Figure 10.28   *Dermatomes of the upper limb and trunk.*

Adapted from and used with kind permission of Lance JW, McLeod JG. A physiological approach to clinical neurology. 3rd ed. London: Butterworths, 1981.

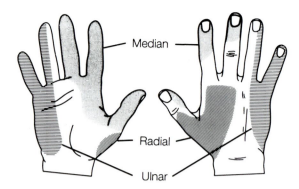

Figure 10.29 *Average loss of pain sensation (pin-prick) with lesions of the major nerves of the upper limbs.*

The Median Nerve (C6–T1)

This nerve contains the *motor* supply to all the muscles on the front of the forearm except the flexor carpi ulnaris and the ulnar half of the flexor digitorum profundus. It also supplies the following short muscles of the hand (LOAF)—the **L**ateral two lumbricals, **O**pponens pollicis, **A**bductor pollicis brevis and **F**lexor pollicis brevis.

Lesion at the wrist (carpal tunnel): use the pen-touching test to assess for weakness of the abductor pollicis brevis. Ask the patient to lay the hand flat, palm upward on the table and attempt to abduct the thumb vertically to touch the examiner's pen held above it (Figure 10.30). This may be impossible if there is a median nerve palsy at the wrist or above. Remember, however, that most patients with the carpal tunnel syndrome have normal power and may indeed have symptoms but no signs at all.

Lesion in the cubital fossa: Ochsner's* clasping test (for loss of flexor digitorum sublimis). Ask the patient to clasp the hands firmly together—the index finger on the affected side fails to flex with a lesion in the cubital fossa or higher (Figure 10.31).

For the *sensory* component of the median nerve, test pin prick sensation over the hand. The constant area of loss includes the palmar aspect of the thumb, index, middle and lateral half of the ring fingers (Figure 10.29).

The Ulnar Nerve (C8–T1)

This nerve contains the *motor* supply to all the small muscles of the hand (except the LOAF muscles), flexor carpi ulnaris and ulnar half of flexor digitorum profundus. Look for wasting of the small muscles of the hand and for partial clawing of the little and ring fingers (a claw-like hand). Clawing is hyperextension at the metacarpophalangeal joints and flexion of the interphalangeal joints. Note that clawing is more pronounced with an ulnar nerve lesion at the wrist, as a lesion at or above the elbow also causes loss of the flexor digitorum profundus, and therefore less flexion of the interphalangeal joints. This is the 'ulnar nerve paradox' in that a more distal lesion causes greater deformity.

---

* Albert Ochsner (1858–1925), American surgeon of Swiss extraction who claimed descent from Andreas Vesalius, the great anatomist.

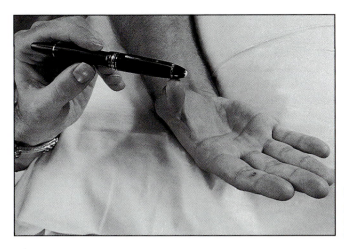

Figure 10.30
Pen touching test for loss of abductor pollicis brevis function.

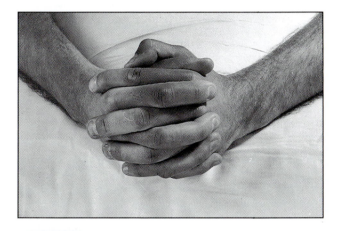

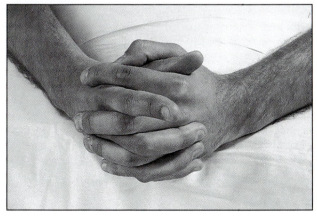

Figure 10.31   *Ochsner's clasping test—upper normal, lower abnormal due to loss of function of the flexor digitorum (simulated demonstration).*

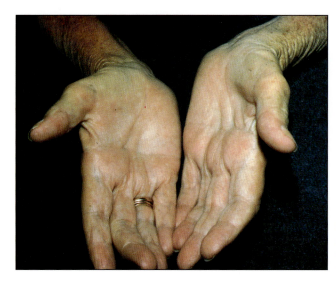

Figure 10.32

Motor neurone disease. Wasting of the small muscles of the hand.

Table 10.11   *Causes of a True Claw Hand (All Fingers Clawed)*

Ulnar and median nerve lesion (ulnar nerve palsy alone causes a claw-like hand)
Brachial plexus lesion (C8—T1)
Other neurological disease—e.g., syringomyelia, polio
Ischaemic contracture (late and severe)
Rheumatoid arthritis (advanced, untreated disease)

Causes of a true claw hand are shown in Table 10.11, while causes of wasting of the small muscles of the hand are shown in Table 10.12 (Figure 10.32).

Froment's* sign: Ask the patient to grasp a piece of paper between the thumb and lateral aspect of the forefinger with each hand. The affected thumb will flex because of loss of the adductor of the thumb.

For the *sensory* component of the ulnar nerve, test for pin prick loss over the palmar and dorsal aspects of the little finger and the medial half of the ring finger (Figure 10.29).

The Brachial Plexus

This is shown in Figure 10.33.

Lesions of the brachial plexus, complete and partial, and the cervical rib syndrome are described in Table 10.13.

Examination of the shoulder girdle from the front and the back is described in Table 10.14.

The Lower Limbs

Begin by testing *gait* if this is possible (see page 390).

---

*   Jules Froment (1878–1946), Professor of Medicine, Lyons, described the sign in 1915.

Table 10.12 *Causes of Wasting of the Small Muscles of the Hand*

Spinal Cord Lesions
- Syringomyelia
- Cervical spondylosis with compression of the C8 segment
- Tumour

Anterior Horn Cell Disease
- Motor neurone disease, poliomyelitis
- Spinal muscular atrophies, e.g., Kugelberg-Welander* disease

Root Lesion
- C8 compression by a disc lesion

Brachial Plexus Lesion
- Thoracic outlet syndromes
- Trauma, radiation, infiltration

Peripheral Nerve Lesions
- Median and ulnar nerve lesions
- Peripheral motor neuropathy

Myopathy
- Dystrophia myotonica—forearms are more affected than the hands
- Distal myopathy

Trophic Disorders
- Arthropathies (disuse)
- Ischaemia, including vasculitis
- Shoulder-hand syndrome

NB: Distinguishing an ulnar nerve lesion from a C8 root/lower trunk brachial plexus lesion depends on remembering that sensory loss with a C8 lesion extends proximal to the wrist, and the thenar muscles are involved with a C8 root or lower trunk brachial plexus lesion. Distinguishing a C8 root from a lower trunk brachial plexus lesion is difficult clinically, but the presence of a Horner's syndrome or an axillary mass suggests that the brachial plexus is affected.
* E Kugelberg and L Welander described this in 1956.

Inspect the legs with the patient lying in bed with the legs and thighs entirely exposed (place a towel over the groin). Note if there is a urinary catheter present, which may indicate that there is spinal cord compression or other spinal cord disease, particularly multiple sclerosis.

The Motor System

Fasciculations and Muscle Wasting

Inspect for fasciculations. Look for muscle wasting. Feel the muscle bulk of the quadriceps and calves. Then run a hand along each shin feeling for wasting of the anterior tibial muscles.

Tone

Test tone at the knees and ankles. Place one hand under a chosen knee and then flick the knee upwards causing flexion. When the patient is relaxed this should occur without resistance. Then, supporting the thigh, flex and extend the knee at increasing velocity feeling for resistance to muscle stretch (tone).

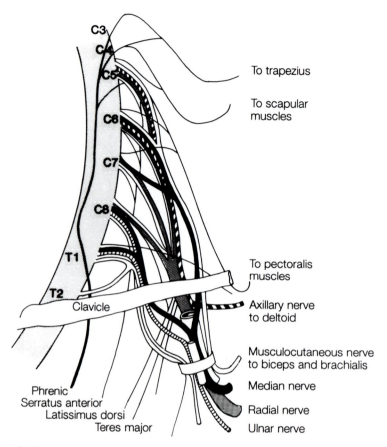

To trapezius

To scapular
muscles

To pectoralis
muscles

Axillary nerve
to deltoid

Musculocutaneous nerve
to biceps and brachialis

Median nerve

Radial nerve

Ulnar nerve

C3
C4
C5
C6
C7
C8
T1
T2
Clavicle

Phrenic
Serratus anterior
Latissimus dorsi
Teres major

Figure 10.33 *The brachial plexus.*

Adapted from Chusid JG. Correlative neuroanatomy and functional neurology. 19th ed. Los Altos: Lange
Medical, 1985. Published with permission.

Next test for *clonus* of the ankle and knee. This is a sustained rhythmical
contraction of the muscles when put under sudden stretch. It is due to hypertonia
from an upper motor neurone lesion. It represents an increase in reflex excitability
(from increased alpha motor neurone activity).

Sharply dorsiflex the foot with the knee bent and the thigh externally rotated.
When ankle clonus is present, recurrent ankle plantar flexion movement occurs.
This may persist for as long as the examiner sustains dorsiflexion of the ankle. Test
for patellar clonus (which is not as common) by resting the hand on the lower part
of the quadriceps with the knee extended and moving the patella down sharply.
Sustained rhythmical contraction of the quadriceps occurs as long as the downward stretch is maintained.

Power

Test power next.

Hip. *Flexion* (L2, L3): ask the patient to lift up the straight leg and not let you
push it down (having placed your hand above the knee). *Extension* (L5, S1, S2):

Table 10.13 *Brachial Plexus Lesions (Figure 10.33)*

Complete Lesion
1. Lower motor neurone signs affect the whole arm
2. Sensory loss (whole limb)
3. Horner's syndrome (an important clue)
NB: This is often painful.

Upper Lesion (Erb* Duchenne) (C5, C6)
1. Loss of shoulder movement and elbow flexion—the hand is held in the waiter's tip position
2. Sensory loss over the lateral aspect of the arm and forearm

Lower Lesion (Klumpke†) (C8, T1)
1. True claw hand with paralysis of all the intrinsic muscles
2. Sensory loss along the ulnar side of the hand and forearm
3. Horner's syndrome

Cervical Rib Syndrome
1. Weakness and wasting of the small muscles of the hand (claw hand)
2. C8 and T1 sensory loss
3. Unequal radial pulses and blood pressure
4. Subclavian bruits on arm manoeuvring (may be present in normal persons)
5. Palpable cervical rib in the neck (uncommon)

* Wilhelm Heinrich Erb (1840–1921), German neurologist.
† Auguste Déjérine-Klumpke (1859–1927), French neurologist, described this lesion as a student. She was an American but was educated in Switzerland. As a final year student she married the great French neurologist Jules Déjérine.

Table 10.14 *Shoulder Girdle Examination*

Method
Abnormalities are likely to be due to a muscular dystrophy, single nerve or a root lesion. Inspect each muscle, palpate its bulk and test function as follows.

From the Back
1. Trapezius (XI, C3, C4): Ask the patient to elevate the shoulders against resistance and look for winging of the upper scapula.
2. Serratus anterior (C5—C7): Ask the patient to push the hands against the wall and look for winging of the lower scapula.
3. Rhomboids (C4, C5): Ask the patient to pull both shoulder blades together with the hands on the hips.
4. Supraspinatus (C5, C6): Ask the patient to abduct the arms from the sides against resistance.
5. Infraspinatus (C5, C6): Ask the patient to rotate the upper arms externally against resistance with the elbows flexed at the sides.
6. Teres major (C5—C7): Ask the patient to internally rotate the upper arms against resistance.
7. Latissimus dorsi (C7, C8): Ask the patient to cough and palpate on both sides.

From the Front
1. Pectoralis major, clavicular head (C5-C8): Ask the patient to lift the upper arms above the horizontal and push them forward against resistance.
2. Pectoralis major, sternocostal part (C6-T1) and pectoralis minor (C7): Ask the patient to adduct the upper arms against resistance.
3. Deltoid (C5, C6) (and axillary nerve): Ask the patient to abduct the arms against resistance.

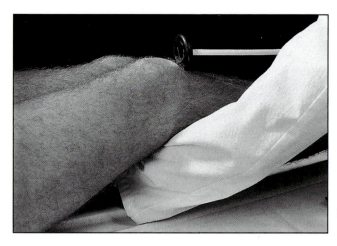

Figure 10.34
The knee jerk.

ask the patient to keep the leg down and not let you pull it up from underneath the calf or ankle. *Abduction* (L4, L5, S1): ask the patient to abduct the leg and not let you push it in. *Adduction* (L2, L3, L4): ask the patient to keep the leg adducted and not let you push it out.

Knee. *Flexion* (L5, S1): ask the patient to bend the knee and not let you straighten it. *Extension* (L3, L4): with the knee slightly bent, ask the patient to straighten the knee and not to let you bend it.

Ankle. *Plantar flexion* (S1, S2): ask the patient to push the foot down and not let you push it up. *Dorsiflexion* (L4, L5): ask the patient to bring the foot up and not let you push it down. *Eversion* (L5, S1): with the foot in complete plantar flexion, ask the patient to evert the foot against resistance. *Inversion* (L5, S1): ask the patient to invert the foot against resistance.

Reflexes

Knee jerk (L3, L4): slide one arm under the knees so they are slightly bent and supported. The tendon hammer is allowed to fall on to the infrapatellar tendon (Figure 10.34). Normally, contraction of the quadriceps causes extension of the knee. Compare the two sides. If the knee jerk appears to be absent on one or both sides it should be tested again following a reinforcement manoeuvre. Ask the patient to interlock the fingers and then pull apart hard at the moment before the hammer strikes the tendon (Jendrassik's* manoeuvre). A reinforcement manoeuvre such as this or teeth clenching or grasping an object should be used if one has difficulty eliciting any of the deep tendon reflexes.

Ankle jerk (S1, S2): have the foot in the mid-position at the ankle with the knee bent, the thigh externally rotated on the bed, and the foot held in dorsiflexion by the examiner. The hammer is allowed to fall on the Achilles tendon. The normal response is plantar flexion of the foot with contraction of the gastrocnemius muscle. Again test with reinforcement if appropriate. This reflex can also be tested with the patient kneeling (page 387, Figure 10.35).

Plantar reflex (L5, S1, S2): after telling the patient about what is to occur, use a blunt object such as the key to an expensive motor car to stroke up the lateral

---

* Ernst Jendrassik (1858–1921), Budapest physician.

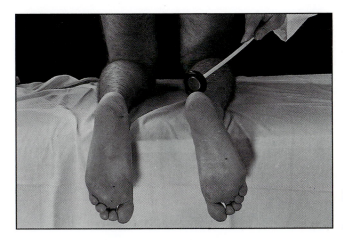

Figure 10.35
The ankle jerk (second method).

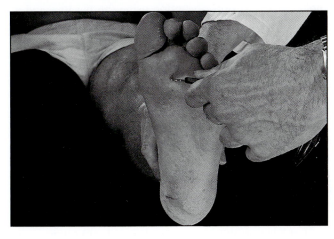

Figure 10.36
The plantar reflex.

aspect of the sole, and curve inwards before it reaches the toes moving towards the middle metatarsophalangeal (MTP) joint (Figure 10.36). The patient's foot should be in the same position as for testing the ankle jerk. The normal response is flexion of the big toe at the MTP joint in patients over one year of age. The extensor (Babinski*) response is abnormal and is characterised by extension of the big toe at the MTP joint (the upgoing toe) and fanning of the other toes. This indicates an upper motor neurone (pyramidal) lesion. Bilateral upgoing toes may also be found after a generalised seizure, or in a patient in coma.

Coordination

Test for cerebellar disease with three manoeuvres.

Heel-shin test: ask the patient to run the heel of one foot up and down the opposite shin at a moderate pace and as accurately as possible. In cerebellar disease the heel wobbles all over the place with oscillations from side to side and

---

*   Josef Babinski (1857–1932), Parisian neurologist of Polish extraction, described this sign in 1896.

overshooting. Closing the eyes makes little difference to this in cerebellar disease, but if there is posterior column loss the movements are made worse when the eyes are shut, that is, there is 'sensory ataxia'.

Toe-finger test: unfortunately, a toe-nose test is not a practical way of assessing the lower limbs, so a toe-finger test is used. Ask the patient to lift the foot (with the knee bent) and touch the examiner's finger with the big toe. Look for intention tremor.

Foot-tapping test: rapidly alternating movements are tested by getting the patient to tap the sole of the foot quickly on the examiner's hand or tap the heel on the opposite shin.

The Sensory System

As for the upper limb, test for pain sensation first in each dermatome, comparing the right with the left side. Map out any abnormality and decide on the pattern of loss.

Then test vibration sense over the ankles, and if necessary on the knees and the anterior superior iliac spines. Next test proprioception using the big toes and, if necessary, the knees and hips.

Finally, test light touch.

Dermatomes

Memorise the following rough guide (Figure 10.37): L2 supplies the upper thigh; L3 supplies the area around the knees; L4 supplies the medial aspect of the leg; L5 supplies the lateral aspect of the leg and the medial side of the dorsum of the foot; S1 supplies the heel and most of the sole; S2 supplies the posterior aspect of the thigh; S3, S4 and S5 supply concentric rings around the anus.

Sensory Levels

If there is peripheral sensory loss attempt to map out the upper level (Figure 10.38). This may involve testing over the abdominal or even the chest dermatomes. Establishing a sensory level on the trunk indicates the spinal cord level that is affected. Remember, a level of hyperaesthesia (increased sensitivity) often occurs above the sensory level and it is the upper level of this that should be determined as it usually indicates the highest affected spinal segment. Also remember that the level of a vertebral body only corresponds to the spinal cord level in the upper cervical cord because the spinal cord is shorter than the spinal canal. The C8 spinal segment lies opposite the C7 vertebra. In the upper thoracic cord there is a difference of about two segments and in the mid-thoracic cord three segments. All the lumbosacral segments are opposite the T11 to L1 vertebrae.

The Abdominal Reflexes (epigastric T6–T9, mid-abdominal T9–T11, lower abdominal T11—L1)

Test these by lightly stroking the abdominal wall diagonally towards the umbilicus in each of the four quadrants of the abdomen. Reflex contractions of the abdominal wall are absent in upper motor neurone lesions above the segmental level and also in patients who have had surgical operations interrupting the nerves. They are usually difficult to elicit in obese patients and can also be absent in some normal people.

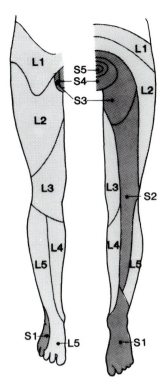

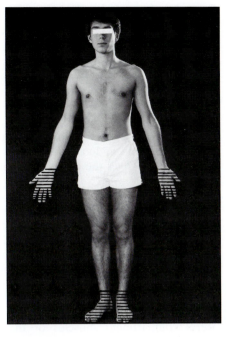

Figure 10.38

Peripheral neuropathy: glove and stocking sensory loss.

Figure 10.37

Dermatomes of the lower limb.

Adapted from and used with permission of Lance JW, McLeod JG. A physiological approach to clinical neurology. 3rd ed. London: Butterworths, 1981.

The Cremasteric Reflexes (L1–L2)

Stroke the inner part of the thigh in a downward direction; normally contraction of the cremasteric muscle pulls up the scrotum and testis on the side stroked.

Saddle Sensation and Anal Reflex

Test now for saddle sensation if a cauda equina lesion is suspected (e.g., because of urinary incontinence). The only sensory loss may be on the buttocks or around the anus (S3 to S5). In this case also test the anal reflex (S2, S3, S4): normal contraction of the external sphincter in response to scratching the perianal skin is abolished in patients with a lesion of the sacral segments of the cauda equina. If, however, the lowest sacral segments are spared but the higher ones are involved this suggests that there is an intrinsic cord lesion.

Spine

Examine the spine and perform the straight leg raising test (page 265).

Examination of the Peripheral Nerves of the Lower Limb

Lateral Cutaneous Nerve of the Thigh

Test for sensory loss. A lesion of this nerve, which usually occurs because of entrapment at the inguinal ligament, causes a sensory loss over the lateral aspect of the thigh with no motor loss detectable. If painful it is called meralgia paraesthetica.

Femoral Nerve (L2, L3, L4)

Test for weakness of knee extension (quadriceps paralysis). Hip flexion weakness is only slight, and adductor strength is preserved. The knee jerk is absent. The sensory loss involves the inner aspect of the thigh and leg.

Sciatic Nerve (L4, L5, S1, S2)

This nerve supplies all the muscles below the knee and some of the hamstrings. Test for loss of power below the knee resulting in a foot drop and for weakness of knee flexion. Test the reflexes: with a sciatic nerve lesion the knee jerk is intact but the ankle jerk and plantar response are absent. Test sensation on the posterior thigh, lateral and posterior calf, and on the foot (lost with a proximal nerve lesion).

Common Peroneal Nerve (L4, L5, S1)

This is a major terminal branch of the sciatic nerve. It supplies the anterior and lateral compartment muscles of the leg. On inspection one may notice a plantarflexed foot (footdrop) (Table 10.15). Test for weakness of dorsiflexion and eversion. Test the reflexes which will all be intact. Test for sensory loss. There is only minimal sensory loss over the lateral aspect of the dorsum of the foot. Note that these findings can be confused with an L5 root lesion, but the latter includes weakness of knee flexion and loss of foot inversion, as well as sensory loss in the L5 distribution.

Gait

Method

Make sure the patient's legs are clearly visible. Now ask the patient to walk normally for a few metres and then turn around quickly and walk back. Then ask the patient to walk heel-to-toe to exclude a midline cerebellar lesion. Ask the patient to then walk on the toes (an S1 lesion will make this difficult) and then on the heels (an L4 or L5 lesion causing footdrop will make this difficult).

Test for proximal myopathy by asking the patient to squat and then stand up, or sit in a low chair and then stand.

Table 10.15 *Causes of Footdrop*

Common peroneal nerve palsy
Sciatic nerve palsy
Lumbosacral plexus lesion
L4, L5 root lesion
Peripheral motor neuropathy
Distal myopathy
Motor neurone disease
Stroke—anterior cerebral artery or lacunar syndrome ('ataxic hemiparesis')

Table 10.16 *Gait Disorders*

Hemiplegia: the foot is plantar flexed and the leg is swung in a lateral arc
Spastic paraparesis: scissors gait
Parkinson's disease: hesitation in starting
                shuffling
                freezing
                festination
                propulsion
                retropulsion
Cerebellar: a drunken gait which is wide based or reeling on a narrow base; the patient
    staggers towards the affected side if there is a unilateral cerebellar hemisphere lesion
Posterior column lesion: clumsy slapping down of the feet on a broad base
Footdrop: high stepping gait
Proximal myopathy: waddling gait
Prefrontal lobe (apraxic): feet appear glued to floor when erect, but move more easily
    when the patient is supine
Hysterical: characterised by a bizarre, inconsistent gait

To test *station*, ask the patient to stand erect with the feet together and the eyes open. Once the patient is stable ask him or her to close the eyes. Compare the steadiness shown with the eyes open then closed. Even in the absence of neurological disease a person may be slightly unsteady with the eyes closed. Marked unsteadiness with the eyes closed is seen with cerebellar or vestibular dysfunction.

The Romberg* test is positive when unsteadiness increases with eye closure. This is usually seen with the loss of proprioceptive sensation.

Gait disorders are summarised in Table 10.16.

Correlation of Physical Signs and Neurological Disease

Upper Motor Neurone Lesions

In neurology a clinical diagnosis is made by defining the deficit which is present, deciding on its anatomical level and then considering the likely causes. It is important to be able to distinguish *upper motor neurone* signs from *lower motor neurone* signs (Figure 10.39). The former occur when a lesion has interrupted a neural pathway at a level above the anterior horn cell; for example, motor pathways in the cerebral cortex, internal capsule, cerebral peduncles, brainstem or spinal cord. When this occurs there is weakness of abductors and extensors in the upper limb, and flexors and abductors in the lower limb, as the normal function of this pathway is to mediate voluntary contraction of the antigravity muscles. Muscle wasting is slight or absent, probably because there is no loss of trophic factors normally released from the lower motor neurone.

Spasticity occurs because of destruction of the corticoreticulospinal tract resulting in stretch reflex hyperactivity.

Monoplegia is paralysis affecting only one limb, when there is a motor cortex or partial internal capsule lesion. *Hemiplegia* affects one side of the body due to a

---

*   Mortz Heinrich Romberg (1795–1873), Berlin professor, wrote the first modern neurology textbook.

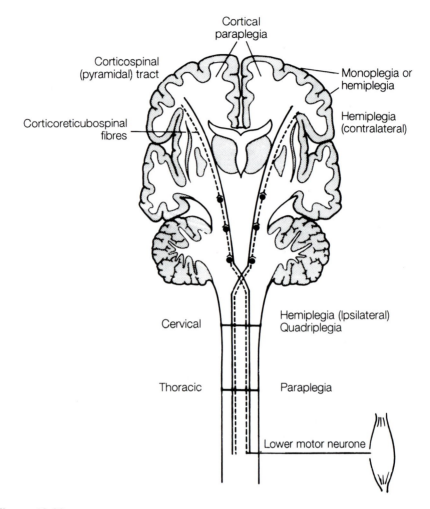

Figure 10.39 *Upper and lower motor neurone lesions.*

Adapted from Lance JG, McLeod JW. A physiological approach to clinical neurology. 3rd ed. London: Butterworths, 1981. Published with permission.

lesion affecting projection of pathways from the contralateral motor cortex. *Para-plegia* affects both legs, while *quadriplegia* affects all four limbs, and is the result of spinal cord trauma or, less often, a brainstem lesion (e.g., basilar artery thrombosis).

Causes of Hemiplegia (Upper Motor Neurone Lesion)

Vascular disease: thrombosis, embolism or haemorrhage occur in specific vascular territories (Figure 10.40). Lesions in the territory of the *internal carotid artery* result in hemiplegia on the opposite side of the body if a large area of the internal capsule or hemisphere is involved. Homonymous hemianopia, hemianaesthesia

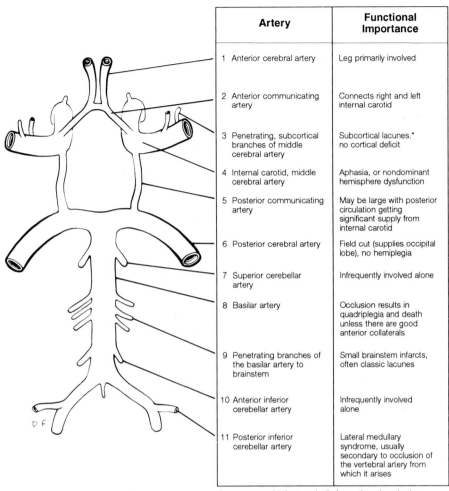

Artery	Functional Importance
1 Anterior cerebral artery	Leg primarily involved
2 Anterior communicating artery	Connects right and left internal carotid
3 Penetrating, subcortical branches of middle cerebral artery	Subcortical lacunes.* no cortical deficit
4 Internal carotid, middle cerebral artery	Aphasia, or nondominant hemisphere dysfunction
5 Posterior communicating artery	May be large with posterior circulation getting significant supply from internal carotid
6 Posterior cerebral artery	Field cut (supplies occipital lobe), no hemiplegia
7 Superior cerebellar artery	Infrequently involved alone
8 Basilar artery	Occlusion results in quadriplegia and death unless there are good anterior collaterals
9 Penetrating branches of the basilar artery to brainstem	Small brainstem infarcts, often classic lacunes
10 Anterior inferior cerebellar artery	Infrequently involved alone
11 Posterior inferior cerebellar artery	Lateral medullary syndrome, usually secondary to occlusion of the vertebral artery from which it arises

*Lacunes: small infacts typically from atherothrombotic occlusive disease of the penetrating branches.

Figure 10.40 *Anatomy of the circle of Willis. The functional importance of the arterial blood supply is shown.*

Adapted, with permission, from Weiner HL, Levitt LP. Neurology for the house officer. 4th ed. Baltimore: Williams & Wilkins, 1989.

and dysphasia may occur (Table 10.17). Stenosis of the internal carotid artery in the neck may be associated with a bruit.

Lesions in the territory of the *vertebrobasilar artery* may produce cranial nerve palsies, cerebellar signs, Horner's syndrome and sensory loss, as well as upper motor neurone signs (often bilateral because of the close proximity of structures in the brainstem). For example, a lesion in the midbrain may be associated with a third nerve paralysis and upper motor neurone signs on the opposite side. Hemianaesthesia and homonymous hemianopia may occur if the posterior cerebral arteries are affected.

Table 10.17   *Intracerebral Thrombosis or Embolism: Clinical Features*

Middle Cerebral Artery	Posterior Cerebral Artery	Anterior Cerebral Artery
Main Branch	Main Branch*	
Infarction middle third of hemisphere: UMN face, arm > leg; homonymous hemianopia; aphasia or non-dominant hemisphere signs (depends on side); cortical sensory loss	Infarction of thalamus and occipital cortex: hemianaesthesia (loss of all modalities); homonymous hemianopia (complete)	UMN leg > arm; cortical sensory loss leg only; urinary incontinence
Perforating Artery		
Internal capsule infarction: UMN VII, UMN arm > leg		

UMN = upper motor neurone lesion
* Effects variable because of anastomoses with distal middle cerebral artery branches and supply from posterior communicating artery, but one would examine particularly for occipital and temporal lobe dysfunction.

Compressive and infiltrative lesions: tumours tend to occur in the lobes of the brain, and focal signs will depend on the tumour site. Signs localised to the parietal, temporal, occipital or frontal lobe suggest this disease process (Table 10.3). There may, however, be false localising signs in the presence of raised intracranial pressure; for example, a unilateral or bilateral sixth nerve palsy (because of the nerve's long intracranial path). Papilloedema is usually associated if there is raised intracranial pressure.

Demyelinating disease: multiple sclerosis results in lesions in different areas usually with a relapsing and remitting course.

Infection: human immunodeficiency virus infection.

Lower Motor Neurone Lesions

Lower motor neurone lesions interrupt the spinal reflex arc and therefore cause muscle wasting, reduced or absent reflexes and often fasciculations. This results from a lesion of the spinal motor neurones, motor root or peripheral nerve (Table 10.18).

Motor Neurone Disease

This disease of unknown aetiology results in pathological changes in the anterior horn cells, the motor nuclei of the medulla and the tracts. It therefore causes a combination of upper motor neurone and lower motor neurone signs, although one type may predominate. Importantly, fasciculations are almost always present. The deep tendon reflexes are usually present (often increased) until late in the course of the disease and there are rarely any objective sensory changes (15% to 20% of patients report sensory symptoms).

Peripheral Neuropathy

Distal parts of the nerves are usually involved first because of their distance from the cell bodies, causing a distal loss of sensation or motor function or both in the

Table 10.18 *Upper and Lower Motor Neurone Lesions (Figure 10.39)*

Signs of Upper Motor Neurone Lesions

1. Weakness is present which in the lower limb is more marked in the flexor and abductor muscles. In the upper limb, weakness is most marked in the abductors and extensors. There is very little muscle wasting.
2. Spasticity: increased tone is present (may be clasp-knife) and often associated with clonus.
3. The reflexes are increased except for the superficial reflexes (e.g., abdominal) which are absent.
4. There is an extensor (Babinski) plantar response (upgoing toe).

Signs of Lower Motor Neurone Lesions

1. Weakness may be more obvious distally than proximally, and the flexor and extensor muscles are equally involved. Wasting is a prominent feature.
2. Tone is reduced.
3. The reflexes are reduced and the plantar response is normal or absent.
4. Fasciculation may be present.

limbs. A typical sensory change is a symmetrical glove and stocking loss to all modalities (Figure 10.38). This is unlike the pattern found with individual nerve or nerve root disease which should be suspected if sensory loss is asymmetrical or confined to one limb. Peripheral muscle weakness may be present due to motor nerve involvement. Occasionally motor neuropathy may occur without sensory change. In the latter case, reflexes are reduced but may not be absent in the distal parts of the limbs (Table 10.19).

Guillain-Barré Syndrome (Acute Inflammatory Polyradiculoneuropathy)

This disease, thought to have an immune basis, may begin seven to ten days after an infective illness. It results in flaccid proximal and distal muscle paralysis, which typically ascends from the lower to the upper limbs. Wasting is rare. The cranial nerves can be affected; occasionally disease is confined to these. Sensory loss is minimal or absent. Unlike transverse myelitis, the sphincters are little affected. Weakness of the respiratory muscles can be fatal but the disease is usually self-limiting. HIV infection can cause a similar syndrome.

Thickened Peripheral Nerves

If there is evidence of a peripheral nerve lesion, peripheral neuropathy or a mononeuritis multiplex (Table 10.20), palpate for thickened nerves. The median nerve at the wrist, the ulnar nerve at the elbow, the greater auricular nerve in the neck and the common peroneal nerve at the head of the fibula are the most easily accessible. If nerves are thickened consider the following diagnoses:

Acromegaly (page 308)
Amyloid
Chronic inflammatory demyelinating polyradiculoneuropathy
Leprosy
Hereditary motor and sensory neuropathy (autosomal dominant) (Table 10.26)
Other—e.g., sarcoid, diabetes mellitus, neurofibromatosis.

Table 10.19 *Peripheral Neuropathy (Figure 10.38)*

Causes of Peripheral Neuropathy
1. Drugs—e.g., isoniazid, vincristine, phenytoin, nitrofurantoin, cisplatinum, heavy metals, amiodarone
2. Alcohol abuse (with or without vitamin B_1 deficiency)
3. Metabolic—e.g., diabetes mellitus, chronic renal failure
4. Guillain-Barré syndrome
5. Malignancy—e.g., carcinoma of the lung (paraneoplastic neuropathy), leukaemia, lymphoma
6. Vitamin deficiency (e.g., B_{12}) or excess (e.g., B_6)
7. Connective tissue disease or vasculitis—e.g., PAN, SLE
8. Hereditary—e.g., hereditary motor and sensory neuropathy
9. Others—e.g., amyloid, HIV infection
10. Idiopathic

Causes of a Predominant Motor Neuropathy
1. Guillain-Barré syndrome, chronic inflammatory polyradiculoneuropathy
2. Hereditary motor and sensory neuropathy
3. Diabetes mellitus
4. Others—e.g., acute intermittent porphyria, lead poisoning, diphtheria, multifocal conduction block neuropathy

Causes of a Painful Peripheral Neuropathy
1. Diabetes mellitus
2. Alcohol
3. Vitamin B_1 or B_{12} deficiency
4. Carcinoma
5. Porphyria
6. Arsenic or thallium poisoning

PAN = polyarteritis nodosa   SLE = systemic lupus erythematosus   HIV =human immunodeficiency virus

Table 10.20 *Mononeuritis Multiplex*

Definition: Mononeuritis multiplex refers to the separate involvement of more than one peripheral (or less often cranial) nerve by a single disease

Acute Causes (usually vascular)
- Polyarteritis nodosa
- Diabetes mellitus
- Connective tissue disease—e.g., rheumatoid arthritis, systemic lupus erythematosus

Chronic Causes
- Multiple compressive neuropathies
- Sarcoidosis
- Acromegaly
- HIV infection
- Leprosy
- Lyme disease
- Others—e.g., carcinoma (rare)

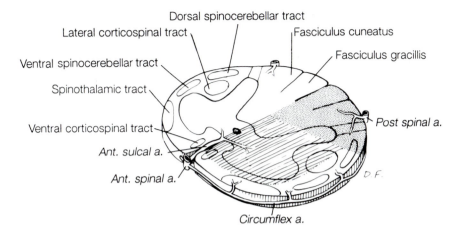

Dorsal spinocerebellar tract

Lateral corticospinal tract

Fasciculus cuneatus

Ventral spinocerebellar tract

Fasciculus gracillis

Spinothalamic tract

Ventral corticospinal tract

Post spinal a.

Ant. sulcal a.

Ant. spinal a.

D.F.

Circumflex a.

Figure 10.41 *Anatomy and vascular supply of the spinal cord. Note anterior spinal artery occlusion spares posterior column function.*

Spinal Cord Compression (Figures 10.41 to 10.45)

It is important to remember that a spinal cord lesion causes lower motor neurone signs at the level of the lesion and upper motor neurone signs below that level (Table 10.21). Don't forget the spinal cord's anatomy and vascular supply (Figure 10.41). Examine any suspected case as follows.

After carefully examining the lower limbs (see above) determine the level of any sensory impairment (Table 10.22). Then examine the back for signs of a local lesion. Look for deformity, scars and neurofibromas. Palpate for vertebral tenderness and auscultate down the spine for bruits. Next examine the upper limbs and cranial nerves to determine the upper level if this is not already obvious.

Important Spinal Cord Syndromes

Brown-Séquard Syndrome*

Clinical features are shown in Figure 10.46. These signs result from hemisection of the cord.

Motor changes: (i) upper motor neurone signs below the hemisection on the *same* side as the lesion; (ii) lower motor neurone signs at the level of the hemisection on the *same* side.

Sensory changes: (i) pain and temperature loss on the *opposite* side to the lesion—NB: the upper level of sensory loss is usually a few segments below the

---

*   Charles Edouard Brown-Séquard (1817–1894) succeeded Claude Bernard at the College de France. He was the son of an American sea captain and a French woman. He was born in Mauritius at a time when it was under British rule. With this background he roved around the world, working in Paris, Mauritius, London and New York. His syndrome usually arose from failed murder attempts. Traditionally Mauritian cane cutters, when trying to murder someone, used a very long thin knife which was slipped between the ribs from behind, to cut the aorta or penetrate the heart. Only such a knife could have caused a cord hemitransection.

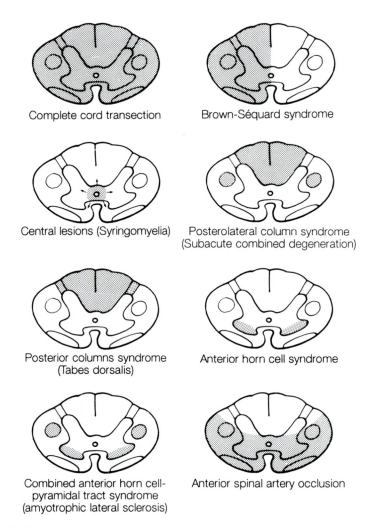

Complete cord transection

Brown-Séquard syndrome

Central lesions (Syringomyelia)

Posterolateral column syndrome
(Subacute combined degeneration)

Posterior columns syndrome
(Tabes dorsalis)

Anterior horn cell syndrome

Combined anterior horn cell-
pyramidal tract syndrome
(amyotrophic lateral sclerosis)

Anterior spinal artery occlusion

Figure 10.42 *Spinal cord syndromes.*

From Brazis PW, Masdeu JC, Biller J. Localisation in clinical neurology. Boston: Little Brown, 1985, with permission.

level of the lesion; (ii) vibration and proprioception loss occur on the *same* side; (iii) light touch is often normal.

   Causes: (i) multiple sclerosis; (ii) angioma; (iii) trauma; (iv) myelitis; (v) post-radiation myelopathy.

Subacute Combined Degeneration of the Cord
(Vitamin B$_{12}$ Deficiency)

Clinical features: (i) posterior column loss symmetrically (vibration and joint position sense), causing an ataxic gait; (ii) upper motor neurone signs in the lower

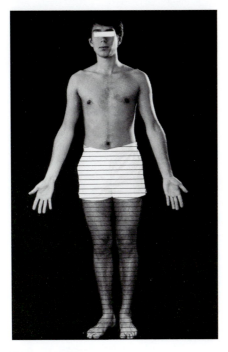

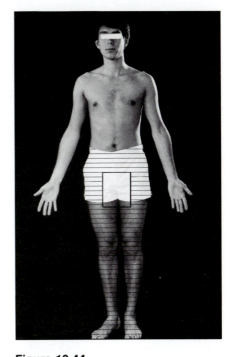

Figure 10.43

Sensory loss with transverse section of the spinal cord.

Figure 10.44

Pattern of sensory loss with intrinsic spinal cord disease, e.g., central tumour or less commonly with extrinsic compression of the spinal cord—sacrum is spared.

limbs symmetrically with absent ankle reflexes; knee reflexes may be absent or, more often, exaggerated. There may also be (iii) peripheral sensory neuropathy (less common and mild); (iv) optic atrophy; (v) dementia.

Dissociated Sensory Loss

This usually indicates spinal cord disease but may occur with a peripheral neuropathy.

Causes of spinothalamic loss only: (i) syringomyelia; (ii) Brown-Séquard syndrome (contralateral leg); (iii) anterior spinal artery thrombosis; (iv) lateral medullary syndrome (contralateral to the other signs) (Figure 10.47); (v) peripheral neuropathy (e.g., diabetes mellitus, amyloid).

Causes of dorsal column loss only: (i) subacute combined degeneration; (ii) Brown-Séquard syndrome (ipsilateral leg); (iii) spinocerebellar degeneration (e.g., Friedreich's ataxia); (iv) multiple sclerosis; (v) tabes dorsalis; (vi) peripheral neuropathy (e.g., diabetes mellitus, hypothyroidism); (vii) sensory neuropathy (a predominant sensory neuropathy which may be caused by carcinoma, diabetes mellitus or Sjögren's syndrome).

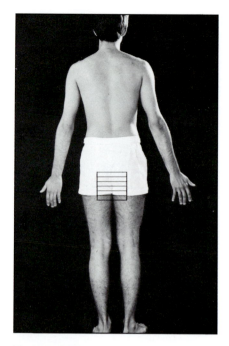

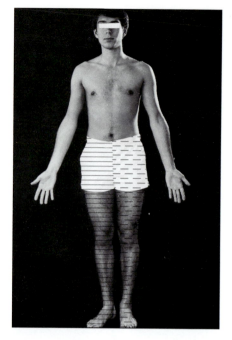

Figure 10.45

Conus medullaris or cauda equina lesion—saddle anaesthesia.

Figure 10.46

Brown-Séquard syndrome—loss of pain and temperature on the side opposite to the lesion, with loss of vibration and proprioception on the same side as the lesion.

Table 10.21   *Important Motor and Reflex Changes of Spinal Cord Compression*

See Figures 10.41 to 10.45 for sensory changes.

Upper Cervical:

Upper motor neurone signs in the upper and lower limbs.

C5:

Lower motor neurone weakness and wasting of rhomboids, deltoids, biceps and brachioradialis.

Upper motor neurone signs affect the rest of the upper and all the lower limbs. The biceps jerk is lost. The brachioradialis jerk is inverted.

C8:

Lower motor neurone weakness and wasting of the intrinsic muscles of the hand.
Upper motor neurone signs in the lower limbs.

Midthoracic:

Intercostal paralysis.
Upper motor neurone signs in the lower limbs.
Loss of upper abdominal reflexes at T7 and T8.

T10–T11:

Loss of the lower abdominal reflexes and upward displacement of the umbilicus.
Upper motor neurone signs in the lower limbs.

—continued

Table 10.21 *Important Motor and Reflex Changes of Spinal Cord Compression (continued)*

L1:

Cremasteric reflex is lost (normal abdominal reflexes).
Upper motor neurone signs in the lower limbs.

L4:

Lower motor neurone weakness and wasting of the quadriceps.
Knee jerks lost.
Ankle jerks may be hyper-reflexic with extensor plantar response (upgoing toes), but more
    often the whole conus is involved, causing a lower motor neurone lesion.

L5–S1:

Lower motor neurone weakness of knee flexion and hip extension (S1) and abduction
    (L5) plus calf and foot muscles.
Knee jerks present.
No ankle jerks or plantar responses.
Anal reflex present.

S3–S4:

No anal reflex.
Saddle sensory loss.
Normal lower limbs.

Causes of Spinal Cord Compression

1. Vertebral
   - Spondylosis
   - Trauma
   - Prolapse of a disc
   - Tumour
   - Infection
2. Outside the dura
   - Lymphoma, metastases
   - Infection—e.g., abscess
3. Within the dura but extramedullary
   - Tumour—e.g., meningioma, neurofibroma
4. Intramedullary*
   - Tumour—e.g., glioma, ependymoma
   - Syringomyelia
   - Haematomyelia

*   Lower motor neurone signs may extend for several segments, and spastic paralysis occurs late, unlike the
    situation with extramedullary lesions.

Syringomyelia (a central cavity in the spinal cord)

Clinical triad: (i) loss of pain and temperature over the neck, shoulders and arms (a 'cape' distribution); (ii) amyotrophy (atrophy and areflexia) of the arms; (iii) upper motor neurone signs in the lower limbs.

There may also possibly be thoracic scoliosis due to asymmetrical weakness of the paravertebral muscles.

An Extensor Plantar Response Plus Absent Knee and Ankle Jerks

Causes: (i) subacute combined degeneration of the cord (B_{12} deficiency); (ii) conus medullaris lesion; (iii) combination of an upper motor neurone lesion with cauda

Table 10.22   *Important Patterns of Abnormal Sensation*

Sign	Location of Lesion
Total unilateral loss of all forms of sensation	Thalamus or upper brainstem (extensive lesion)
Pain and temperature loss on one side of face and *opposite* side of body	Medulla involving descending nucleus of spinal tract of the fifth nerve and ascending spinothalamic tract (lateral medullary lesion) (Figure 10.47)
Bilateral loss of all forms of sensation below a definite level	Spinal cord lesion (if only pain and temperature affected: anterior cord lesion)
Unilateral loss of pain and temperature below a definite level	Partial unilateral spinal cord lesion on opposite side (Brown-Séquard syndrome) (Figure 10.46)
Loss of pain and temperature over several segments but normal sensation above and below	Intrinsic spinal cord lesion near its centre anteriorly (involves the crossing fibres), e.g., syringomyelia, intrinsic cord tumour (NB: more posterior lesions cause proprioceptive loss)
Loss of sensation over many segments with sacral sparing	Intrinsic cord compression more likely
Saddle sensory loss (lowest sacral segments)	Cauda equina lesion (touch preserved in conus medullaris lesions)
Loss of position and vibration sense only	Posterior column lesion
Glove and stocking loss (hands and feet)	Peripheral neuropathy
Loss of all forms of sensation over a well-defined body part only	Posterior root lesion (purely sensory) or peripheral nerve (often motor abnormality associated)

equina compression or peripheral neuropathy, e.g., stroke in an alcoholic; (iv) syphilis (tabo-paresis); (v) Friedreich's ataxia; (vi) motor neurone disease; (vii) diabetes mellitus (uncommon); (viii) human T-cell lymphoma virus (HTLV-I) infection.

A summary of the features that differentiate intramedullary from extra-medullary cord lesions is presented in Table 10.23.

Myopathy

Muscle weakness can be due to individual peripheral nerve lesions, mononeuritis multiplex, peripheral neuropathy or spinal cord disease. Each of these has a characteristic pattern. Primary disease of muscle (myopathy) also causes weakness. There is no sensory loss with myopathy, which is an important clue. The motor weakness is similar to that of the lower motor neurone type. There are two major patterns: proximal myopathy and distal myopathy.

Proximal myopathy is the more common form. On examination there is proximal muscle wasting and weakness (Tables 10.24 and 10.25) (Figure 10.48). Reflexes involving these muscles may be reduced. This can be caused by genetic (e.g.,

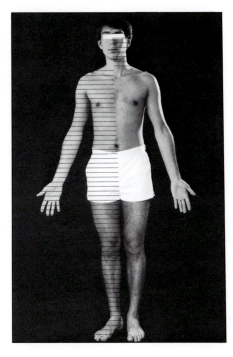

Figure 10.47
Pattern of sensory loss in the lateral medullary syndrome.

Table 10.23   *Differentiating Intramedullary from Extramedullary Cord Lesions*

Intramedullary	Extramedullary
Root pains rare	Root pains common
Late onset of corticospinal signs	Early onset of corticospinal signs
Lower motor neurone signs extend for several segments	Lower motor neurone signs localised
Dissociated sensory loss (pain and temperature) may be present	Brown-Séquard syndrome if lateral cord compression
Normal or minimally altered cerebrospinal fluid findings	Early, marked cerebrospinal fluid abnormalities
May have sacral sparing	

muscular dystrophy) or acquired disease. Distal myopathy also occurs, although peripheral neuropathy is a much more common cause of distal muscle weakness. If the distal limbs are affected, consider hereditary motor and sensory neuropathy (Table 10.26). Motor neurone disease also causes weakness without any sensory loss.

Dystrophia Myotonica

If this disease (which is inherited as an autosomal dominant condition) is suspected because of an inability on the part of the patient to let go when shaking hands (myotonia), or because general inspection reveals the characteristic appearance (Figure 10.49), examine as follows.

Table 10.24   *Causes of Proximal Weakness and Myopathy*

Causes of Proximal Weakness
- Myopathy (see below)
- Neuromuscular junction disease, e.g., myasthenia gravis
- Neurogenic, e.g., motor neurone disease, polyradiculopathy, Kugelberg-Welander disease (proximal muscle wasting and fasciculation due to anterior horn cell disease—autosomal recessive)

Causes of Myopathy
- Hereditary muscular dystrophy (Table 10.25)
- Congenital myopathies (rare)
- Acquired myopathy (mnemonic, PACHE, PODS)
  Polymyositis or dermatomyositis (Figure 10.48)
  Alcohol
  Carcinoma
  HIV infection
  Endocrine—e.g., hyperthyroidism, hypothyroidism, Cushing's syndrome, acromegaly, hypopituitarism
  Periodic paralysis (hyperkalaemic, hypokalaemic or normokalaemic)
  Osteomalacia
  Drugs—e.g., clofibrate, chloroquine, steroids, zidovudine
  Sarcoidosis
NB: Causes of *proximal myopathy with a peripheral neuropathy* include:
Paraneoplastic syndrome
Alcohol
Hypothyroidism
Connective tissue diseases

Table 10.25   *Muscular Dystrophies*

1. Duchenne's* (pseudohypertrophic)
   - Affects only males (sex-linked recessive)
   - Calves and deltoids: hypertrophied early, weak later
   - Proximal weakness: early
   - Dilated cardiomyopathy
2. Becker†
   - Affects only males (sex-linked recessive)
   - Similar clinical features to Duchenne's except for less heart disease, a later onset and less rapid progression
3. Limb girdle
   - Males or females (autosomal recessive), onset in the third decade
   - Shoulder or pelvic girdle affected
   - Face and heart usually spared
4. Facioscapulohumeral
   - Males or females (autosomal dominant)
   - Facial and pectoral weakness with hypertrophy of deltoids
5. Dystrophia myotonica (autosomal dominant)

* Guillaume Duchenne (1806–1875), brilliant eccentric who founded French neurology.
† Peter Becker (b. 1908), German Professor of Genetics.

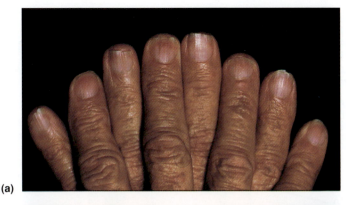

(a)

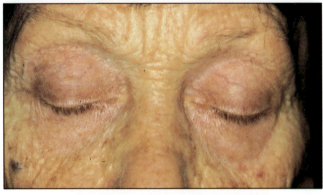

(b)

Figure 10.48 *(a) Gottren's sign in dermatomyositis—heliotrope (lilac-coloured) flat topped papules which occur over the knuckles but may also be seen over the elbows or knees and may ulcerate.*

(b) Dermatomyositis and the closely related condition polymyositis are idiopathic myopathies. Dermatomyositis may also cause a heliotrope rash on the face (especially on the eyelids, upper cheeks and forehead), periorbital oedema, erythema, maculopapular eruptions and scaling dermatitis. Up to 10% of adult patients with dermatomyositis may have an underlying malignancy.

Table   10.26 *Features   of   Hereditary   Motor   and   Sensory   Neuropathy (Charcot-Marie-Tooth* Disease)*

1. Pes cavus (short arched feet)
2. Distal muscle atrophy due to peripheral nerve degeneration. This does not usually extend above the elbows or above the middle third of the thighs
3. Absent reflexes
4. Slight or no sensory loss in the limbs
5. Thickened nerves
6. Optic atrophy, Argyll-Robertson pupils (rare)

*   Jean Martin Charcot (1825–1893), Parisian physician and neurologist; Pierre Marie (1853–1940), Parisian neurologist and Charcot's greatest pupil; and Howard Henry Tooth (1856–1926), London physician, who described the condition independently in 1886. Type I is usually autosomal dominant.

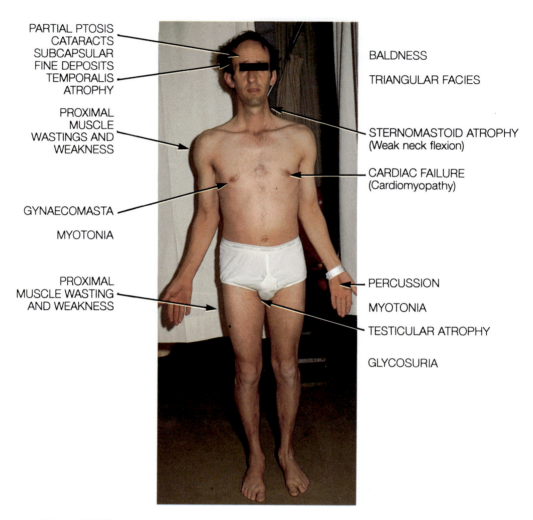

PARTIAL PTOSIS
CATARACTS
SUBCAPSULAR
FINE DEPOSITS
TEMPORALIS
ATROPHY

PROXIMAL
MUSCLE
WASTINGS AND
WEAKNESS

GYNAECOMASTA

MYOTONIA

PROXIMAL
MUSCLE WASTING
AND WEAKNESS

BALDNESS

TRIANGULAR FACIES

STERNOMASTOID ATROPHY
(Weak neck flexion)

CARDIAC FAILURE
(Cardiomyopathy)

PERCUSSION

MYOTONIA

TESTICULAR ATROPHY

GLYCOSURIA

Figure 10.49 *Dystrophia myotonica.*

Observe the face for frontal baldness (the patient may be wearing a wig), the expressionless triangular facies, atrophy of the temporalis muscle and partial ptosis. Note: thick spectacles, a traditional sign of this disease, are not often seen now because of lens surgery. One should still examine the eyes as these patients can develop senile cataracts and subcapsular fine deposits.

Look at the neck for atrophy of the sternomastoid muscles and then test neck flexion (neck flexion is weak while extension is normal).

Go to the upper limbs. Shake hands and test for percussion myotonia. Tapping over the thenar eminence causes contraction and then slow relaxation of abductor pollicis brevis. Examine the arm now for signs of wasting and weakness distally (forearms are usually affected first) and proximally. There are no sensory changes.

Go to the chest and look for gynaecomastia (uncommon). Examine the cardio-vascular system for cardiomyopathy. Next palpate the testes for atrophy. Examine the lower limbs. The tibial nerves are affected first. Always ask to test the urine for sugar (diabetes mellitus is associated with this disease).

NB: Muscle myotonia can also occur in the hereditary diseases myotonia congenita (autosomal dominant or recessive) and hereditary paramyotonia (autosomal dominant cold-induced myotonia).

Myasthenia Gravis

Myasthenia gravis is an autoimmune disease of the neuromuscular junction. There are circulating antibodies against acetylcholine receptors. It differs from the proximal myopathies in that muscle power decreases with use. There is little muscle wasting and no sensory change.

It is necessary to test for muscle fatigue. Test the oculomotor muscles by asking the patient to sustain upward gaze by looking up at the examiner's finger for one minute, and watch for progressive ptosis (Figure 10.21). Then test the proximal limb girdle muscles—ask the patient to hold the arms above the head. Power will decrease with repeated muscle contraction.

Look for a thymectomy scar (over the sternum)—thymectomy is often undertaken as treatment for generalised myasthenia.

The Cerebellum (Figure 10.50)

If the patient complains of clumsiness or problems with coordination of movement, a cerebellar examination is indicated. Signs of cerebellar disease occur on the same side as the lesion in the brain. This is because most cerebellar fibres cross twice in the brainstem. Proceed as follows with the examination.

Look first for nystagmus, usually jerky horizontal nystagmus with an increased amplitude on looking towards the side of the lesion. Assess speech next. Ask the patient to say 'British Constitution' and 'West Register Street' (Figure 10.51). Cerebellar speech is jerky, explosive and loud, with an irregular separation of syllables (page 335).

Go to the upper limbs. Ask the patient to extend the arms and look for arm drift and static tremor due to hypotonia of the agonist muscles. Test tone. Hypotonia* is due to loss of a facilitatory influence on the spinal motor neurones.

Next perform the finger-nose test. The patient touches the nose, then rotates the finger and touches the examiner's finger. Note any intention tremor (tremor which increases as the target is approached—this is due to loss of cerebellar connections in the brainstem) and past-pointing (the patient overshoots the target). Test rapidly alternating movements: the patient taps alternately the palm and back of one hand on the other hand or thigh. Inability to perform this movement smoothly is called dysdiadochokinesis. Now test rebound*—ask the patient to lift the arms quickly from the sides then stop (incoordination of antagonist and agonist action causes the patient to be unable to stop the arms). Always demonstrate these movements for the patient's benefit.

Go on to examine the legs. Again, test tone here. Then perform the heel-shin test looking for accuracy of fine movement when the patient slides the heel down

---

*   The concepts of hypotonia, rebound and pendular jerks in cerebellar disease are currently being reassessed. They stem from Gordon Holmes' 1917 description of signs in acute unilateral cerebellar disease. They may well not exist in other cerebellar problems. Students will, however, still be expected to know how to test for these signs.

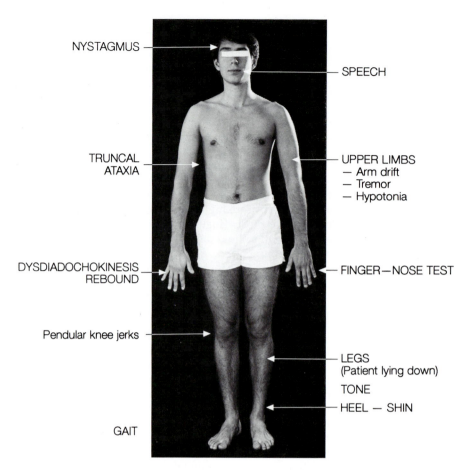

NYSTAGMUS

SPEECH

TRUNCAL
ATAXIA

UPPER LIMBS
— Arm drift
— Tremor
— Hypotonia

DYSDIADOCHOKINESIS
REBOUND

FINGER—NOSE TEST

Pendular knee jerks

LEGS
(Patient lying down)

TONE

HEEL — SHIN

GAIT

Figure 10.50   *The cerebellar examination.*

the shin slowly on each side for several cycles. Then ask the patient to lift the big toe up to touch the examiner's finger, and look for intention tremor and past-pointing. Ask the patient then to tap each heel on the other shin.

Look for truncal ataxia by asking the patient to fold the arms and sit up. While sitting, ask the patient to put the legs over the side of the bed and test for pendular knee jerks (the lower leg continues to swing a number of times before coming to rest—this is evidence of hypotonia).

Test gait (the patient will stagger towards the affected side if there is a unilateral cerebellar hemisphere lesion).

If there is an obvious unilateral cerebellar problem examine the cranial nerves for evidence of a cerebellopontine angle tumour (fifth, seventh and eighth nerves affected) or the lateral medullary syndrome, and auscultate over the cerebellum. Always look in the fundi for papilloedema. Next examine for peripheral signs of malignant disease and for vascular disease (carotid bruits).

If there is evidence of a midline lesion, such as truncal ataxia or abnormal heel-toe walking or abnormal speech, consider either a midline tumour or a paraneoplastic syndrome (Table 10.27). If there is bilateral disease look for signs

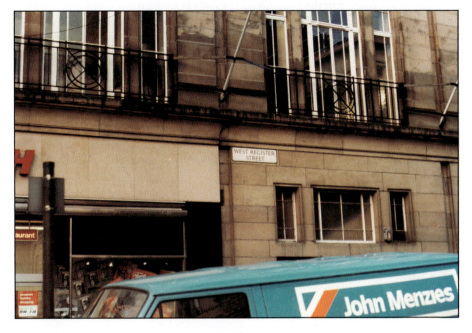

Figure 10.51   *West Register Street, Edinburgh.*

Table 10.27   *Causes of Cerebellar Disease*

Rostral Vermis Lesion (only lower limbs affected)

Usually due to alcohol

Unilateral
1. Space-occupying lesion (tumour, abscess, granuloma)
2. Ischaemia (vertebrobasilar disease)
3. Multiple sclerosis
4. Trauma

Bilateral
1. Drugs—e.g., phenytoin
2. Alcohol (both acutely and chronically, possibly due to thiamine deficiency)
3. Friedreich's ataxia
4. Hypothyroidism
5. Paraneoplastic syndrome
6. Multiple sclerosis
7. Trauma ('punch drunk')
8. Arnold-Chiari malformation
9. Large space-occupying lesion, cerebrovascular disease

Midline
1. Paraneoplastic syndrome
2. Midline tumour

of multiple sclerosis, Friedreich's ataxia (pes cavus is the most helpful initial clue (Table 10.28)) and hypothyroidism (rare). Alcoholic cerebellar degeneration (which affects the anterior lobe of the cerebellar vermis) classically spares the arms. If there are, in addition, upper motor neurone signs, consider the causes in Table 10.29.

Parkinson's Disease

This is a common extrapyramidal disease of middle to old age where there is degeneration of the substantia nigra and its pathways. This results in dopamine deficiency and a relative excess of cholinergic transmission in the caudate nucleus and putamen which causes excessive supraspinal excitatory drive.

Examine as follows.

Inspection

Note the lack of facial expression which leads to a mask-like facies. The posture is characteristically flexed and there are few spontaneous movements.

Table 10.28 *Clinical Features of Friedreich's Ataxia (Autosomal Recessive)*

This is usually a young person with:
1. Cerebellar signs (bilateral) including nystagmus
2. Pes cavus,* cocking of the toes, kyphoscoliosis
3. Upper motor neurone signs in the limbs (although reflexes are absent)
4. Peripheral neuropathy
5. Posterior column loss in the limbs
6. Cardiomyopathy (ECG abnormalities occur in more than 50% of cases)
7. Diabetes mellitus (common)
8. Optic atrophy (uncommon)
9. Normal mentation

* Other causes of pes cavus include hereditary motor and sensory neuropathy, spinocerebellar degeneration or neuropathies in childhood.

Table 10.29 *Causes of Spastic and Ataxic Paraparesis (upper motor neurone and cerebellar signs combined)*

In Adolescence

Spinocerebellar degeneration—e.g., Marie's spastic ataxia

In Young Adults

Multiple sclerosis
Syphilitic meningomyelitis
Spinocerebellar degeneration
Arnold-Chiari malformation or other lesion at the craniospinal junction

In Later Life

Multiple sclerosis
Syringomyelia
Infarction (in upper pons or internal capsule on one side—'ataxic hemiparesis')
Lesion at the craniospinal junction—e.g., meningioma

NB: Unrelated diseases that are relatively common (e.g., cervical spondylosis and cerebellar degeneration from alcohol) may cause a similar clinical picture.

Gait

Ask the patient to rise from a chair, walk, turn quickly, stop and start.

The characteristic gait is described as shuffling—there are small steps, and the patient hardly raises the feet from the ground. There is often difficulty in initiating walking, but once it begins the patient hurries (festination) and has difficulty stopping. The patient seems always to be trying to catch up with the centre of gravity. There is a lack of the normal arm swing. Don't test for propulsion or retropulsion (propulsion involves pushing the patient from behind and retropulsion pushing from in front; the patient may be unable to stop and may fall over).

Kinesia paradoxica is the striking ability of a patient to perform rapid movements (especially if startled) but not slow ones; for example, the patient may be able to run down the stairs in response to a fire alarm but be unable to stop at the bottom—this is *not* a recommended test.

Bradykinesia may be the result of a lesion in the nigro-striatal pathway (a dopaminergic pathway) which affects connections between the caudate nucleus, putamen and the motor cortex, causing abnormal movement programming and abnormal recruitment of single motor units.

Tremor

Have the patient return to bed. Look for a resting tremor. The characteristic movement is described as pill-rolling. Movement of the fingers at the metacarpophalangeal joints is combined with the movements of the thumb at a rate of 4 to 8Hz. Various attending movements may also occur at the wrist. On finger-nose testing the resting tremor decreases, but a faster action tremor (7 to 12Hz) may supervene.

Tremor can be facilitated by getting the patient to perform 'serial 7s' (mental stimulation) or moving the contralateral limb (e.g., by rapidly opposing the contralateral thumb and fingers). Other causes of tremor are summarised in Table 10.30.

Tone

Test tone at both wrists. The characteristic increase in tone is called cogwheel rigidity. Tone is increased with an interrupted nature, the muscles giving way with a series of jerks. If hypertonia is not obvious, obtain reinforcement by asking the patient to turn the head from side to side or wave the contralateral arm. Cogwheel rigidity occurs because the exaggerated stretch reflex is interrupted by tremor.

Remember, the signs are often asymmetrical early in the course of Parkinson's disease.

Face

There may be titubation (tremor) of the head, absence of blinking, dribbling of saliva and lack of facial expression. Test the glabellar tap—keeping your finger out of the patient's line of vision, tap the middle of the forehead (glabella) with your middle finger. This sign is positive when the patient continues to blink as long as the examiner taps. Normal people only blink a couple of times and then stop.

Assess speech, which is typically monotonous, soft and faint, lacking intonation. Sometimes palilalia is present; this is repetition of the end of a word (the opposite of stuttering).

Table 10.30 *A Classification of Tremor**

1. Parkinsonian (4 to 6 Hertz)—resting tremor.
2. Postural/action tremor. Present throughout movement.
Most often a static or postural tremor of the outstretched arms.
(a) idiopathic (most common)
(b) anxiety
(c) drugs
(d) familial
(e) thyrotoxicosis
3. Intention tremor (cerebellar disease). Increases towards the target.
4. Midbrain ('red nucleus') tremor—abduction-adduction movements of upper limbs with flexion-extension of wrists (usually associated with intention tremor).

* Tremor is a rhythmic oscillation of a part of the body around a fixed point.
NB: Flapping (asterixis) is not strictly a tremor but a sudden brief loss of tone in hepatic failure, cardiac failure, respiratory failure or renal failure (metabolic encephalopathies).

Now test the ocular movements, particularly for weakness of upward gaze. Isolated failure of upward gaze is a feature of Parkinson's disease. There is a separate group of patients with marked rigidity and paralysis of gaze who should be diagnosed as having progressive supranuclear palsy (page 352) rather than Parkinson's disease. These people develop loss first of downward gaze then of upward gaze and finally of horizontal gaze.

Feel the brow for greasiness (seborrhoea) or sweatiness, due to associated autonomic dysfunction. Orthostatic hypotension may also be present for the same reason.

Writing

Ask the patient to write his or her name and address. Micrographia (small writing) is characteristic. The patient may also be unable to do this because of the development of dementia, a late manifestation. Test the higher centres if appropriate.

Causes of Parkinson's Syndrome

These are shown in Table 10.31.

Other Extrapyramidal Movement Disorders (Dyskinesia)

Chorea

Here there is a lesion of the corpus striatum which causes non-repetitive, abrupt, involuntary jerky movements. These are commonly unilateral. Often the patient attempts to disguise this by completing the involuntary movements with a voluntary one. In this disease, dopaminergic pathways dominate over cholinergic transmissions.

Chorea must be distinguished from hemiballismus, athetosis and pseudo-athetosis. *Hemiballismus* is due to a subthalamic lesion on the side opposite to the movement disorder. It causes unilateral wild rotatory movements of the proximal joints. There may be skin excoriation due to limb trauma. These movements may persist during sleep.

Athetosis is due to a lesion of the outer segment of the putamen and causes slow sinuous writhing distal movements which are present at rest. *Pseudoathetosis* is a

Table 10.31 *Causes of Parkinson's Syndrome*

Idiopathic: Parkinson's disease
Drugs: e.g., phenothiazines, methyldopa
Post-encephalitis (now very rare)
Other: toxins (carbon monoxide, manganese), Wilson's disease, progressive supranuclear
    palsy, Steele-Richardson syndrome, Shy Drager syndrome, syphilis, tumour (e.g.,
    giant frontal meningioma)
Atherosclerosis is a controversial possible cause.

Table 10.32 *Causes of Chorea*

Huntington's disease (autosomal dominant)
Sydenham's chorea (rheumatic fever) and other post-infectious states (both rare)
Senility
Wilson's disease
Drugs: e.g., phenothiazines, the contraceptive pill, phenytoin, levodopa
Kernicterus (rare)
Vasculitis or connective tissue disease—e.g., systemic lupus erythematosus (very rare)
Thyrotoxicosis (very rare)
Polycythaemia or other hyperviscosity syndromes (very rare)
Viral encephalitis (very rare)

description given to athetoid movements in the fingers in patients with severe proprioceptive loss (these are especially prominent when the eyes are shut).

If the patient has chorea, proceed as follows. First shake hands. There may be tremor and dystonia superimposed on lack of sustained hand grip ('milkmaid's grip'). Ask the patient to hold out hands, look for a choreic (dystonic) posture. This typically involves finger and thumb hyperextension and wrist flexion.

Go to the face and look at the eyes for exophthalmos (thyrotoxicosis), Kayser-Fleischer rings (Wilson's disease) and conjunctival injection (polycythaemia). Ask the patient to poke out the tongue and note frequent retraction of the tongue (serpentine movements). Look for skin rashes (e.g., systemic lupus erythematosus, vasculitis). If the patient is young examine the heart for signs of rheumatic fever (Sydenham's* chorea).

Test the reflexes. The abdominal reflexes are usually brisk, but tendon reflexes are reduced and may be pendular (due to hypotonia).

Assess the higher centres for dementia (Huntington's[†] chorea).

Causes of chorea are shown in Table 10.32.

Dystonia

The patient manifests an involuntary abnormal posture with excessive co-contraction of antagonist muscles. Dystonia may be focal (e.g., spasmodic torticollis), segmental or generalised. Other forms of movement disorder may be present (e.g.,

---

*   Thomas Sydenham (1624–1684), English physician, gave clinical descriptions of gout, fevers, hysteria
    and venereal disease.

†   George Huntington (1850–1916), American general practitioner, described this disease in 1872.

myoclonic dystonia). The acute onset of dystonia is seen most commonly as a side effect of various drugs (e.g., levodopa, phenothiazines, metoclopramide).

The Unconscious Patient

The rapid and efficient examination of the unconscious patient is important. The word COMA provides a mnemonic for four major groups of causes of unconsciousness.

C—CO_2 narcosis (respiratory failure: uncommon).

O—Overdose of drugs: tranquillisers, alcohol, salicylates, carbon monoxide, antidepressants.

M—Metabolic: hypoglycaemia, diabetic ketoacidosis, uraemia, hypothyroidism, hepatic coma, hypercalcaemia, adrenal failure.

A—Apoplexy: head injury, cerebrovascular accident (infarction or haemorrhage), subdural or extradural haematoma, meningitis, encephalitis, epilepsy.

Coma occurs when the reticular formation is damaged by a lesion or metabolic abnormality, or when the cortex is diffusely damaged.

General Inspection

Look to see if the patient is breathing, as indicated by chest wall movement. If not, urgent attention is required, including clearing the airway and providing ventilation. Note particularly the pattern of breathing (Table 4.4). Cheyne-Stokes respiration (which may indicate diencephalic injury, but is not specific), irregular ataxic breathing (Biot's breathing, from an advanced brainstem lesion) and deep rapid respiration (e.g., Kussmaul breathing, secondary to a metabolic acidosis, as in diabetes mellitus) are important things to look for.

Circulation

Look for signs of shock, dehydration and cyanosis. A typical cherry red colour occurs in cases of carbon monoxide poisoning. Take the pulse rate and blood pressure.

Posture

Look for signs of trauma. Note any neck hyperextension (from meningism in children or cerebellar tonsillar herniation).

Look for:

1. A *decerebrate* or extensor posture which may be held spontaneously or occur in response to stimuli, and which suggests severe midbrain disease. The arms are held extended and internally rotated and the legs are extended.

2. A *decorticate* or flexor posture suggests a lesion above the brainstem. It can be unilateral or bilateral. There is flexion and internal rotation of the arms and extension of the legs.

Involuntary Movements

Recurrent or continuous convulsions which may be focal or generalised suggest status epilepticus. Myoclonic jerks can occur after hypoxic injury and as a result of metabolic encephalopathy. Remember that complex partial seizure status epilepticus can cause a reduced level of consciousness without convulsive movements.

Level of Consciousness

Press your knuckles over the sternum firmly to cause pain. Determine the level of consciousness. *Coma* is unconsciousness with a reduced response to external stimuli. Coma in which the patient responds semi-purposefully is considered light. In deep coma there is no response to any stimuli and no reflexes are present (it is usually due to a brainstem or pontine lesion though drug overdosage, for example with barbiturates, can be responsible).

Stupor is unconsciousness, but the patient can be aroused with a considerable amount of effort. Purposeful movements occur in response to painful stimuli.

Drowsiness resembles normal sleepiness. The patient can be fairly easily roused to normal wakefulness, but when left alone falls asleep again.

The Neck

If there is no evidence of neck trauma, assess for neck stiffness and Kernig's sign (for meningitis or subarachnoid haemorrhage).

The Head and Face

Inspect and palpate for head injuries, including Battle's* sign, bruising behind the ear indicating a fracture of the base of the skull. Look for facial asymmetry (i.e., facial weakness). The paralysed side of the face will be sucked in and out with respiration. A painful stimulus (e.g., pressing the supraorbital notch) may produce grimacing and make facial asymmetry more obvious. Note jaundice (e.g., hepatic coma) or manifestations of myxoedema.

The Eyes

Inspect the pupils. Very small pupils occur in pontine lesions and with narcotic overdoses. One dilated pupil suggests a subdural haematoma, raised intracranial pressure (unilateral tentorial herniation) or a subarachnoid haemorrhage from a posterior communicating artery aneurysm. Conjunctival haemorrhage with no posterior limit suggests skull fracture. Widely dilated pupils may occur when increased intracranial pressure and coning cause secondary brainstem haemorrhage or with atropine-like drugs. Look in the fundi for papilloedema, diabetic or hypertensive retinopathy, or subhyaloid haemorrhage.

Look at the position of the eyes. Particular cranial nerve palsies may cause deviation of an eye in various directions. The sixth nerve is particularly vulnerable to damage because of its long intracranial course. Deviation of both eyes to one side in the unconscious patient may be due to a destructive lesion in a cerebral hemisphere which causes fixed deviation towards the side of the lesion. An irritative (epileptic) focus causes the direction of gaze to be away from the lesion. Upward or downward eye deviation suggests a brainstem problem. Trapping of the globe or extraocular muscles by fracture may also lead to an abnormal eye position or to an abnormal eye movement.

---

* William Battle (1855–1936), surgeon, St Thomas Hospital, London.

Perform *doll's eye testing* by lifting the patient's eyelids and rolling the head from side to side. When vestibular reflexes are intact (i.e., an intact brainstem), the eyes maintain their fixation as if looking at an object in the distance, but change their position relative to the head. This is the normal 'doll's eye phenomenon'. Brainstem lesions or drugs affecting the brainstem cause the eyes to move with the head so that fixation is not maintained.

Ears and Nostrils

Look for any bleeding or drainage of cerebrospinal fluid (the latter indicating a skull fracture). A watery discharge can be simply tested for glucose. The presence of glucose confirms that it is cerebrospinal fluid.

The Tongue and Mouth

Trauma may indicate a previous seizure, and corrosion around the mouth may indicate ingestion of a corrosive poison. Gum hyperplasia suggests that the patient may be taking phenytoin for epilepsy. Smell the breath for evidence of alcohol ingestion, diabetic ketosis, hepatic coma or uraemia. Remember that alcohol ingestion may be associated with head injury. Test the gag reflex; its absence may indicate brainstem disease or deep coma.

The Upper and Lower Limbs

Look for injection marks (drug addiction, diabetes mellitus). Test tone in the normal way and by picking up the arm and letting it fall. Compare each side, assessing for evidence of hemiplegia. Test the deep tendon reflexes, which may be absent on a paralysed side in coma.

Test for pain sensation by placing a pen over a distal finger or toe just below the nail bed. Press firmly and note if there is arm or leg withdrawal. Test all limbs. There will be no response to pain if sensation is absent or if the coma is deep. If sensation is intact but the limb is paralysed, there may be grimacing with movement of the other limbs.

The presence of grimacing or purposeful movements is important. Segmental reflexes alone can cause the limb to move in response to pain.

The Body

Look for signs of trauma. Examine the heart, lungs and abdomen.

The Urine

Note if there is incontinence. Test the urine for glucose, ketones (diabetic ketoacidosis), protein (uraemia), and blood (trauma).

The Blood Glucose

Always prick the finger, place a drop of blood on an impregnated test strip, and test for hypoglycaemia or hyperglycaemia. If this cannot be done immediately, give the patient a bolus of intravenous glucose anyway (which will not harm the patient in diabetic ketoacidosis, but will save the life of a patient with hypoglycaemia). If there is any possibility of Wernicke's encephalopathy thiamine must be given as well.

Table 10.33 *Glasgow Coma Scale*

** Add up the score for 1, 2 and 3.			
1. Eyes	Open	Spontaneously	4
		To loud verbal command	3
		To pain	2
	No response		1
2. Best Motor Response	To verbal command	Obeys	6
	To painful stimuli	Localises pain	5
		Flexion—withdrawal	4
		Flexion—abnormal (decorticate rigidity)	3
		Extension (decerebrate rigidity)	2
		No response	1
3. Best Verbal Response		Oriented and converses	5
		Disoriented and converses	4
		Inappropriate words	3
		Incomprehensible sounds	2
		No response	1

The Temperature

Hypothermia (as in hypothyroidism) or fever (as in meningitis) must be looked for.

Stomach Contents

While protecting the airway examine these by inserting a nasogastric tube and washing out the stomach if a drug overdose is suspected, or if no other diagnosis is obvious.

Coma Scale

It is most useful to score the depth of coma, as changes in the level of consciousness can then be judged more objectively (Table 10.33).

Summary

Examining the Nervous System: A Suggested Method (Figure 10.52)

Handedness, Orientation and Speech

Ask the patient if he or she is right or left handed. As a screening assessment, ask for the patient's name, present location and the date. Next ask the patient to name an object pointed at and have them point to a named object in the room. Ask him or her to say 'British Constitution'.

1. HANDEDNESS
   AND CONSCIOUS
   LEVEL
2. NECK STIFFNESS
   AND KERNIG'S
   SIGN
3. CRANIAL NERVES
   II   Visual acuity and
        fields
        Fundoscopy
   III IV VI Pupils and
        eye movements
   V   Corneal reflexes
        Facial sensation
   VII Facial muscles
   VIII Hearing
   IX X Palate
        and gag
   XI   Trapezius and
        sternomastoids
   XII Tongue

4. UPPER LIMBS
5. LOWER LIMBS
   Motor system
   (Tone, power,
   reflexes)
   Co-ordination
   Sensation
6. SADDLE REGION
7. BACK
8. GAIT

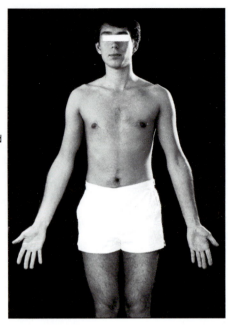

Figure 10.52   *The nervous system examination.*

Neck Stiffness and Kernig's Sign
Cranial Nerves

The patient should be sat over the edge of the bed. Begin by general inspection of the head and neck looking for craniotomy scars, neurofibromas, facial asymmetry, ptosis, proptosis, skew deviation of the eyes or inequality of the pupils.

The first nerve: examination of this is rarely required. Each nostril is tested separately using non-pungent substances in a series of sample bottles.

The second nerve: test visual acuity with the patient wearing his or her spectacles. Each eye is tested separately, while the other is covered with a small card.

Examine the visual fields by confrontation using a hat pin. The examiner's head should be level with the patient's head. Each eye is tested separately. If visual acuity is very poor, the fields are mapped using the fingers.

Look into the fundi.

The third, fourth and sixth nerves: look at the pupils, noting the shape, relative sizes and any associated ptosis. Use a pocket torch and shine the light from the side to gauge the reaction of the pupils to light. Assess quickly both the direct and consensual responses. Look for an afferent pupillary defect by moving the torch in an arc from pupil to pupil. Test accommodation by asking the patient to look into the distance and then at the hat pin placed about 30cm from the nose.

Assess eye movements with both eyes first, getting the patient to follow the pin in each direction. Look for failure of movement and for nystagmus. Ask about diplopia.

The fifth nerve: test the corneal reflexes gently and ask the patient if the touch of the cotton wool on the cornea can be felt. The sensory component of this reflex is V and the motor component VII.

Test facial sensation in the three divisions: ophthalmic, maxillary and mandibu-lar. Test pain sensation with the pin first and map any area of sensory loss from dull to sharp. Test light touch as well so that sensory dissociation can be detected if present.

Examine the motor division of the fifth nerve by asking the patient to clench the teeth while you feel the masseter muscles. Then get the patient to open the mouth while you attempt to force it closed; this is not possible if the pterygoid muscles are working. A unilateral lesion causes the jaw to deviate towards the weak (affected) side.

Test the jaw jerk. This is increased in cases of pseudobulbar palsy.

The seventh nerve: test the muscles of facial expression. Ask the patient to look up and wrinkle the forehead. Look for loss of wrinkling and feel the muscle strength by pushing down on each side. This is preserved in upper motor neurone lesions because of bilateral cortical representation of these muscles.

Next ask the patient to shut the eyes tightly and compare the two sides. Tell the patient to grin and compare the nasolabial grooves.

Examining for taste on the anterior two-thirds of the tongue is not usually required.

The eighth nerve: whisper softly a number 60 cm away from each ear. Perform Rinné's and Weber's tests with a 256 Hertz tuning fork if there is deafness. Examine the external auditory canals and the eardrums if this is indicated.

The ninth and tenth nerves: look at the palate and note any uvular displacement. Ask the patient to say 'Ah' and look for symmetrical movement of the soft palate. With a unilateral lesion the uvula is drawn towards the unaffected (normal) side. Test gently for a gag reflex (the ninth nerve is the sensory component and the tenth nerve the motor component). Ask the patient to speak to assess hoarseness, and to cough and swallow. A bovine cough suggests bilateral recurrent laryngeal nerve lesions. Taste on the posterior third of the tongue is not routinely tested.

The twelfth nerve: while examining the mouth inspect the tongue for wasting and fasciculation. Next ask the patient to protrude the tongue. With a unilateral lesion the tongue deviates towards the weaker (affected) side.

The eleventh nerve: ask the patient to shrug the shoulders and feel the trapezius as you push the shoulders down. Then ask the patient to turn the head against resistance and also feel the bulk of the sternomastoid.

Then examine the skull and auscultate for carotid bruits.

Upper Limbs

Shake the patient's hand firmly. Ask him or her to sit over the side of the bed facing you.

Examine the *motor system* systematically every time. Inspect first for wasting (both proximally and distally) and fasciculations. Don't forget to include the shoulder girdle in your inspection.

Ask the patient to hold both hands out with the arms extended and close the eyes. Look for drifting of one or both arms (upper motor neurone weakness, cerebellar lesion or posterior column loss).

Also note any tremor, or pseudoathetosis due to proprioceptive loss. Feel the muscle bulk next, both proximally and distally, and note any muscle tenderness.

Test tone at the wrists and elbows by passively moving the joints at varying velocities.

Assess power at the shoulders, elbows, wrists and fingers.

If indicated, test for an ulnar nerve lesion (Froment's sign) and a median nerve lesion (pen touching test).

Examine the reflexes: biceps (C5, C6), triceps (C7, C8) and brachioradialis (C5, C6).

Assess coordination with finger-nose testing and look for dysdiadochokinesis and rebound.

Motor weakness can be due to an upper motor neurone lesion, a lower motor neurone lesion or a myopathy. If there is evidence of a lower motor neurone lesion, consider anterior horn cell, nerve root or brachial plexus lesions, peripheral nerve lesions or a motor peripheral neuropathy.

Examine the *sensory system* after motor testing, because this can be time-consuming.

First test the spinothalamic pathway (pain and temperature). Demonstrate to the patient the sharpness of a pin on the anterior chest wall or forehead. Then ask him or her to close the eyes and tell you if the sensation is sharp or dull. Start proximally and test each dermatome. As you are assessing, try to fit any sensory loss into dermatomal (cord or nerve root lesion), peripheral nerve, peripheral neuropathy (glove) or hemisensory (cortical or cord) distribution. It is not usually necessary to test temperature.

Next test the posterior column pathway (vibration and proprioception). Use a 128 Hertz tuning fork to assess vibration sense. Place the vibrating fork on a distal interphalangeal joint when the patient has the eyes closed and ask if it can be felt. If so, ask the patient to tell you when the vibration ceases and then, after a short wait, stop the vibrations. If the patient has deficient sensation, test at the wrist, then elbow, then at the shoulder.

Examine proprioception first with the distal interphalangeal joint of the index finger. When the patient has the eyes open grasp the distal phalanx from the sides and move it up and down to demonstrate, then ask the patient to close the eyes; repeat the manoeuvre. Normally, movement through even a few degrees is detectable, and the patient can tell if it is up or down. If there is an abnormality, proceed to test the wrist and elbows similarly.

Test light touch with cotton wool. Touch the skin lightly (do not stroke) in each dermatome.

Feel for thickened nerves—the ulnar at the elbow, the median at the wrist and the radial at the wrist—and feel the axillae if there is evidence of a proximal lesion. Note any scars, and finally examine the neck if relevant.

Lower Limbs

Test the stance and gait first if possible. Then put the patient in bed with the legs entirely exposed. Place a towel over the groin—note whether a urinary catheter is present.

Look for muscle wasting and fasciculations. Note any tremor. Feel the muscle bulk of the quadriceps and run your hand up each shin, feeling for wasting of the anterior tibial muscles.

Test tone at the knees and ankles. Test clonus at this time. Push the lower end of the quadriceps sharply down towards the knee. Sustained rhythmical contractions indicate an upper motor neurone lesion. Also test the ankle by sharply dorsiflexing the foot with the knee bent and the thigh externally rotated.

Assess power next at the hips, knees and ankles.

Elicit the reflexes: knee (L3, L4), ankle (S1, S2) and plantar response (L5, S1, S2).

Test coordination with the heel-shin test, toe-finger test and tapping of the feet.

Examine the sensory system as for the upper limbs: pin prick, then vibration and proprioception, and then light touch. If there is a peripheral sensory loss attempt to establish a sensory level on the trunk and abdomen. Examine sensation in the saddle region and test the anal reflex (S2, S3, S4).

Go to the back. Look for deformity, scars and neurofibromas. Palpate for tenderness over the vertebral bodies and auscultate for bruits. Perform the straight leg raising test.

Suggested Reading

Original and Review Articles

Consensus Development Panel. Differential diagnosis of dementing diseases. *JAMA* 1987; 258: 3411–3416.

Dalessio DJ, Diagnosing the severe headache. *Neurology* 1994; 44(5 Suppl 3): S6–12.

Damasio AR. Aphasia. *N Engl J Med* 1992; 326: 531–539.

Froehling DA, Silverstein MD, Mohr DN, Beatty CW. Does this dizzy patient have a serious form of vertigo? *JAMA* 1994; 271: 385–388.

Gilman S. Advances in neurology. *N Engl J Med* 1992; 326: 1608–1616, 1671–1676.

Goldstein LB, Matchar DB, Clinical assessment of stroke. *JAMA* 1994; 271: 1114–20.

Headache Classification Committee of the International Headache Society. Classification and diagnostic criteria for headache disorders, cranial neuralgia and facial pain. *Cephalalgia* 1988; 8: 1–96.

Petch MC. Syncope. An accurate history tells all. *BMJ* 1994; 308: 1251–1252.

Massey EW, Scherokman B. Soft neurologic signs. *Postgrad Med* 1981; 70: 66–70.

Sauve JS, Thorpe KE, Sackett DL, et al. Can bruits distinguish high-grade from moderate symptomatic carotid stenosis? The North American Symptomatic Carotid Endarterectomy Trial. *Ann Intern Med* 1994; 120: 633–637.

Textbooks

Bickerstaff ER, Spillane JA. Neurological examination in clinical practice. 5th ed. Oxford: Blackwell, 1989.

Caplan LR. The effective clinical neurologist. London: Blackwell, 1990.

Hopkins A. Clinical neurology: A modern approach. Oxford: Oxford University Press, 1993.

Khaw PT, Gikinton AR. ABC of eyes. London: BMJ Publishing Group, 1994.

Kritzinger EE, Wright BE. Colour atlas of the eye and systemic disease. Chicago: Year Book, 1984.

Medical Research Council Memorandum No. 45. Aids to the examination of the peripheral nervous system. London: Her Majesty's Stationery Office, 1976.

Morris JGL. The neurological short case. London: Edward Arnold, 1992.

Walton J. Brain's diseases of the nervous system. 9th ed. Oxford: Oxford University Press, 1985.

Weiner HL, Levitt LP. Neurology: house officer series. 5th ed. Baltimore: Williams & Wilkins, 1994.

Chapter 11

THE PSYCHIATRIC HISTORY AND MENTAL STATE EXAMINATION

Law number four: the patient is the one with the disease.

House of God: Samuel Shem

This chapter deals with the psychiatric history and the mental state examination. The practising clinician must have an understanding of psychiatric illness and know how to perform a psychiatric interview and a mental state examination. This is because there is considerable overlap between psychiatric and physical illness.

Psychiatric disorders (especially anxiety and depression) are common, and persons suffering from these conditions often have medical problems. Appropriate management of these patients will require an understanding of the intercurrent psychiatric disorder and the effect of that disorder on the primary medical problem. A medical illness may, in some instances, present as a psychiatric illness. For example, some endocrine disorders, such as myxoedema, may present with depression. On the other hand, some psychiatric disorders may present medically. Panic disorder (or acute anxiety) may be mistaken for an acute myocardial infarction. Furthermore, a patient's psychological state may interfere with the course of a medical illness; it may lead in some cases to exaggeration of the symptoms or in others to denial of the severity of physical symptoms.

The psychiatric history generally follows the same format as the standard medical history, and the principles described in Chapter 1 apply just as much here as in any history taking. One should inquire about the history of the present illness, the past psychiatric and medical history and the social and family history. However, the psychiatric history aims to elicit more detail about the patient's illness from a broad perspective, focusing not only on symptoms but also on the patient's social background, psychological functioning and life circumstances (a biopsychosocial approach). There is, therefore, more attention paid to the developmental, personal and social history than is normal for a standard medical history.

The method of psychiatric history taking is somewhat different from the standard medical interview. The psychiatric interview aims to be therapeutic as well as diagnostic. In the course of the interview it is hoped that the patient will be able to talk about his or her problems and their context. In doing so, patients will gain some relief from their distress by airing their problems. For this to take place, the clinician's attitude needs to be unhurried, patient and understanding. The psychiatric history also aims to gain an understanding of how the patient's problem arose from a biological, interpersonal, social and psychological perspective so that the best management plan can be worked out.

Obtaining the History

The clinician taking a psychiatric history wants the patient to tell his or her story in his or her own words. In this way the patient will be more likely to report the most important aspects of the illness. This is best achieved using a non-directive approach with open-ended questions. Open-ended questions are those to which the patient will respond with narrative (or a description about what has been happening) rather than a simple factual response. They give the patient an opportunity to talk about his or her problems. Closed questions are more likely to elicit 'yes' or 'no' responses. For example, in the assessment of a patient with depression, a closed question would be: 'Have you been depressed?' An open-ended question would be: 'Tell me about how you have been feeling'. At first glance it might appear that the open-ended question is less efficient, as it could take a longer time to find out about a range of symptoms. However, with a careful and judicious approach, open-ended questioning, by permitting the patient to tell the story, will enable the clinician to get a comprehensive history efficiently. This is not to say that targeted, more closed questions, must not be used—they are necessary to elicit certain symptoms.

While the patient is telling his or her story, the clinician should begin to formulate hypotheses about the problem or diagnosis. These hypotheses are tested by asking more focused questions later in the interview, at which point a diagnostic hypothesis can be rejected or pursued further. For example, a patient may describe tiredness and lethargy, an inability to concentrate and loss of appetite. These symptoms will suggest a diagnosis of depression. Follow-up questions should focus on this possibility. The clinician should ask questions about other symptoms of depression such as: 'How have you been feeling in yourself?' 'What has your mood been like?' and 'How have you been sleeping?'

Introductory Questions

The psychiatric interview should start off with non-threatening questions. After introducing yourself, it is best to begin by asking about basic demographic information (age, marital state, occupation, whom the patient lives with) and then making the patient feel at ease by discussing some neutral topic.

History of the Presenting Illness

In assessing the history of the presenting illness one needs to cover a number of areas.

1. The Problem

Find out the nature of the patient's problem, and the patient's perception of his or her difficulties. This can, of course, be difficult if the patient is psychotic and does not believe a problem exists at all. In these cases it is essential that a corroborative history be taken. For example, a manic patient may consider that there is nothing wrong and that his or her behaviour is reasonable, whereas his or her partner is able to recognise that spending $5000 taking the family out for the day, when the family is impoverished, is a problem.

A range of symptoms commonly found in psychiatric disorders needs to be reviewed in the course of assessing the history of the present illness. These include mood change, anxiety, worry, sleep pattern, appetite, hallucinations and delusions. A set of simple screening questions for each of the major diagnoses is listed in Table 11.1. It is especially useful to ask about symptoms of anxiety and depression (the most common psychiatric disorders). The definitions of other symptoms are given in Table 11.2. It is important to ask about drug usage (legal and illegal) as well as alcohol and caffeine (which may be associated with anxiety disorders).

2. Precipitating Events

Psychiatric illness rarely occurs for no reason and there is generally an event that has precipitated the illness. Such events include a range of experiences which may have affected the patient, or a member of the patient's social network. Events such as physical illness, drug treatment, or treatment non-compliance may be implicated as precipitants. The last-mentioned is important, as patients with psychiatric illness are often non-compliant, a major contribution to relapse.

3. Risk

An assessment of the patient's risk of harm, either to others or to him or herself, is essential: this will indicate whether the patient needs to be treated involuntarily. Patients with psychotic illness may, in some circumstances, need to be treated involuntarily under the Mental Health Act. While the exact details for involuntary treatment are different under individual mental health acts the essential features are generally that: (a) a person has a mental illness; and (b) the person is a danger to self or to others. Assessment of danger to others is difficult, with the best predictor being a history of past threat or harm to others. It is best to err on the side of caution in such cases. Assessment of suicide risk needs to be made with sensitivity and using a direct approach, as shown in Table 11.3.

The Past History

Both the past psychiatric and medical history should be assessed. The past medical history should be evaluated in the same way as in the general medical history. For the past psychiatric history it is important to obtain not only the diagnosis but also the treatment the patient has had and its outcome. An assessment should be made of stresses that may have contributed to past episodes of illness, and that may have led to relapse.

The Family History

There is a familial component in many psychiatric disorders. Two aspects must be assessed in the family history.

First, the patient should be asked tactfully if anyone in the family has had any psychiatric or mental illness or has committed suicide. He or she should also be asked if anyone in the family has had any treatment for psychological problems, such as anxiety, depression, agoraphobia, eating disorders or drug and alcohol problems (these last few areas are often not considered by patients to be psychiatric or mental illnesses).

Table 11.1 *Screening Questions for the Common Psychiatric Disorders*

Mood Disorders

Mood disorders have a pathological disturbance in mood (depression or mania) as the predominant feature. They are distinguished from 'normal' mood changes by their persistence, duration and severity, together with the presence of other symptoms and impairment of functioning.

Screening Questions

Manic-depressive Illness—Bipolar Disorder

Bipolar disorder is a broad term to describe a recurrent illness characterised by episodes of either mania or depression, with a return to normal functioning between episodes of illness.

Mania

A disorder demonstrated by change in mood (*elation*), thought form (*grandiosity*) and behaviour disturbance (*increased energy and disinhibition*). Frequently associated symptoms: increased talkativeness, distractability, decreased need for sleep, loss of inhibition (e.g., engaging in reckless behaviour such as spending sprees, sexual indiscretion, or social over-familiarity).	Have you felt especially good about yourself? Have you been needing less sleep than usual? Do you feel that you are special or that you have special powers? Have you been spending more than usual?

Depression

A disorder characterised by depressed mood (or loss of pleasure) and the presence of somatic (*sleep disturbance, change in appetite, fatigue and weight*), psychological (*low self-esteem, worry-anxiety, guilt, suicidal ideation*), affective (*sadness, irritability, loss of pleasure and interest in activities*) and psychomotor (*retardation or agitation*) symptoms.	How have you been feeling in yourself? What has your mood been like? Have you been feeling sad, blue, down or depressed? Have you lost interest in things you usually enjoy? How have you been sleeping?

Anxiety Disorders

Anxiety disorders are those in which the person experiences excessive levels of anxiety. Anxiety may be somatic (*palpitations, difficulty breathing, dry mouth, nausea, frequency of micturition, dizziness, muscular tension, sweating, abdominal churning, tremor, cold skin*) or psychological (*feelings of dread and threat, irritability, panic, anxious anticipation, inner (psychic) tension, worrying over trivia, difficulty concentrating, initial insomnia, inability to relax*).

Generalised Anxiety Disorder (GAD)

A chronic disorder characterised by a tendency to worry excessively about everyday things. It is accompanied by: symptoms of anxiety or tension; mental tension (*feeling tense or nervous, poor concentration, on edge*); physical tension.	Have you been feeling nervy or tense? Do you worry a lot about things? Do you worry about things most other people would not worry about?

—continued

Table 11.1 *Screening Questions for the Common Psychiatric Disorders (continued)*

Panic Disorder

A disorder characterised by episodes of panic occurring spontaneously in situations where most people would not be afraid. A panic attack is characterised by the presence of physical symptoms (*palpitations, chest pain, a choking feeling, a churning stomach, dizziness, feelings of unreality*) or fear of some disaster (*losing control or going mad, heart attack, sudden death*). They begin suddenly, build up rapidly, and may last only a few minutes.

Have you ever had an attack of acute anxiety or panic?
Did this occur in a situation in which most people would not feel afraid?
Can these attacks happen at any time?

Agoraphobia

A disorder in which an individual avoids places (such as supermarkets or trains) in which they fear they may have a panic attack and cannot escape.

Do you avoid going out?
Do you avoid going to places because you fear you may have an anxiety attack?

Obsessive Compulsive Disorder

A disorder in which the person has either obsessions or compulsions which interfere with everyday life.

Are there any rituals or habits that you have to carry out every day?
Do they cause you problems?
Do you ever have a thought going round in your head that you can't get rid of?

Severe Stress Disorders

Individuals may present shortly after a traumatic event with a range of symptoms, such as *anxiety, depression, disturbed sleep, problems with memory or concentration*. Images, dreams or flashbacks of the traumatic event may also occur.

Have you been having any problems following . . .?
Have you been feeling worried?
. . . or depressed?
. . . had trouble sleeping?
. . . bad memories?

Post-traumatic Stress Disorder (PTSD)

Onset of persistent problems within six months of a traumatic event of exceptional severity. The individual experiences *repetitive and intrusive re-enactments* of the trauma in images, dreams or flashbacks. *Sleep, concentration, memory, mood and attention may be disturbed.* Individuals may feel emotionally detached and avoid things that act as reminders of the traumatic event.

Since . . . happened, have you been troubled by bad memories of it?
Have you been having nightmares?
Have you had trouble with sleep?
Have you had trouble with your memory?
Are you jumpy?

—continued

Table 11.1 *Screening Questions for the Common Psychiatric Disorders (continued)*

Schizophrenia

A disorder characterised by disorders of content (*presence of delusions*), thought form (*shown by difficulty understanding the connections between the patient's thoughts*), perception (*hallucinations— predominantly auditory*), behaviour (*erratic or bizarre*) and/or volition (*apathy and withdrawal*).	Have you ever heard people speaking when there is no-one around? Do you ever hear voices? Have you heard your thoughts out loud? Do you have any thoughts or beliefs that others might find unusual or strange? Have you felt people may be against you? Have you felt that the TV or radio sends you messages? Do you ever feel as if someone is spying on you or plotting to hurt you? Do you have any ideas that you don't like to talk about because you're afraid other people will think you're mad?

Organic Brain Disorders

These are disorders in which there is brain dysfunction manifest by cognitive disturbances such as memory loss or disorientation; there may be behavioural disturbance as well.

Delirium (Acute Brain Syndrome)

A disorder characterised by the acute onset of disturbed consciousness plus changes in cognition that are not due to a pre-existing dementia. It is a direct physiological consequence of a *general medical condition* (*substance intoxication or withdrawal, use of a medication, exposure to a toxin, or a combination of these factors*). Delirium is characterised by *confusion* and *clouding of consciousness*. This may be accompanied by *poor memory, disorientation, inattention, agitation, emotional upset, hallucinations, visions or illusions, suspiciousness and disturbed sleep (reversal of sleep pattern).*	What day is it today? How long have you been here? What is the name of the place we are in? Do you remember my name? Mental state examination.

Dementia (Chronic Brain Syndrome)

A generalised impairment of intellect, memory and personality with no impairment of consciousness. Characterised by *loss of memory* (especially short-term memory), *loss of orientation and deterioration in social functioning and behaviour and emotional control* (may be easily upset (tearful or irritable)).	What day is it today? How long have you been here? What is the name of the place we are in? Do you remember my name? Mental state examination.

—continued

Table 11.1   *Screening Questions for the Common Psychiatric Disorders (continued)*

Other Disorders

There are a number of other psychiatric disorders which may present with physical problems, or may be seen in an emergency department with some complication (particularly after attempted suicide).

Eating Disorders

(Anorexia Nervosa and Bulimia Nervosa)

Here the sufferer (generally female) has a disturbed body image with an unreasonable fear of being fat, and makes extensive efforts to lose weight (strict dieting, vomiting, use of purgatives, excessive exercise). She may deny that weight or eating habits are problems. *Bulimia nervosa* is characterised by binge eating followed by vomiting or purging. *Anorexia nervosa* is characterised by excessive dieting, but there may also be binges followed by vomiting or purging. Anorexic patients will be grossly underweight and may show signs of malnutrition. Amenorrhoea is generally present.

Do you worry about your weight?
Do you think that you are fat?
Do you diet?
Have you ever made yourself sick after a meal?

Somatisation Disorder

A disorder characterised by multiple physical complaints which cannot be satisfactorily explained by physical disease. An individual with this disorder will have complaints in several bodily systems (e.g., gastrointestinal, cardiac, respiratory, musculoskeletal, menstrual).

Do you have any other medical problems?
Have you had symptoms which your doctor has not been able to find a cause for?
Are you often sick?

Personality Disorders

In these disorders the individual, while not having specific symptoms, has behavioural disturbances and problems with impulse control, interpersonal relationships and mood. Individuals who repeatedly attempt suicide often have a personality disorder. They may also have stormy illnesses causing frequent problems for staff.

Have you ever tried to harm yourself?
Have you ever had problems with relationships?

Second, one should try to determine what sort of family the patient grew up in. Drawing up a family tree is a useful way of finding this out. Factual details about each family member can be included in this family tree (age, mental state, health). In the psychiatric history we also need to know about what type of person each family member is, and how family members get on with each other. It is worth exploring how much care (or neglect) the patient received from each parent, and how controlling or protective each was. These two things have been shown to be important in contributing to psychiatric illness. One needs to ask about the quality of the parental relationship and the general family atmosphere. Childhood abuse (physical or sexual) may be an important predisposing event for many illnesses, and should be inquired about. This can be elicited by saying something like 'Sometimes children can have had some unpleasant experiences—I wonder if you had any? Did anyone ever harm you? ... or hit you? ... how about interfering with you sexually? ... could you tell me more about that and what happened?'

Taking a detailed family history in this way sets the scene for the patient's developmental history, which should be taken next.

Table 11.2 *Symptoms of Psychiatric Illness*

Affect	The observable behaviour by which a person's internal emotional state is judged.
Agitation (psychomotor agitation)	Excessive motor activity associated with a feeling of inner tension. The activity is usually non-productive and repetitious and consists of such behaviour as pacing, fidgeting, wringing the hands, pulling the clothes and inability to sit still.
Anxiety	The apprehensive anticipation of future danger or misfortune. It is associated with feelings of tension and symptoms of autonomic arousal.
Conversion symptom (hysteria)	A loss of, or alteration in, motor or sensory function. Psychological factors are judged to be associated with the development of the symptom, which is not fully explained by anatomical or pathological conditions. The symptom is the result of unconscious conflict and is not feigned.
Delusion	A false unshakable idea or belief which is out of keeping with the patient's educational, cultural and social background.
Depersonalisation	An alteration in the awareness of the self—the individual feels as if he or she is unreal.
Derealisation	An alteration in the perception or experience of the external world so that it seems unreal.
Disorientation	Confusion about the time of day, date, or season (time), where one is (place), or who one is (person).
Flight of ideas	A nearly continuous flow of accelerated speech with abrupt changes from topic to topic that are usually based on understandable associations, distracting stimuli, or plays on words. When severe, speech may be disorganised or incoherent.
Grandiosity	An inflated appraisal of one's worth, power, knowledge, importance or identity. When extreme, grandiosity may be of delusional proportions.
Hallucination	A sensory perception that seems real, but occurs without external stimulation of the relevant sensory organ. The term *hallucination* is not ordinarily applied to the false perceptions that occur during dreaming, while falling asleep (*hypnagogic*) or when awakening (*hypnopompic*).
Ideas of reference	The feeling that casual incidents and external events have a particular significance and unusual meaning that is specific to the person.

—continued

Table 11.2 *Symptoms of Psychiatric Illness (continued)*

Illusion	A misperception or misinterpretation of a real external stimulus.
Mood	A pervasive and sustained emotion that colours the perception of the world.
Overvalued idea	An unreasonable belief that is held, but not as strongly as a delusion (i.e., the person is able to acknowledge the possibility that the belief may not be true). The belief is not one that is ordinarily accepted by other members of the person's culture or subculture.
Personality	Enduring patterns of perceiving, relating to, and thinking about the environment and oneself.
Phobia	A persistent irrational fear of a specific object, activity or situation (the phobic stimulus) that results in a compelling desire to avoid it.
Pressured speech	Speech that is increased in amount, accelerated, and difficult or impossible to interrupt. Usually it is also loud and emphatic. Frequently the person talks without any social stimulation and may continue to talk even though no-one is listening.
Psychomotor retardation	Visible generalised slowing of movements and speech.
Psychotic	Psychotic can be used to mean a loss of contact with reality, but is generally used to imply the presence of delusions or hallucinations.

Based on DSMIV, APA 1994

Table 11.3 *Assessment of Suicide Risk*

Suicide is the unfortunate outcome of psychiatric illness. Assessing the risk of suicide is an essential part of the psychiatric interview. Asking about this does not increase the risk or put the idea into the patient's head. It may reduce the risk, as the patient may feel relief in talking about his or her fears. The risk of suicide is assessed by asking directly whether the person has ever contemplated it.
Have you thought that life was not worth living?
   or
Have you felt so bad that you have considered ending it all?
   If 'yes' . . .
Have you thought of killing yourself?
Have you thought how you might do this?
Have you made any plans for doing this?

The Social and Personal History

Open-ended questions are again the best way to obtain the personal and social history. Ask the patient something like, 'Could you tell me a bit about your background, your development, what sort of childhood you had, what are the important things you remember from your childhood?' and then allow the patient to tell his or her own story. During the course of this narrative the patient may require some prompting to add information about important issues such as the birth history (schizophrenia is known to be associated with perinatal morbidity) and early development, and whether there were significant problems in early childhood, such as head injuries or serious infections. How did the patient cope with early separations, particularly when starting primary school and going on to secondary school (difficulty in separation may be a risk factor for panic disorder or abnormal illness behaviour). The patient should be asked about peer relationships, friendships, school, academic ability, adolescence and teenage relationships. The adult history should focus predominantly on the quality of intimate relationships and the social support network, especially whether there are people in whom the patient can confide.

The patient's living circumstances should be asked about in the same way as for a medical history. There should also be a focus on the patient's occupation; not only on the type of job but also on how he or she copes with work or, if he or she does not work, how that is coped with.

Premorbid Personality

An assessment should be made of the patient's premorbid personality. Ask the patient to describe him or herself. The personality can be described using the predominant trait, such as obsessional, nervy or highly strung; it is not necessary to use official systems to describe a patient's personality. In the assessment of premorbid personality it is important to evaluate both positive and negative aspects of the person, how he or she copes adaptively and maladaptively to life stress, what type of interests he or she has, and what other strengths and weaknesses are present.

The Mental State Examination

While assessing the patient, one should carefully make observations about appearance, behaviour, patterns of speech, attitude to the examiner and ways of interacting. These observations are brought together in a systematic fashion in the Mental State Examination. This is not something that is 'done' at the conclusion of taking a history; it is an essential part of the total process of assessing the patient.

However, there are a number of tests that need to be conducted in a formalised way as part of the Mental State Examination. These include assessing the cognitive state (orientation, memory, attention, registration) and inquiring about perceptual disturbances and, in some cases, disorders of thought. The Mental State Examination provides valuable diagnostic information; with some disorders, it is this examination which gives most of the diagnostic clues.

The headings under which the mental state is recorded are shown in Table 11.4, together with some simple bedside tests for assessing cognitive function. Also shown in the Table are some abnormal features of the Mental State Examination which are commonly found in psychiatric disorders.

When cognitive dysfunction is suspected, as in patients with dementia, a more detailed examination of cognitive function should be carried out. A widely used tool for doing this is the Mini-Mental State Examination, which assesses aspects of orientation, memory and concentration. Details of this examination are shown in Table 11.5. Some of the common causes of delirium and dementia are listed in Table 11.6.

Table 11.4 *The Mental State Examination*

Item	What is Assessed, Described or Observed	Common Findings indicating Psychopathology	Types of Illness
General Description			
Appearance	A general description of the patient's appearance, including body build, posture, clothing (appropriateness), grooming (e.g., make-up) and hygiene. Note any physical stigmata (e.g., tattoos) and facial expression (depression, apprehension, worry etc.).	Bizarre appearance.	Psychotic disorders (schizophrenia, mania). Personality disorder.
		Unkempt, poorly groomed.	Schizophrenia, depression.
		Apprehensive, anxious.	Anxiety disorders.
		Over bright clothing	Mania, personality disorder.
		Scarred wrists, tattoos.	Personality disorder.
Behaviour	All aspects of the patient's behaviour. Note the appropriateness of the patient's behaviour within the interview context.	Uncooperative behaviour.	Psychotic disorder, personality disorder.
	Abnormal motor behaviour: mannerisms, stereotyped movements, tics.	Manneristic behaviour.	Psychotic disorder.
	Variants of normal motor behaviour: restlessness, psychomotor change (agitation, retardation).	Stereotypic behaviour.	Psychotic disorders, developmental disability, organic syndromes.
		Bizarre behaviour.	Psychotic disorders.
		Assaultive, threatening.	Personality disorders. intoxication, neurological disorders.
		Restlessness.	Akathisia from antipsychotic medication.
		Psychomotor change.	Depression.

Attitude towards examiner	The way the patient responds to the interviewer, the level of cooperation, willingness to disclose information. A range of attitudes and deviation from appropriateness may occur, ranging from hostility to seductiveness.	Uncooperative attitude, belligerence. Seductiveness.	Psychotic disorder, personality disorder. Personality disorder.
Mood and Affect			
Mood	A relatively persistent emotional state: describe the depth, intensity, duration and fluctuations of mood. Mood may be neutral, euphoric, depressed, anxious or irritable.	Depressed. Anxious/irritable.	Depression. Depression/anxiety disorders.
Affect	The way a patient conveys his or her emotional state. Affect may be full, blunted, restricted or inappropriate.	Depressed. Blunted, restricted.	Depression. Schizophrenia.
Appropriateness	Are the patient's responses appropriate to the matter being discussed?	Inappropriate.	Schizophrenia.
Speech	The tempo, modulation and quality of the patient's speech should be described here. Note should be made of dysphasia or dysarthria (see Chapter 10).	Increased tempo. Slowed.	Mania, acute schizophrenia. Depression.
Perceptual disturbances	The presence of hallucinations (auditory, visual, gustatory or tactile) should be noted. It is important to check whether they occurred with a clear sensorium. Hypnagogic or hypnopompic hallucinations are normal experiences. Other perceptual disturbances (e.g., illusions, depersonalisation or derealisation) should be noted.	Visual hallucinations. Auditory. Tactile/gustatory.	Acute brain syndrome. Epilepsy. Alcohol withdrawal. Drug intoxication. Schizophrenia. Epilepsy, schizophrenia.

—continued

Table 11.4 *The Mental State Examination (continued)*

Thought		
Thought form	The process of the patient's thinking. This involves the quantity of ideas (pressured thought, poverty of ideas) and the way in which the ideas (thoughts) are produced. Are they logical and relevant, or are they fragmented and irrelevant? The link between ideas should be assessed—do they flow logically, or are they disconnected and 'fragmented'? Are ideas connected by spurious concepts (rhyming, the way they sound—'clang' associations)?	Disorder of thought form. Flight of ideas. Poverty of ideas.	Schizophrenia. Mania, schizophrenia. Schizophrenia, mania, depression.
Thought content	The content of the patient's thought. Abnormalities range from precoccupation, obsessions, overvalued ideas to delusions. Themes should also be assessed: suicidal or homicidal thoughts or paranoid ideas. In the medical setting, preoccupation with illness (hypochondriacal thoughts) should be assessed, as well as thoughts of omnipotence—denying illness when it is present.	Delusions.	Schizophrenia, mania, depression.

Sensorium and Cognition
Listed below are bedside tests for a basic assessment of cognitive function.
If abnormalities are detected, a full Mini-Mental State Examination (Table 11.5) should be carried out.

Alertness and level of consciousness	The level of consciousness should be assessed. Clouding or fluctuating levels of consciousness should be noted.	Clouding.	Delirium.

Orientation	Orientation to time, place and person. Ask the day, date, month and year. Ask where he or she is, and if he or she knows who he or she is.	Disorientation.	Dementia, delirium.
Short-term memory	Short-term memory refers to the ability to retain information over a period of 3–5 minutes. Less than this refers to immediate recall. Ask the patient to recall a list of 3 objects after 3–5 minutes.	Loss of short-term memory.	Dementia, delirium.
Long-term memory	This refers to memory of remote events. Ask the patients to recall events of the previous few days, as well as events of a year ago.	Loss of long-term memory.	Dementia.
Concentration	Subtract 7 from 100 and keep subtracting 7, or spell 'world' backwards.	Poor concentration.	Delirium, acute psychosis.
General knowledge and intelligence	Ask about some recent events. Intelligence can be gauged from the language used. Ask the patient to do some simple arithmetical tasks. Literacy should be assessed.	Poor general knowledge.	Dementia, delirium.
Judgment and Insight			
Judgment	The capacity to behave appropriately. Describe a hypothetical situation, and ask how the patient would behave in it (e.g., 'What would you do if you smelt smoke while sitting in a cinema?').	Impaired judgment.	Psychoses. Dementia. Personality disorders.
Insight	Determine whether the patient is aware that he or she has a problem, and the level of understanding of this.	Lack of insight.	Psychoses. Dementia.

Table 11.5 *The Mini-Mental State Examination*

	Score	Max
Orientation		
'What is the (year) (season) (date) (day) (month)?' Ask for the date, then specifically inquire about parts omitted (e.g., season). Score 1 point for each correct answer.	☐	5
'Where are we (country) (state) (town) (hospital) (ward)?' Ask in turn for each place. Score 1 point for each correct answer.	☐	5
Registration		
'May I test your memory?' Repeat three objects (e.g., pen, watch, book). Score 1 point for each correct answer. Then repeat until the patient learns all three. Count trials and record (up to six).	☐	3
Attention and Calculation		
'Count backwards from 100 by sevens' (Serial 7s). One point for each answer, up to five (93, 86, 79, 72, 65) *or* Spell 'world' backwards. Score 1 point for each letter in correct order.	☐	5
Recall		
Ask the patient to recall the three objects in 'registration', above. Score 1 point for each correct answer.	☐	3
Language		
Ask the patient to name two objects shown (e.g., pen and watch). Score 0–2 points.	☐	2
'Repeat the following: 'No ifs, ands or buts '.' Score 1 point.	☐	1
Ask the patient to follow a three stage command: e.g., 'Take this paper in your right hand, fold it in half and put it on the table.' Score 1 point for each step.	☐	3
Read and obey the following: CLOSE YOUR EYES. Score 1 point.	☐	1
WRITE A SENTENCE. Do not dictate—must be sensible, but punctuation and grammar not essential. Score 1 point.	☐	1 ·
'Copy this design.'	☐	1

All ten angles must be present, and the two must intersect.
Score 1 point.

	TOTAL ☐	30

Assess patient's level of consciousness along a continuum

Alert	Drowsy	Stuporose	Coma

Scores of 21 to 29 indicate mild cognitive impairment.

Scores below 20 indicate more severe cognitive impairment, and are highly likely to be due to dementia, especially if obtained on repeated examinations.

Table 11.6   *Some Common Causes of Delirium and Dementia*

Delirium	
Drug intoxication	Anticholinergics Anxiolytics Digoxin L-dopa Alcohol 'Street drugs'
Withdrawal states	Alcohol (delirium tremens) Anxiolytic sedatives
Metabolic disturbance	Uraemia Liver failure Anoxia Cardiac failure Electrolyte imbalance Postoperative states
Endocrine disturbance	Diabetic ketosis Hypoglycaemia
Systemic infections	Pneumonia Urinary tract infection Septicaemia Viral infections
Intracranial infection	Encephalitis Meningitis
Other intracranial causes	Space-occupying lesions Raised intracranial pressure
Head injury	Subdural haemorrhage Cerebral contusion Concussion
Nutritional and vitamin deficiency	Thiamine (Wernicke's encephalopathy) Vitamin B_{12} Nicotinic acid
Epilepsy	Status epilepticus Post-ictal states
Dementia	
Degenerative	Senile dementia of Alzheimer's type Pick's disease Huntington's chorea Parkinson's disease Normal-pressure hydrocephalus Multiple sclerosis
Intracranial space-occupying lesions	Tumour Subdural haematomas
Traumatic	Head injuries Boxing encephalopathy

—continued

Table 11.6 *Some Common Causes of Delirium and Dementia (continued)*

Infections and related conditions	Encephalitis Neurosyphilis HIV (AIDS dementia) Jacob-Creutzfeldt disease
Vascular	Multi-infarct dementia Carotid artery occlusion
Metabolic	Uraemia Hepatic failure
Toxic	Alcoholic dementia Heavy metal poisoning
Anoxia	Anaemia Carbon monoxide poisoning Cardiac arrest Chronic respiratory failure
Vitamin deficiency	Vitamin B$_{12}$ Folic acid Thiamine (Wernicke–Korsakoff's syndrome)
Endocrine	Myxoedema Addison's disease

The Diagnosis

At the conclusion of the psychiatric history, which should include a general physical examination, a provisional diagnosis and formulation should be made. Essentially, the diagnostic formulation is a means of pulling together, in a succinct yet comprehensive manner, your understanding of the patient's problem. Psychiatric disorders generally arise through a combination of biological, psychological and psychosocial factors, and each of these needs to be considered when a patient's problem is being assessed (a biopsychosocial approach). The patient's problem needs to be understood longitudinally, by defining biophysical factors that may have predisposed to the illness and, more immediately, may have precipitated the illness, and factors that may be contributing to the person remaining ill (perpetuating factors). A simple grid can be used for assessing the patient in this manner (Table 11.7). Here biological, psychological or psychosocial factors which either predispose to, precipitate or perpetuate the psychiatric illness are identified. Perpetuating factors are very important, particularly among medically ill patients, as it may be the medical or physical illness which maintains the patient's psychiatric problem. By the same token, psychological factors may perpetuate a patient's medical illness.

An example of such a grid is shown for a 53-year-old man who becomes depressed after a myocardial infarction. He has a family history of depression (a genetic predisposing factor) and chronic low self-esteem (a psychological predisposing factor) which he coped with by succeeding in business. He has few friends and his marriage is unsatisfactory (a psychosocial factor). He had his infarct one

Table 11.7   *A Formulation Grid*

	Predisposing	Precipitating	Perpetuating
Biological			
Psychological			
Psychosocial			

Table 11.8   *A Completed Formulation Grid*

	Predisposing	Precipitating	Perpetuating
Biological	Genetic predisposition	Acute myocardial infarct	Neurotransmitter changes
Psychological	Low self-esteem	Not promoted	Low self-esteem and insecurity
Psychosocial	Poor social support. Dysfunctional marriage		Dysfunctional marriage

week after he heard that he would not be promoted at work (a psychological factor) and his job was at risk (a psychosocial precipitant). His insecurity about work and his failing marriage, together with his low self-esteem, is maintaining his illness, as are the biological changes to the neurotransmitter system. A formulation grid for this patient is shown in Table 11.8.

Understanding the patient in this manner helps to plan an effective management approach which will focus on all the relevant factors, so that a combination of antidepressants, marital counselling and assertiveness training (to build self-esteem) can be organised.

A good psychiatric history will provide a comprehensive understanding of the patient and will permit one to plan appropriate management.

This is immensely rewarding for the clinician, and will also be of considerable benefit to the patient.

Reference

American Psychiatric Association. Diagnostic and Statistical Manual of Mental Disorders, 4th ed. Washington DC: APA, 1994.

Suggested Reading

Original Articles

Folstein MF, Folstein SE, McHugh PR. Mini Mental State. A practical method for grading the cognitive state of patients for the clinician. *J Psychiatr Res* 1975; 12: 189–198.

Kopelman MD, Structured psychiatric interview: psychiatric history and assessment of the mental state. *Brit J Hosp Med* 1994; 52: 93–8.

Rossor MN, Management of neurological disorders: dementia. *J Neurol Neurosurg Psych* 1994; 57: 1451–6.

Textbooks

Balint M. The doctor, his patient and the illness. 2nd ed. London: Pitman, New York: International Universities Press, 1964.

Block S, Singh BS. Foundations of clinical psychiatry. Melbourne: Melbourne University Press, 1994.

Cassem NH. Massachusetts General Hospital handbook of general hospital psychiatry. 3rd ed. St Louis: Mosby Year Book Inc, 1991.

Kaplan HI, Sadock BJ. Synopsis of psychiatry. Behavioural sciences clinical psychiatry. 6th ed. Baltimore: Williams & Wilkins, 1991.

Lishman WA. Organic psychiatry. The psychological consequences of cerebral disorder. Oxford: Blackwell Scientific Book Distributors, 1987.

Nurcombe B, Gallagher RM. The clinical process in psychiatry. Diagnosis and management planning. Cambridge: Cambridge University Press, 1986.

Sim A. Symptoms in the mind: an introduction to descriptive psychopathology. London: Baillière Tindall, 1988.

Chapter 12

THE SKIN

For one mistake made for not knowing,
ten mistakes are made for not looking.

J A Lindsay

The Dermatological History

With any rash or skin condition, it is important to determine when and where it began, its distribution, whether it has changed over time, its relationship to sun exposure or heat or cold, and any response to treatment. Ask if pruritus is associated; localised pruritus is usually due to dermatological disease. Determine if pain or disturbed sensation has occurred; for example, inflammation and oedema can produce pain in the skin, while disease involving neurovascular bundles or nerves can produce anaesthesia (e.g., leprosy, syphilis). Constitutional symptoms such as fever, headache, fatigue, anorexia and weight loss also need to be documented.

It is important to obtain a past history of rashes or allergic reactions. A past history of asthma, eczema or hay fever suggests atopy. Similarly, evidence of systemic disease in the past may be important in a patient with a rash (e.g., diabetes mellitus, connective tissue disease, inflammatory bowel disease).

A detailed social history needs to be obtained regarding occupation and hobbies, as chemical exposure and contact with animals or plants can all induce dermatitis. All medications that have been taken must be documented. Orally ingested or parenteral medications can cause a whole host of cutaneous lesions and can mimic many skin diseases (Table 12.1). Similarly, a family history of atopic dermatitis, hay fever or skin infestation can be helpful.

General Principles of Physical Examination of the Skin

The aim of this chapter is to provide an approach to the diagnosis of skin diseases. Particular emphasis will be placed on cutaneous signs as indications of systemic disease. Other chapters have included the usual clues that can be used to arrive at a particular diagnosis. This chapter tries to unify the concept of 'inspection' as a valuable starting point in the examination of the patient.

Ask the patient to undress. The whole surface of the skin and its appendages should be carefully inspected (Table 12.2).

Table 12.1   *Types of Cutaneous Drug Reactions*

1. Acne, e.g., steroids
2. Hair loss (alopecia), e.g., cancer chemotherapy
3. Pigment alterations: hypomelanosis (e.g., hydroxyquinone, chloroquine, topical steroids), hypermelanosis (page 453)
4. Exfoliative dermatitis or erythroderma (page 450)
5. Urticaria (hives), e.g., non-steroidal anti-inflammatory drugs, radiographic dyes, captopril, penicillin
6. Maculopapular (morbilliform) eruptions, e.g., ampicillin, allopurinol
7. Photosensitive eruptions, e.g., sulphonamides, sulphonylureas, chlorothiazides, phenothiazines, tetracycline, nalidixic acid, anticonvulsants
8. Drug-induced lupus erythematosus, e.g., procainamide, hydralazine
9. Vasculitis, e.g., propylthiouracil, allopurinol, thiazides, penicillin, phenytoin
10. Skin necrosis, e.g., warfarin
11. Drug-precipitated porphyria, e.g., alcohol, barbiturates, sulphonamides, contraceptive pill
12. Lichenoid eruptions, e.g., gold, antimalarials, beta-blockers, captopril
13. Fixed drug eruption, e.g., sulphonamides, tetracycline, phenylbutazone, barbiturates
14. Bullous eruptions, e.g., frusemide, nalidixic acid, penicillamine, clonidine
15. Erythema nodosum or erythema multiforme (page 451)
16. Toxic epidermal necrolysis, e.g., allopurinol, phenytoin, sulphonamides, non-steroidal anti-inflammatory drugs
17. Pruritus (page 443)

Table 12.2   *Considerations When Examining the Skin*

1. Hair
2. Nails
3. Sebaceous glands—oil producing and present on the head and neck and back
4. Eccrine glands—sweat producing and present all over the body
5. Apocrine glands—sweat producing and present in the axillae and groin
6. Mucosa

Table 12.3   *Dermatological Terms*

Macule: a circumscribed alteration of skin colour
Papule: a circumscribed palpable elevation, less than 1cm diameter
Nodule: a circumscribed palpable mass greater than 1cm diameter
Plaque: a palpable disc-shaped lesion
Weal: an area of dermal oedema
Vesicle: a small collection of fluid below the epidermis
Bulla: a larger collection of fluid below the epidermis
Pustule: a visible collection of pus
Ulcer: a circumscribed loss of tissue
Scales: an accumulation of excess keratin
Crust: dried serum and exudate
Atrophy: thinning of epidermis with loss of normal skin markings
Sclerosis: induration of subcutaneous tissues which may involve the dermis
Pigment alterations: increased (hyperpigmentation) or decreased (hypopigmentation)
Excoriations: lesions caused by scratching that results in loss of the epidermis

When one is examining actual skin lesions a number of features should be documented. First, each lesion should be *described* precisely, including colour and shape. Use the appropriate dermatological terminology (Table 12.3), even though this may seem to make dermatological diseases more, rather than less, mysterious. Since many dermatological diagnoses are purely descriptive, a good description will often be of considerable help in making the diagnosis. Second, the *distribution* of the lesions should be noted, as certain distributions suggest specific diagnoses. Third, the *pattern* of the lesions (e.g., linear, annular, reticulated (net-like), serpiginous (snake-like) arciform or grouped) also helps establish the diagnosis. Then *palpate* the lesions noting consistency, tenderness, temperature, depth and mobility. A clinical algorithm for diagnosis is presented in Figure 12.1.

How to Approach the Clinical Diagnosis of a Lump

First, determine the lump's site, size, shape, consistency and tenderness. Next, evaluate in what tissue layer the lump is situated. If it is in the *skin* (e.g., sebaceous cyst, epidermoid cyst, papilloma), it should move when the skin is moved, but if it is in the *subcutaneous tissue* (e.g., neurofibroma, lipoma), the skin can be moved over the lump. If it is in the *muscle* or *tendon* (e.g., tumour), then contraction of the muscle or tendon will limit the lump's mobility. If it is in a *nerve*, pressing on the lump may result in pins and needles being felt in the distribution of the nerve and the lump cannot be moved in the longitudinal axis but can be moved in the transverse axis. If it is in *bone*, the lump will be immobile.

Determine if the lump is *fluctuant* (i.e., contains fluid). Place one forefinger (the 'watch' finger) halfway between the centre and periphery of the lump. The forefinger from the other hand (the 'displacing' finger) is placed diagonally opposite the first at an equal distance from the centre of the lump. Press with the displacing finger and keep the watching finger still. If the lump contains fluid, the watching finger will be displaced in *both* axes of the lump (i.e., fluctuation is present). Place a small torch behind the lump to determine if it can be *transilluminated*.

Note any associated signs of *inflammation* (i.e., redness, swelling, heat and tenderness).

Look for similar lumps elsewhere, e.g., multiple subcutaneous swellings from neurofibromas or lipomas.

If an inflammatory or neoplastic lump is suspected, remember always to examine the regional lymphatic field, and the other lymph node groups.

Correlation of Physical Signs and Skin Disease

There are many different skin diseases with many varied physical signs. With each major sign the groups of common important diseases that should be considered will be listed.

Pruritus

Pruritus simply means itching. It may be either generalised or localised. Scratch marks are usually present. Localised pruritus is usually caused by a dermatological condition such as dermatitis or eczema. Generalised pruritus may be caused by primary skin disease, systemic disease or psychogenic factors.

Figure 12.1 *Diagnosis of Skin Disease: An Algorithm*

Adapted from Lynch PJ. Dermatology for the house officer. 2nd ed. Baltimore: Williams & Wilkins, with permission.

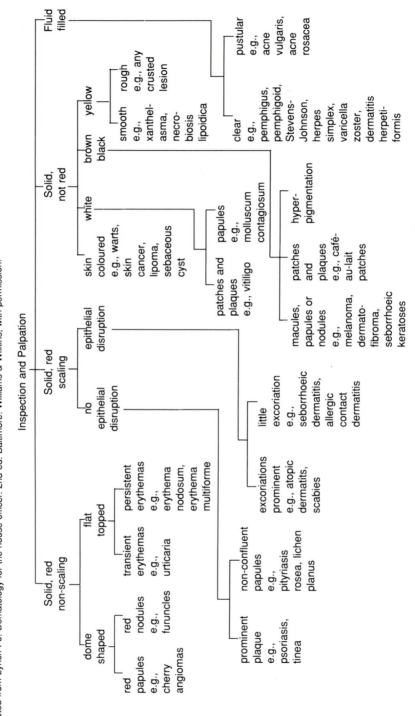

To determine the cause of the pruritus it is essential to examine the skin in detail (Table 12.4). Excoriations are caused by scratching, regardless of the underlying cause. Specific features of cutaneous diseases such as dermatitis, scabies (Figure 12.2) or the blisters of dermatitis herpetiformis (page 150) should be looked for.

When primary skin diseases have been excluded, a detailed history and examination should be undertaken to consider the various systemic diseases which are listed in Table 12.5.

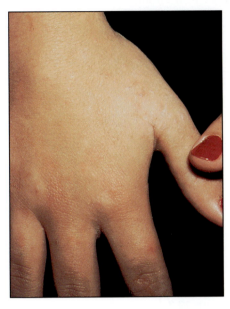

Figure 12.2

Scabies: scattered fine papules with severe itching. Fingerweb involvement is common.

Table 12.4   *Primary Skin Disorders Causing Pruritus*

1. Asteatosis (dry skin)
2. Atopic dermatitis
3. Urticaria
4. Scabies
5. Dermatitis herpetiformis

Table 12.5   *Systemic Conditions Causing Pruritus*

1. Cholestasis—e.g., primary biliary cirrhosis
2. Chronic renal failure
3. Pregnancy
4. Lymphoma and other internal malignancies
5. Iron deficiency, polycythaemia rubra vera
6. Endocrine diseases—e.g., diabetes mellitus, hypothyroidism, hyperthyroidism, carcinoid syndrome

Erythrosquamous Eruptions

Erythrosquamous eruptions are made up of lesions which are red and scaly. They may be well demarcated or have diffuse borders. They may be itchy or asymptomatic.

When one is attempting to establish a diagnosis of an erythrosquamous eruption the history is very important. First ask about the time course of the eruption, about a family history of similar skin diseases and whether or not there is a family history of atopy.

The presence or absence of itching and the distribution of the lesions also give clues about the diagnosis.

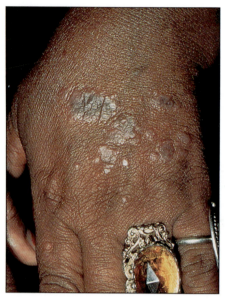

Figure 12.3

Lichen planus with polygonal flat-topped violaceous lesions.

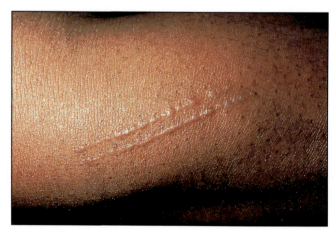

Figure 12.4

Lichen planus, with development of lesions in an area of trauma— the 'Koebner' phenomenon.

Asymptomatic lesions on the palms and soles are suggestive of secondary syphilis, whereas itchy lesions in the same location would be more suggestive of lichen planus (Figures 12.3 and 12.4). Lichen planus is occasionally associated with primary biliary cirrhosis and other liver diseases, chronic graft-versus-host disease and drugs (e.g., gold, penicillamine). Scattered lesions of recent origin on the trunk would be more suggestive of pityriasis rosea (Figure 12.5), whereas more widespread diffuse intensely itchy lesions would be more suggestive of nummular eczema (Figure 12.6) (Table 12.6).

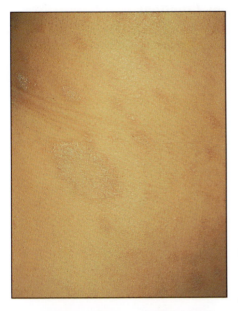

Figure 12.5
Pityriasis rosea, with scattered scaly oval lesions on the trunk and a larger 'herald' patch.

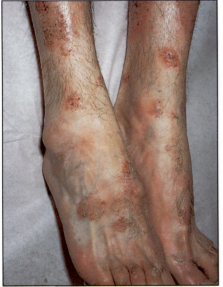

Figure 12.6
Nummular eczema: typical scattered coin-like lesions of indolent dermatitis.

Scaly lesions with a well demarcated edge over the extensor surfaces are usually due to psoriasis (Figures 12.7 and 12.8).

Blistering Eruptions

There are a number of different diseases which will present with either vesicles or blisters. Dermatitis can present as a blistering eruption, particularly acute contact dermatitis (Figure 12.9) (Table 12.7).

Clinical Features of Different Bullous Eruptions

Viral blisters such as those of herpes simplex virus infection (Figure 12.10) have a distinctive morphology (grouped vesicles on an erythematous background).

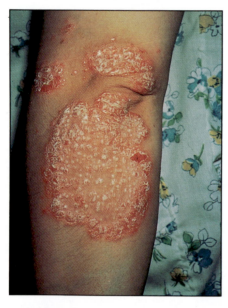

Figure 12.7

Psoriasis: typical bright red scaly plaque with silvery scale, over a joint.

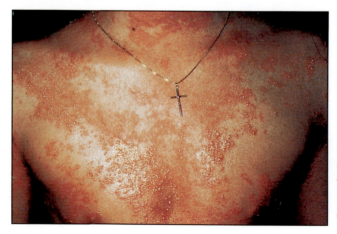

Figure 12.8

Acute widespread pustular psoriasis. Often the eruption is bright red with bizarre patterns and pustules predominantly at the margins.

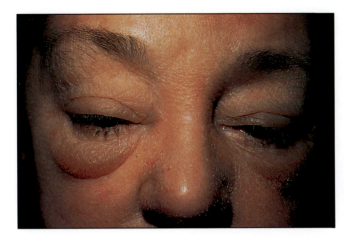

Figure 12.9

Allergic contact dermatitis from over-the-counter topical medication rubbed over congested sinuses.

Table 12.6   *Causes of Erythrosquamous Eruptions*

1. Psoriasis (bright pink plaques with silvery scale)
2. Atopic eczema (diffuse erythema with fine scaling)
3. Pityriasis rosea (paler pink scaly macular lesions)
4. Nummular eczema (round patches of subacute dermatitis)
5. Contact dermatitis (irritant or allergic)
6. Dermatophyte infections (ringworm)
7. Lichen planus (violet-coloured, small, polygonal papules)
8. Secondary syphilis (flat, red hyperkeratotic lesions)

Table 12.7   *Causes of Blistering Eruptions*

1. Traumatic blisters and burns
2. Bullous impetigo
3. Viral blisters (e.g., herpes simplex, varicella)
4. Bullous erythema multiforme
5. Bullous pemphigoid
6. Dermatitis herpetiformis
7. Pemphigus
8. Porphyria
9. Epidermolysis bullosa
10. Dermatophyte infections

Bullous pemphigoid is a rare disease usually affecting older patients. Blisters are widespread, have a thick roof and tend not to rupture easily.

Pemphigus vulgaris is much more severe. It has thin-roofed blisters that readily rupture and form crusts. The affected superficial skin can be moved over the deeper layer (Nikolsky's* sign). Oral ulcers are common.

Dermatitis herpetiformis is characterised by a very itchy widespread vesicular or bullous eruption.

---

* Pyotr Vasilyevich Nikolsky (b. 1858), Kiev and Warsaw dermatologist.

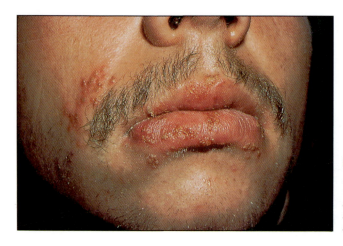

Figure 12.10
Primary herpes simplex virus infection in an adult—typical widespread distribution around the mouth.

Porphyria cutanea tarda is characterised by clear or haemorrhagic blisters on the hands (page 151).

Erythroderma

Erythroderma is best thought of as the end stage of numerous skin conditions (Table 12.8). The erythrodermic patient has involvement of nearly all the skin with an erythematous inflammatory process, often with exfoliation. There is usually associated oedema and loss of muscle mass.

An attempt should be made to determine the underlying cause of the erythroderma and this is best done based on history and examination. Specific treatment can then be directed at the underlying cause. Some patients with erythroderma will develop profound metabolic changes (including hypoalbuminaemia and extrarenal water loss), and these patients require constant supervision and monitoring until they have recovered from the acute phase of their illness.

The most common cause is eczema, which is usually of the atopic variety. These patients often have an intense pruritus. Some of them will develop a chronic unremitting erythroderma.

Pustular and Crusted Lesions

The clinical appearance of a *pustular* lesion results from accumulation of neutrophils. Such collections usually indicate an infectious process; however, sterile pustules may form as part of a number of skin diseases due to the release of chemotactic factors following an immunological reaction.

A *crust* is a yellowish crystalline material that is found on the skin; it is made up of desiccated serum.

It is essential to determine whether or not a pustular lesion (or a group of pustular lesions) represents a primarily infectious process or an inflammatory dermatological condition.

For example, pustular lesions on the hands and feet may either be due to tinea infection, or be a primary pustular psoriasis or palmoplantar pustulosis (Table 12.9).

Table 12.8   *Causes of Erythroderma*

1. Eczema
2. Psoriasis
3. Drugs—e.g., phenytoin, allopurinol
4. Pityriasis rubra pilaris
5. Mycosis fungoides, leukaemia, lymphoma
6. Lichen planus
7. Pemphigus foliaceus
8. Hereditary disorders
9. Dermatophytosis

Table 12.9   *Causes of Pustular and Crusted Lesions*

1. Acne vulgaris
2. Impetigo
3. Folliculitis
4. Acne rosacea
5. Viral lesions
6. Pustular psoriasis
7. Drug eruptions
8. Dermatophyte infections

Table 12.10   *Causes of Dermal Plaques*

1. Granuloma annulare
2. Necrobiosis lipoidica
3. Sarcoidosis
4. Erythema nodosum
5. Lupus erythematosus
6. Morphoea and scleroderma
7. Tuberculosis
8. Leprosy

Dermal Plaques

Plaques are localised thickenings of the skin which are usually caused by changes in the dermis or subcutaneous fat. These may be due to chronic inflammatory processes or scarring sclerotic processes (Table 12.10).

The pattern of involvement of the plaques, the age of the patient and other clinical features should enable a diagnosis to be established.

Erythema Nodosum

This is the best known of the group of diseases classified as nodular vasculitis. The lesions of erythema nodosum are usually found below the knee in the pretibial area and are erythematous, palpable and tender (Figure 5.20, page 192). There may be an associated fever (Table 12.11).

Table 12.11   *Causes of Erythema Nodosum*

1. Streptococcal infections (β haemolytic)
2. Drugs, e.g., sulphonamides, penicillin, sulphonylurea, oestrogen, iodides, bromides
3. Inflammatory bowel disease
4. Sarcoidosis
5. Tuberculosis
6. Other infections—e.g., lepromatous leprosy, toxoplasmosis, histoplasmosis, *Yersinia, Chlamydia*
7. Systemic lupus erythematosus
8. Behçet's syndrome

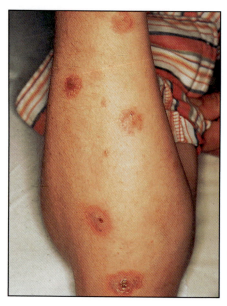

Figure 12.11

Erythema multiforme: classic iris or target lesions, secondary to herpes simplex virus infection of the lips.

Erythema Multiforme

This is a distinctive inflammatory reaction of skin and mucosa. It is not a systemic disease. Characteristic discrete target lesions occur, particularly on the distal extremities (Figure 12.11). The periphery of these lesions is red, whereas the centre becomes bluish or even purpuric. The lesions can become bullous, and severe cases of this syndrome involve widespread desquamation of the mucosal surfaces (the Stevens-Johnson* syndrome). In many cases the condition is precipitated by clinical or subclinical herpes simplex virus infection. Other causes include *Mycoplasma pneumoniae*, histoplasmosis, malignancy, sarcoidosis and drugs (including those that can cause toxic epidermal necrolysis). Sometimes no underlying cause of the erythema multiforme will be established.

---

*   Albert Mason Stevens (b. 1884), New York paediatrician, and FC Johnson (b. 1894), American physician.

Erythema multiforme is not the same as toxic epidermal necrolysis, which is a systemic condition and usually a drug reaction. The major causes include penicillin, sulphonamides, phenytoin and non-steroidal anti-inflammatory drugs.

Hyperpigmentation

The presence of hyperpigmentation can be a clue to underlying systemic disease (Table 12.12).

Flushing and Sweating

Flushing of the skin may sometimes be observed, especially on the face, by the examiner. Some of the causes of this phenomenon are presented in Table 12.13.

Excessive sweating (hyperhidrosis) can occur with thyrotoxicosis, phaeochromocytoma, acromegaly, hypoglycaemia, autonomic dysfunction, stress, fever and menopause.

Table 12.12   *Causes of Diffuse Hyperpigmentation*

Endocrine Disease

Addison's disease (excess ACTH)
Ectopic ACTH secretion (e.g., carcinoma)
The contraceptive pill or pregnancy
Thyrotoxicosis, acromegaly, phaeochromocytoma

Metabolic

Malabsorption or malnutrition
Liver diseases—e.g., haemochromatosis, primary biliary cirrhosis, Wilson's disease
Chronic renal failure
Porphyria
Chronic infection—e.g., bacterial endocarditis
Connective tissue disease, e.g., systemic lupus, scleroderma, dermatomyositis

Other

Drugs—e.g., chlorpromazine, busulphan, arsenicals
Radiation

Racial or Genetic

Table 12.13   *Causes of Facial Flushing*

1. Menopause
2. Drugs and foods, e.g., nifedipine, monosodium glutamate (MSG)
3. Alcohol after taking the drug disulfiram (or alcohol alone in some people)
4. Systemic mastocytosis
5. Rosacea
6. Carcinoid syndrome (secretion of serotonin and other mediators by a tumour may produce flushing, diarrhoea and valvular heart disease)
7. Autonomic dysfunction
8. Medullary carcinoma of the thyroid

Skin Tumours

Skin tumours are very common and are usually benign (Table 12.14). Most malignant skin tumours can be cured if they are detected early and treated appropriately (Table 12.15).

Skin cancer occurs in those individuals predisposed (fair skin of Celtic or Northern European origin) who undergo chronic exposure to ultraviolet light.

Skin cancers may present as flat scaly lesions or as raised scaly or smooth lesions. They may be large or small and they may eventually ulcerate. All non-healing ulcers should be considered to be skin cancer, until proved otherwise.

Table 12.14   *Benign Skin Tumours*

1. Warts
2. Molluscum contagiosum
3. Seborrhoeic keratoses
4. Dermatofibroma
5. Neurofibroma
6. Angioma
7. Xanthoma

Table 12.15   *Malignant Skin Tumours*

1. Basal cell carcinoma
2. Squamous cell carcinoma
3. Bowen's* disease
4. Malignant melanoma
5. Secondary deposits

*   John Templeton Bowen (b. 1857), Boston dermatologist.

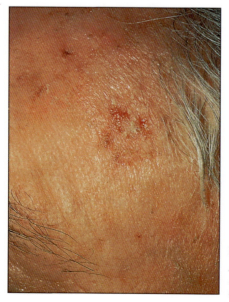

Figure 12.12

Actinic keratosis, slightly eroded and scaly. Higher on the forehead additional granular keratoses could be easily palpated.

The earliest lesions are actinic (solar) keratoses, which are pink macules or papules surmounted by adherent scale (Figure 12.12). Basal cell carcinoma is characteristically a translucent papule with a depressed centre and a rolled border with ectatic capillaries (Figure 12.13). Squamous cell carcinoma is typically an opaque papule or plaque which is often eroded or scaly (Figure 12.14).

Malignant melanomas are usually deeply pigmented lesions which are enlarging and have an irregular notched border (Figure 12.15). There is often variation of pigment within the lesion. Patients with numerous large and unusual pigmented naevi (dysplastic naevus syndrome) are at an increased risk of developing malignant melanoma.

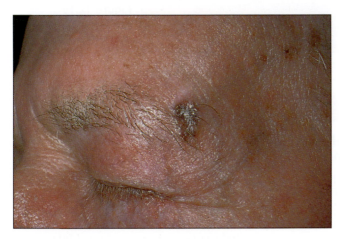

Figure 12.13

Pigmented basal cell carcinoma with pearly quality and depressed centre, in a patient with sun-damaged skin.

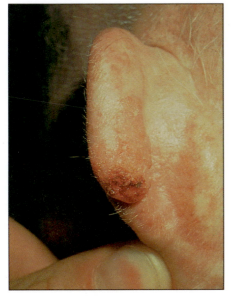

Figure 12.14

Squamous cell carcinoma.

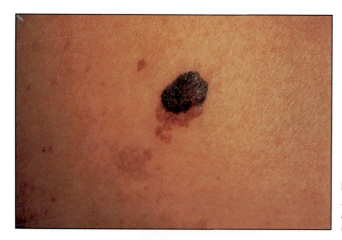

Figure 12.15
Superficial spreading melanoma, still confined to the upper dermis.

Summary

The Dermatological Examination in Internal Medicine:
A Suggested Method (Figure 12.16)

Even if the patient only shows the examiner a small single area of abnormality, proceed to examine all the skin.

After obtaining good lighting conditions and asking the patient to disrobe, begin by looking at the *nails and hands*. Paronychia is an infection of the skin surrounding the nails. Other changes to note include pitting (psoriasis, fungal infections) and onycholysis (e.g., thyrotoxicosis, psoriasis). Dark staining under the nail may indicate a subungual melanoma. Linear splinter haemorrhages (e.g., vasculitis) or telangiectasiae (e.g., systemic lupus erythematosus) may be seen in the nail bed.

A purplish discoloration in streaks over the knuckles may indicate dermatomyositis. Also look at the backs of the hands and forearms for the characteristic blisters of porphyria, which occur on the exposed skin. Papules and scratch marks on the backs of the hands, between the fingers and around the wrists may indicate scabies. Viral warts are common on the hands.

Look at the palms for Dupuytren's contracture, pigmented flat junctional moles (which have a high risk of becoming malignant) and xanthomata in the palmar creases.

Go on to look at the *forearms*, where lichen planus may occur on the flexor surfaces (characterised by small shiny, purple-coloured papules) and psoriasis may be present on the extensor surfaces. Acanthosis nigricans can occur in the axillae.

Inspect the patient's *hair and scalp*. Decide whether or not the hair is dry and whether the distribution is normal. Alopecia may indicate male pattern baldness, recent severe illness, hypothyroidism or thyrotoxicosis. Patches of alopecia occur in the disease alopecia areata. Short broken-off hairs occur typically in systemic lupus erythematosus. In psoriasis there are silvery scales which may be seen on the skin of the scalp. Metastatic deposits may rarely be felt as firm nodules within the skin of the scalp. Sebaceous cysts are common. The unfortunate examiner may find nits sticking to the head hairs.

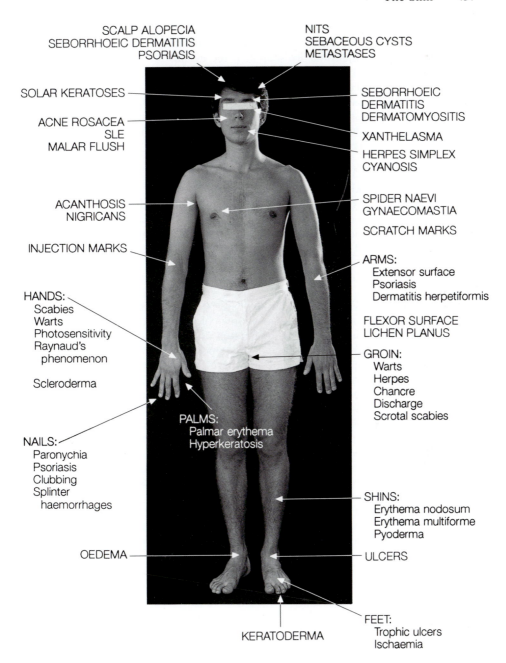

SCALP ALOPECIA
SEBORRHOEIC DERMATITIS
PSORIASIS

NITS
SEBACEOUS CYSTS
METASTASES

SOLAR KERATOSES

SEBORRHOEIC
DERMATITIS
DERMATOMYOSITIS

ACNE ROSACEA
SLE
MALAR FLUSH

XANTHELASMA

HERPES SIMPLEX
CYANOSIS

ACANTHOSIS
NIGRICANS

SPIDER NAEVI
GYNAECOMASTIA

SCRATCH MARKS

INJECTION MARKS

ARMS:
    Extensor surface
    Psoriasis
    Dermatitis herpetiformis

FLEXOR SURFACE
LICHEN PLANUS

HANDS:
    Scabies
    Warts
    Photosensitivity
    Raynaud's
        phenomenon

Scleroderma

GROIN:
    Warts
    Herpes
    Chancre
    Discharge
    Scrotal scabies

PALMS:
    Palmar erythema
    Hyperkeratosis

NAILS:
    Paronychia
    Psoriasis
    Clubbing
    Splinter
        haemorrhages

SHINS:
    Erythema nodosum
    Erythema multiforme
    Pyoderma

OEDEMA

ULCERS

FEET:
    Trophic ulcers
    Ischaemia

KERATODERMA

Figure 12.16 *Sites of some important skin lesions of the limbs, face and trunk. SLE = systemic lupus erythematosus.*

Move down now to the *eyebrows* and look for scaling and greasiness which are found in seborrhoeic dermatitis. A purplish erythema occurs around the eyelids in dermatomyositis. Xanthelasma are seen near the eyelid.

Look at the *face* for rosacea, which causes bright erythema of the nose, cheeks, forehead and chin, and occasionally pustules and rhinophyma (disfiguring swelling of the nose). Acne causes papules, pustules and scars involving the face, neck and upper trunk. The butterfly rash of systemic lupus erythematosus occurs across the cheeks but is rare. Spider naevi may be present. Ulcerating lesions on the face may include basal cell carcinoma, squamous cell carcinoma or rarely tuberculosis (lupus vulgaris).

Benign tumours of the face include keratoacanthoma (a volcano-like lesion from a sebaceous gland) and congenital haemangiomas.

Look for the blisters of herpes zoster, which may occur strictly in the distribution of one of the divisions of the trigeminal nerve.

Inspect the *neck* which is prone to many of the lesions that occur on the face. Rarely, the redundant loose skin of pseudoxanthoma elasticum will be seen around the neck.

Go on to inspect the *trunk* where any of the childhood exanthems produce their characteristic rashes.

Look for spider naevi. Campbell de Morgan spots are commonly found on the abdomen (and chest), as are flat greasy yellow-coloured seborrhoeic warts. Erythema marginatum (rheumatic fever) occurs on the chest and abdomen. Herpes zoster may be seen overlying any of the dermatome distributions. Metastases from internal malignancies may rarely occur anywhere on the skin. Neurofibromas are soft flesh-coloured tumours; when associated with more than five 'café-au-lait' spots (brownish, irregular lesions), they suggest neurofibromatosis (von Recklinghausen's disease). Pigmented moles are seen on the trunk and evidence of malignancy must be looked for with these. The patient's buttocks and sacrum must be examined for bed sores, and the abdomen and thighs may have areas of fat atrophy or hypertrophy from insulin injections.

Go to the *legs* where erythema nodosum or erythema multiforme may be seen on the shins. Necrobiosis lipoidica diabeticorum affects the skin over the tibia in diabetics. Pretibial myxoedema also occurs over the shins. Look for ulcers on either side of the lower part of the leg.

Inspect the *feet* for the characteristic lesion of Reiter's disease called keratoderma blenorrhagica, where crusted lesions spread across the sole because of the fusion of vesicles and pustules. Look at the foot for signs of ischaemia, associated with wasting of the skin and skin appendages. Trophic ulcers may be seen in patients with peripheral neuropathy (e.g., diabetes mellitus).

Suggested Reading

Original and Review Articles

Ashton RE, Teaching non-dermatologists to examine the skin: a review of the literature and some recommendations. *Brit J Derm* 1995; 132: 221–5.

Callen JP. Skin signs of internal malignancy; fact, fancy and fiction. *Semin Dermatol* 1984; 3: 340–357.

Marks R. A diagnostic approach to common dermatology problems. *Aust Fam Phys* 1982;11: 696–702.

Stevens GL, Adelman HM, Wallach PM, Palpable purpura: an algorithmic approach. *Am Fam Phys* 1995; 52: 1355–62.

Textbooks

Buxton PK. ABC of dermatology. 2nd ed. London: BMJ Publishing Group, 1993.

Fitzpatrick TB, Eisen AE, Wolff K, Freedberg IM, Austen KF, editors. Dermatology in general medicine. 4th ed. New York: McGraw-Hill, 1993.

Fitzpatrick TB, Johnson RA, Polano MK, Suurmond D, Wolff K. Color atlas and synopsis of clinical dermatology. 2nd ed. New York: McGraw-Hill, 1992.

Levene GM, Calnan CD. A colour atlas of dermatology. London: Wolfe Medical, 1984.

Sauer GC. Manual of skin diseases. 6th ed. Philadelphia: JB Lippincott, 1991.

Chapter 13

A SYSTEM FOR THE INFECTIOUS DISEASES EXAMINATION

As it takes two to make a quarrel, so it takes two to make a disease, the microbe and its host.

Charles Chaplain (1856–1941)

We have selected two important diseases to be covered in this chapter to show how infectious diseases can be approached in a systematic manner.

Pyrexia of Unknown Origin (PUO)

This condition is defined as documented fever ($>38°C$) of more than three weeks' duration where no cause is found despite basic investigations. In studies of fever of unknown origin, infection is found to be the cause in 30%, neoplasia in 30%, connective tissue disease in 15% and miscellaneous causes in 15%; in 10% the aetiology remains unknown (Table 13.1). Remember, the longer the duration of the fever, the less likely there is an infectious aetiology. The majority of patients do not have a rare disease but rather a relatively common disease presenting in an unusual way.

History

The history may give a number of clues in these puzzling cases. In some patients a careful history may give the diagnosis where expensive tests have failed.

The time course of the fever and any associated symptoms must be uncovered. Symptoms from the various body systems should be sought methodically. Examples include:

1. The gastrointestinal system—diarrhoea, abdominal pain, recent abdominal surgery, inflammatory bowel disease, diverticular disease, cholangitis.
2. The cardiovascular system—heart murmurs, dental procedures, (infective endocarditis), chest pain (pericarditis).
3. Rheumatology—joint symptoms, rashes,.
4. Neurology—headache (meningitis, cerebral abscess).
5. Genitourinary system—history of renal disease or infection, dysuria.

Table 13.1 *Common Causes of Pyrexia of Unknown Origin*

1. **Neoplasms**
   i. Hodgkin's and non-Hodgkin's lymphoma, leukaemia, malignant histiocytosis
   ii. Other tumours: hepatic, renal, lung, disseminated carcinoma, atrial myxoma

2. **Infections**
   i. Bacterial: e.g., tuberculosis, brucellosis and other bacteraemias, abscess formation (especially pelvic or abdominal), endocarditis, pericarditis, osteomyelitis, cholangitis, pyelonephritis, pelvic inflammatory disease, prostatitis, syphilis, Lyme disease, borreliasis, cat scratch disease
   ii. Viral: e.g., infectious mononucleosis, cytomegalovirus infection, hepatitis B or C, human immunodeficiency virus (HIV) infection, Ross River virus
   iii. Parasitic, rickettsial and others: e.g., malaria, Q fever, toxoplasmosis
   iv. Fungal: e.g., histoplasmosis, cryptococcosis, blastomycosis

3. **Connective Tissue Diseases**
   i. Rheumatoid arthritis, systemic lupus erythematosus
   ii. Vasculitis, e.g., polyarteritis nodosa, polymyalgia rheumatica

4. **Miscellaneous**
   Drug fever, inflammatory bowel disease, granulomatous disease (e.g., sarcoid), multiple pulmonary emboli, familial Mediterranean fever, factitious fever

5. **Uncertain**

6. Respiratory system—old tuberculosis (TB) or recent TB contact, chest symptoms.

Details of any recent overseas travel are important. Find out also about hobbies and exposure to pets. Occupational exposure may be important. Take a drug history. Find out if the patient is involved in behaviour posing a risk of HIV infection. Patients who are already in hospital may have infected cannulas or old cannula sites.

Examination

General

Look at the temperature chart to see if there is a pattern of fever that is identifiable (page 23). Inspect the patient and decide how seriously ill he or she appears. Look for evidence of weight loss (indicating a chronic illness). Note any skin rash (Table 13.2).

Hands

Look for the stigmata of infective endocarditis or vasculitic changes. Note if there is clubbing. The presence of arthropathy or Raynaud's phenomenon may point to a connective tissue disease.

Arms

Inspect for drug injection sites suggesting intravenous drug abuse (Figure 3.22). Feel for the epitrochlear and axillary nodes (e.g., lymphoma, other malignancy, sarcoidosis, focal infections).

Table 13.2 *Some Causes of Prolonged Fever and Rash*

1. Viral: e.g., infectious mononucleosis, rubella, dengue fever
2. Bacterial: e.g., syphilis, Lyme disease
3. Non-infective: e.g., drugs, systemic lupus erythematosus, erythema multiforme (which may also be related to an underlying infection)

Head and Neck

Feel the *temporal arteries* (over the temples). In temporal arteritis these may be tender and thickened.

Examine the *eyes* for iritis or conjunctivitis (connective tissue disease—e.g., Reiter's syndrome) or jaundice (e.g., ascending cholangitis, blackwater fever in malaria). Look in the fundi for choroidal tubercles in miliary tuberculosis, Roth's spots in infective endocarditis, and retinal haemorrhages or the infiltrates of leukaemia or lymphoma.

Inspect the *face* for a butterfly rash (systemic lupus erythematosus) (Figure 8.27) or seborrhoeic dermatitis which is common in patients with HIV infection.

Examine the *mouth* for ulcers, gum disease or candidiasis and the teeth and tonsils for infection (e.g., abscess). Look in the *ears* for otitis media. Feel the *parotid glands* for evidence of infection.

Palpate the cervical lymph nodes. Examine for thyroid enlargement and tenderness (subacute thyroiditis).

Chest

Examine the chest. Palpate for bony tenderness. Carefully examine the respiratory system (e.g., for signs of pneumonia, tuberculosis, empyema, carcinoma) and the heart for murmurs (e.g., infective endocarditis, atrial myxoma) or rubs (e.g., pericarditis).

The Abdomen

Examine the abdomen. Inspect for rashes including rose coloured spots (in typhoid fever—2 to 4mm flat red spots which blanch on pressure and occur on the upper abdomen and lower chest). Feel for evidence of hepatomegaly and ascites (e.g., spontaneous bacterial peritonitis, hepatic carcinoma, metastatic deposits), splenomegaly (e.g., haemopoietic malignancy, infective endocarditis, malaria), renal enlargement (e.g., renal cell carcinoma) or localised tenderness (e.g., collection of pus). Palpate for testicular enlargement (e.g., seminoma, tuberculosis). Feel for inguinal lymphadenopathy.

Perform a rectal examination feeling for a mass or tenderness in the rectum or pelvis (e.g., abscess, carcinoma, prostatitis). Sigmoidoscopy should also be performed for evidence of inflammatory bowel disease or carcinoma. Perform a vaginal examination to detect collections of pelvic pus or evidence of pelvic inflammatory disease. Look at the penis and scrotum for a discharge or rash.

Central Nervous System

Examine the central nervous system for signs of meningism (e.g., chronic tuberculous meningitis, cryptococcal meningitis) or focal neurological signs (e.g., brain abscess, mononeuritis multiplex in polyarteritis nodosa).

Table 13.3   *Revised Centers for Disease Control Classification of AIDS*

Group 1	Acute infection (and HIV seroconversion): sore throat, fever, night sweats, urticaria or maculopapular rashes, arthralgia, myalgia, diarrhoea, headache, photophobia, lymphadenopathy (3 to 6 weeks after primary infection)
Group 2	Asymptomatic infection (seropositive)
Group 3	Persistent generalised lymphadenopathy (PGL): 1cm or more at two or more extrainguinal sites for more than 3 months
Group 4	Other disease
Subgroup A	Constitutional disease: fever, diarrhoea for more than one month, or weight loss of more than 10% (includes AIDS-related complex)*
Subgroup B	Neurological syndromes: encephalopathy (AIDS dementia), aseptic meningitis, myelopathy, peripheral neuropathy, cognitive changes
Subgroup C	Opportunistic infections: oral candidiasis, pneumocystis, toxoplasmosis, cytomegalovirus, cryptosporidia, isospora, cryptococcosis, *Mycobacterium avium intracellulare*, extrapulmonary tuberculosis
Subgroup D	Secondary malignancies: Kaposi's sarcoma, non-Hodgkin's lymphoma
Subgroup E	Other: lymphocytic interstitial pneumonia (usually in children, possibly an Ebstein-Barr virus associated lymphoproliferative lung disease)

*   AIDS-related complex = non-specific symptoms or signs in the absence of full-blown AIDS (e.g. fatigue, fever, weight loss, persistent skin rash, oral hairy leukoplakia, herpes simplex, oral thrush).

HIV Infection and the Acquired Immunodeficiency Syndrome (AIDS)

This syndrome, first described in 1981, is caused by the human immunodeficiency virus (HIV). This is a T-cell lymphotrophic virus, which results in T4 cell destruction and therefore susceptibility to opportunistic infections and the development of tumours, notably Kaposi's* sarcoma and non-Hodgkin's lymphoma. A classification of AIDS is summarised in Table 13.3.

HIV infection should be suspected particularly if the patient falls into a high-risk group (e.g., male homosexual, intravenous drug abuser, haemophiliac, blood transfusion recipient, prostitute, Haitian or Central African origin, or sexual contact of one of these). Examine the patient as follows.

Examination

General Inspection

Take the temperature. The patient may appear ill and wasted due to chronic ill health or chronic opportunistic infection. Look at the skin for rashes. There may be a maculopapular rash of acute infection, herpes zoster (shingles—which may involve more than one dermatome in this disease and is more commonly seen in

---

*   Moritz Kohn Kaposi (1837–1902), Professor of Dermatology, Vienna, described the sarcoma in 1892.

early rather than in advanced HIV infection), herpes simplex (cold sores), flexural candidiasis, seborrhoea or other non-specific exanthem. In particular look for Kaposi's sarcoma: red-purple vascular non-tender tumours. These present typically on the skin but can occur anywhere.

Adverse drug reactions are more common in patients with HIV infection and may be the cause of a rash. Look for hyperpigmentation. Patients taking the drug clofamizine for *Mycobacterium avium* complex infection usually become deeply pigmented.

Hands and Arms

Look for nail changes including onycholysis. Feel for the epitrochlear nodes and note any injection marks.

Face

Inspect the mouth for candidal plaques, angular stomatitis, aphthous ulcers, tongue ulceration (e.g., herpes simplex, cytomegalovirus or candidal infections) or gingivitis. Periodontal disease is very common. Kaposi's sarcoma may also occur on the hard or soft palate (in which case associated lesions are almost always present elsewhere in the gastrointestinal tract). Oral squamous cell carcinoma and non-Hodgkin's lymphoma are more common in AIDS.

Parotidomegaly is sometimes seen as a result of HIV-associated Sjögren's syndrome. These patients may have dry eyes and mouth for this reason.

Hairy leukoplakia is a unique raised or flat, white, often hairy looking lesion typically present on the lateral surface of the tongue; it is associated with Epstein-Barr virus infection in HIV-infected persons.

Palpate over the sinuses for tenderness (sinusitis). Examine the cervical and axillary nodes. There may be generalised lymphadenopathy and all lymph node groups should be examined.

Chest

Note any tachypnoea or dry cough. Chronic cough, either dry or productive of purulent sputum, is common. On auscultation crackles may be present at the bases due to bronchiolitis obliterans. There are often, however, no chest signs despite the presence of pulmonary infiltrates on chest X-ray due to *Pneumocystis carinii* or other opportunistic infections.

Abdomen

Examine for hepatosplenomegaly (e.g., infection, lymphoma). Perform a rectal examination (e.g., perianal ulceration from herpes simplex) and a sigmoidoscopy looking for Kaposi's sarcoma or proctitis (e.g., cytomegalovirus, herpes simplex, amoebic dysentery, pseudomembranous colitis) (from antibiotic use). Examine the genitals for herpes simplex, warts, discharge or chancre.

Nervous System

Look for signs of meningism (e.g., cryptococcal meningitis). There may be focal signs due to a space-occupying intracranial lesion (e.g., toxoplasmosis, non-Hodgkin's lymphoma).

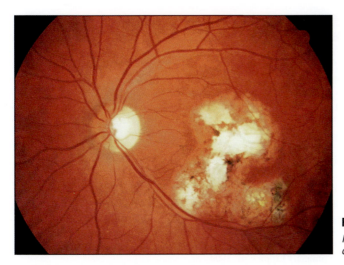

Figure 13.1
*Retinal toxoplasmosis—
old chorioretinal scar.*

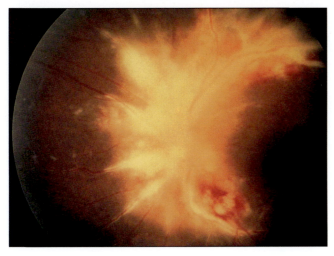

Figure 13.2
Cytomegalovirus retinitis.

A syndrome similar to Guillain-Barré and a pure sensory neuropathy can occur. HIV infection itself, opportunistic infection or the drugs used in treatment can be responsible for peripheral sensorimotor neuropathy, polymyositis, radiculopathy, mononeuritis multiplex or a myelopathy.

Look in the fundi for cotton wool spots (common in AIDS patients), scars (e.g., toxoplasmosis (Figure 13.1)) or retinitis (e.g., cytomegalovirus-induced retinitis with perivascular haemorrhages and fluffy exudates, which can cause blindness of rapid onset (Figure 13.2)). There may be signs of dementia (AIDS encephalopathy).

Suggested Reading

Original and Review Articles

American College of Physicians and Infectious Diseases Society of America. Human Immunodeficiency Virus (HIV) infection. *Ann Intern Med* 1994; 120: 310–319.

Knockaert DC, Vanneste LJ, Vanneste SB, Bobbaers HJ. Fever of unknown origin in the 1980s. An update of the diagnostic spectrum. *Arch Intern Med* 1992; 152: 51–55.

Nandwani R, Human immunodeficiency virus medicine for the MRCP short cases. *Brit J Hosp Med* 1994; 51: 353–6.

Whitby M, The febrile patient. *Aust Fam Phys* 1993; 22: 1753–5, 1758–61.

Textbooks

Adler MW, editor. ABC of AIDS. 3rd ed. BMJ Publishing Group, 1993.

Edmond RTD, Rowland HAK, editors. A colour atlas of infectious diseases. 2nd ed. London: Wolfe Medical, 1987.

Hoeprich PD, Jordan MC, Ronald AR, editors. Infectious diseases. A treatise of infectious processes. 5th ed. Philadelphia: JB Lippincott, 1994.

WRITING AND PRESENTING THE HISTORY AND PHYSICAL EXAMINATION

Experience is never limited,
and it is never complete.

Henry James

It is important that the medical record is kept short and simple. The following approach is one recommended by the authors.

History

Personal Information

Record the name, sex, date of birth and address. Write down the date and time of the examination.

Presenting (Principal) Symptoms (PS)

A short sentence identifies the *major* symptoms and their duration; it is often useful to quote the patient's own words.

History of Present Illness (HPI)

Don't record every detail; rather, prepare short prose paragraphs telling the story of the illness in chronological order. Describe the characteristics of each symptom. Note why the patient presents at this time. Also, describe any past medical problems which are related to the current symptoms. Include the relevant positive and negative findings on the system review here. If there are many seemingly unrelated problems, summarise these in an introductory paragraph and present the history of each problem in separate paragraphs. List current medications and doses and the indications for their use, if they are known, and any side effects. Finally, record your impression of the reliability of the historian and, if the patient was unable to give the history, describe who was the source.

Past History (PH)

List in chronological order past medical or surgical problems, past medication use, if of relevance, and any history of allergy (particularly drug allergy). A history of blood transfusions should be noted.

Social History (SH)

This may include recording the patient's occupation, schooling, hobbies, marital status, family structure, personal support system, living conditions and recent travel. The number and sex of sexual partners may be relevant. Analgesic use, smoking, alcohol and other recreational drug use should also be described.

Family History (FH)

Describe causes of mortality in the first degree relatives and, if indicated, draw a family tree.

Systems Review (SR)

All directly relevant information should be incorporated into the HPI or PH.

Physical Examination (PE)

Under each of the major systems, list the relevant positives and negatives using brief statements. See Appendix II.

Provisional Diagnosis, Problem List and Plans

Using a sentence or two, summarise the most important findings and then give a provisional diagnosis (PD) and differential diagnosis (DD).

Remember Occam's razon: choose the simplest hypothesis to explain observations. Also remember Sutton's law: the famous bank robber said he robbed banks because 'that's where the money is' i.e.—consider a common diagnosis before resorting to a rare one to explain the symptoms and signs.

List all the active problems that require management. Outline the diagnostic tests and therapy planned for each problem.

Sign your name and then put your name and position underneath.

Continuation Notes

Date (and time) each progress note in the record. The SOAP format can be useful (**s**ubjective, **o**bjective, **a**ssessment and **p**lans).

Subjective data refer to what the patient tells you; note any new problems.

Objective data are physical or laboratory findings; relevant data for each active problem are summarised.

Assessment refers to the interpretation of any relevant findings for each problem.

Plans describe any interventions that will be started for each problem.

Presentation

In their formal examinations and less formally on the wards, students and resident medical officers will often be expected to present the history and physical examination of a patient to an examiner or senior colleague. This is excellent training for clinical practice since the need to discuss patients with colleagues or specialists arises frequently in both hospital and non-hospital practice.

A successful case presentation is both *succinct* and *relevant.* The examiner is most interested in what the patient's problems are now. One should aim to convey basic biographical information and an assessment of the patient's presenting problem in the first few sentences. It is often helpful to present the case as a diagnostic or management problem, or both.

The information will have been obtained from the patient by history taking in the way set out above. The examination of the patient should be performed as set out in Appendix II, with particular attention to the areas most likely to be abnormal. This information must then be assembled into a form that can easily be conveyed to others. The following is a suggested method.

1. Begin with a sentence that tells your colleague something about the patient and the clinical problem. For example, one might say 'Mr Jones is a 72-year-old retired cabinet minister who presents with two hours of chest pain which is not typically ischaemic'. This gives an idea about the patient himself and indicates that the problem is likely to be a diagnostic one.

2. One should then go on to explain in what way the pain is atypical of ischaemia and whether it has features suggestive of any other diagnosis.

3. Once the presenting symptom or problem has been described relevant past history should be discussed. In a patient with chest pain this would include any previous cardiac history or investigations, and a summary of the patient's risk factors for ischaemic heart disease.

4. Important previous health problems should be outlined briefly. This retired cabinet minister might also have a history of intermittent claudication and of chronic airflow limitation. These facts will affect possible treatment for ischaemic heart disease, e.g., the use of beta-blockers.

5. Present a list of the patient's current medications.

6. Present the physical examination in two parts. (a) Abnormal and *important* normal examination findings in the presenting system. In this patient's case this would mean giving the pulse rate and blood pressure but not details of normal heart sounds. If there was a history of claudication, as in this case, the examination of the peripheral pulses should be presented even if it is normal. (b) Abnormal findings in the rest of the examination.

7. Offer the most likely diagnosis and the differential diagnosis.

8. Suggest a plan for investigation and treatment.

9. Much more detail will have been obtained in the assessment of the patient than should be presented routinely, but further details may be asked for by your colleague. These may include information about the patient's living conditions and the availability of support from the family. This may determine how soon the patient can be sent home from hospital.

By the end of your presentation your colleague should know what you think is wrong with the patient and what you intend to do about it.

A SUGGESTED METHOD FOR A RAPID SCREENING PHYSICAL EXAMINATION

To all students of medicine who listen, look, touch and reflect: may they hear, see, feel and comprehend.

John B Barlow, 1986

Begin by positioning the appropriately undressed patient in bed at 45 degrees. Use this opportunity to make a spot diagnosis if this is possible. Look particularly for any of the diagnostic facies or body habituses. Decide also whether the patient looks ill or well. Note if there is any dyspnoea or other distress. Take the blood pressure. Repeat the measurement a few minutes later if the first reading is high.

The Hands and Arms

Begin by picking up the patient's right hand and examine the nails for clubbing (RESP, CVS, GIT) and for the stigmata of infective endocarditis (CVS) or chronic liver disease (GIT). The nail changes suggesting chronic renal disease or iron deficiency must also be spotted (RENAL, HAEM). Note any evidence of arthropathy (RHEUM). Examine the other hand.

Take the patient's pulse, and note the rate and regularity or irregularity (CVS). While this is being done the arms can be inspected for bruising or scratch marks (GIT, HAEM, RENAL). Determine the state of hydration (GIT, RENAL, CVS). Go on and examine for axillary lymphadenopathy (HAEM).

The Face

Look at the eyes for jaundice (GIT, HAEM) or exophthalmos (ENDO). Look at the face for evidence of a vasculitic rash (RHEUM). Inspect the mouth for mucosal ulcers (RHEUM, GIT, HAEM, INF) and the tongue for glossitis (nutritional deficiencies) or cyanosis (RESP, CVS).

The Front of the Neck

Feel the carotid pulses and pay careful attention to the state of the jugular venous pressure (CVS). Feel gently for the position of the trachea (RESP). Then palpate the supraclavicular lymph nodes (HAEM, GIT).

The Chest

Examine the front of the chest for scars and deformity. Note any spider naevi (GIT) or hair loss (GIT, ENDO). Palpate the chest wall and auscultate the heart (CVS). Then percuss and auscultate the chest (RESP) and examine the breasts.

The Back

Sit the patient up and lean him or her forward. After inspection test chest expansion of the upper and lower lobes of the lungs. Percuss and auscultate the back of the chest (RESP). Feel for cervical lymphadenopathy (RESP, GIT, HAEM). Then examine formally for a goitre from behind (ENDO). Test for sacral oedema (CVS, RENAL).

The Abdomen

Lie the patient flat on one pillow. Inspect the abdomen from the side and then palpate for organomegaly and other abdominal masses. Percuss for shifting dullness if this is appropriate and auscultate over the renal arteries and liver and spleen. Palpate for inguinal lymphadenopathy and hernias, and in men palpate the testes (GIT, RENAL).

The Legs

Look for peripheral oedema (CVS, RENAL) and leg ulcers (HAEM, RHEUM, CVS, CNS). Feel all the peripheral pulses (CVS).

Neurological Examination

Neurological evaluation should be performed separately. Begin with examination of the higher centres and cranial nerves. Test orientation and note any speech defect. Then examine the visual acuity, visual fields, the fundi (II), the pupils and eye movements (III, IV, VI). Screen for the other cranial nerves by testing pain sensation over the face (V), the strength of upper and lower facial muscles (VII), whispered voice hearing (VIII), the palatal movement ('Ah') (IX, X), poking out the tongue (XII), and rotation of the head (XI).

Next look for wasting and fasciculation in the upper limbs. Test tone, power (shoulders, elbows, wrists and fingers), and the biceps, triceps and brachioradialis reflexes. Assess finger-nose movements. Then test pin prick sensation on the tip of the shoulder, outer and inner forearms, and on the median, ulnar and radial areas of the hands.

Go to the lower limbs. Test gait fully: ask the patient to walk away several paces, turn around rapidly and walk back. Then test heel-toe walking (cerebellum), ability to stand on the toes (S1) and heels (L4, L5), and squatting (proximal muscles). Finally look for Romberg's sign (posterior columns). If gait cannot be assessed, test hip and knee flexion and extension, and dorsiflexion and plantar flexion of the feet in bed. Then do knee, ankle and plantar reflexes, and heel-shin tests. Test pin prick sensation on the middle third of the thighs, both sides of the tibia, the dorsum of the feet, the little toes, on the buttocks, and three levels on the trunk on both sides.

Completing The Examination

Thorough physical examination always requires a rectal and pelvic examination, analysis of the patient's urine, a temperature reading and measurement of weight.

Particular details of the examination will be altered depending on what is found. An important guide to the areas where examination should be particularly directed, apart from the history, is the general inspection. A minute or two spent standing back to inspect the patient before the detailed examination begins is never wasted.

Key

CVS—Cardiovascular system
RESP—Respiratory system
GIT—Gastrointestinal system
HAEM—Haematological system
RENAL—Renal system
RHEUM—Rheumatological system
CNS—Central (and peripheral) nervous system
ENDO—Endocrine system
INF—Infection

Appendix III

THE PRE-ANAESTHETIC MEDICAL EVALUATION (PAME)

An appropriate medical evaluation of the patient who has been admitted for elective surgery is always required. It includes a history and examination which is sufficient to uncover any likely major problems with anaesthesia or the procedure itself.

The History

The first thing to find out, of course, is the presenting problem, what operation is intended, and whether the surgery is expected to be performed under general or local anaesthesia. Clearly the assessment of a patient having a small lesion removed under local anaesthesia can be briefer than the assessment of a patient undergoing extensive bowel resection under general anaesthesia. As a rule, before any patient undergoes surgery under general anaesthesia or spinal anaesthesia, careful attention must be given to identifying if he or she is at higher risk.

The Cardiovascular History

The most important questions here relate to a history of ischaemic heart disease. Patients who have had a myocardial infarct in the preceding six months should not usually undergo elective surgery; the risks of further infarction or malignant arrhythmia are higher during this period. A patient who has symptoms of angina which have recently become unstable is also at greater risk. A history of stable angina which has not changed for months or years is not a contraindication to most forms of surgery. Symptoms of cardiac failure should be sought. Any patient with uncontrolled cardiac failure is at considerable risk of severe cardiac failure postoperatively. This is particularly true if large amounts of intravenous fluids are given during and after surgery while the patient's anti-failure drugs are omitted.

Cardiac drugs should be asked about, particularly anti-anginal and anti-failure drugs. It is important to attempt to ensure that the patient gets these drugs on the day of the operation. Previous coronary artery bypass grafting or angioplasty is not a contraindication to surgery.

A history of infective endocarditis or the presence of a prosthetic cardiac valve may be an indication for antibiotic prophylaxis.

Respiratory History

Inquire about a history of respiratory disease, particularly chronic airflow limitation or severe asthma. Patients who have continued to smoke up to the time of their surgery have a much higher risk of postoperative chest infections than those who have not. Even stopping a few weeks before will reduce this risk. Severe respiratory disease is a relative contraindication to surgery. It may be difficult to reverse the anaesthetic and muscle relaxant drugs in such a patient, and he or she may require ventilation postoperatively. Doctors in charge of intensive care units are always happier to be warned that a patient may require ventilation postoperatively than to have it come as a surprise. Drug therapy for respiratory disease must be asked about. Steroids may impair wound healing, and steroid doses may need to be increased during the operative period because of steroid-induced adrenal suppression.

Other

Inquire about any history of bleeding diathesis, diabetes mellitus, renal disease, hepatitis, jaundice and drug abuse. The blood sugar control in diabetic patients can be difficult in the perioperative period, especially while normal diet is impossible.

Specific inquiries about *previous operations and anaesthetics,* particularly with reference to any complications, should be made. *Allergies* to anaesthetic agents or other drugs must be asked about. Attempt to distinguish a true allergy or anaphylaxis from an adverse effect such as vomiting after a morphine injection. Some operations involve the use of contrast media, and an allergy to iodine may be a contraindication to their use. This risk is now much less with the new non-ionic contrast media. There may occasionally be a *family history of anaesthetic complications* or deaths. This raises the possibility of malignant hyperthermia, which is an inherited disorder leading to fever and muscle destruction in response to muscle relaxants.

The Examination

Examination according to the rapid screening method outlined in Appendix II represents the best approach. Record height, weight and vital signs (pulse rate, blood pressure, respiratory rate). The cardiovascular and respiratory systems must be fully examined.

If a previously undiagnosed symptom or sign of significance is uncovered, some further investigations may be required before surgery, and the operation may have to be deferred. For example, the discovery of a new and significant heart murmur, uncontrolled hypertension, respiratory failure, a bleeding diathesis, uncontrolled diabetes mellitus or renal failure should be brought to the attention of the surgeon and anaesthetist.

Suggested Reading

Wolfsthal SD, editor. Medical perioperative management. Norwalk, Connecticut: Appleton & Lange, 1989.

*Now this is not the end. It is not
even the beginning of the end. But it is,
perhaps, the end of the beginning.*

Winston Churchill

Speech at the Lord Mayor's Day Luncheon, London,

10 November 1942

INDEX